DISEASE & DRUG CONSULT

Psyc
Disc

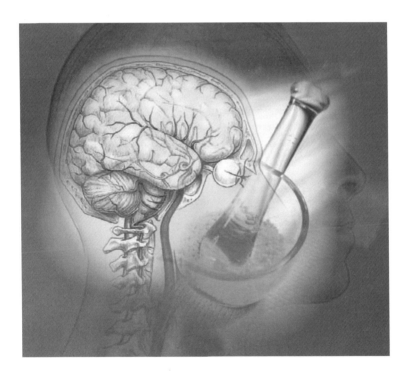

Wolters Kluwer | Lippincott Williams & Wilkins
Health

Philadelphia · Baltimore · New York · London
Buenos Aires · Hong Kong · Sydney · Tokyo

Staff

Executive Publisher
Judith A. Schilling McCann, RN, MSN

Clinical Director
Joan M. Robinson, RN, MSN

Art Director
Elaine Kasmer

Senior Editors
Deborah Grandinetti, Sean Webb

Clinical Project Manager
Lorraine M. Hallowell, RN, BSN, RVS

Editor
Jennifer Kowalak

Copy Editors
Pamela Wingrod, Linda Hager

Designer
Joseph John Clark

Associate Manufacturing Manager
Beth J. Welsh

Editorial Assistants
Karen J. Kirk, Jeri O'Shea, Linda K. Ruhf

Production Project Manager
Cynthia Rudy

Library of Congress Cataloging-in-Publication Data

Disease & drug consult. Psychiatric disorders.
    p. ; cm.
  Includes bibliographical references and index.
  ISBN 978-1-60547-051-1 (alk. paper)
  1. Psychiatric nursing—Handbooks, manuals, etc. 2. Psychology, Pathological—Handbooks, manuals, etc. 3. Psychotropic drugs—Handbooks, manuals, etc. I. Lippincott Williams & Wilkins. II. Title: Psychiatric disorders. III. Title: Disease and drug consult. Psychiatric disorders.
  [DNLM: 1. Mental Disorders—nursing—Handbooks. 2. Drug Therapy—methods—Handbooks. 3. Mental Disorders—drug therapy—Handbooks. WY 49 D6107 2009]

  RC440.D57 2009
  616.89'0231—dc22

2008049841

Contents

Contributors and consultants

Kathleen C. Banks, MSN, CNS
Assistant Professor of Nursing
Kent State University
East Liverpool, Ohio

Anne L. Bateman, EdD, APRN, BC
Assistant Professor
University of Massachusetts Medical School
Worcester

Noreen R. Brady, PhD, APRN-BC, LPCC
Director of Hirsh Institute for Evidence-Based
    Nursing Practice
Assistant Professor
Frances Payne Bolton School of Nursing
Case Western Reserve University
Cleveland

Linda Carman Copel, PhD, APRN, BC, CGP,
    NCC, CNE, FAPA
Associate Professor
Villanova (Pa.) University

Gloria F. Donnelly, PhD, RN, FAAN
Dean and Professor
College of Nursing, and Health Professions
Drexel University
Philadelphia

Donna Scemons, PhD(c), MSN, MA, FNP-BC,
    CNS
President
Health Care Systems, Inc.
Castaic, Calif.

Allison J. Terry, RN, MSN, PhD
Director, Center for Nursing
Alabama Board of Nursing
Montgomery

Kathleen R. Tusaie, PhD, PMHNCNS, BC
Advance Practice Psychiatric Nurse (private
    practice)
Associate Professor
University of Akron (Ohio) College of Nursing

Part

1

Disorders

Alcohol-related disorders

Alcohol-related disorders consist of alcohol abuse or alcohol dependence. Typically, the patient who abuses alcohol drinks too fast, too much, or too often. He often has a recurring pattern of high-risk alcohol use that creates problems for himself or for others as well as in society. An alcohol-dependent patient has lost control over his drinking and demonstrates intense alcohol-seeking behavior with increasing dependence and tolerance. People with these patterns of drinking are usually socially and occupationally impaired.

CAUSES AND INCIDENCE

The alcohol in alcoholic beverages (ethyl alcohol) is produced by the fermentation of sugar. Ethyl alcohol is a potent central nervous system (CNS) depressant, and ingestion results in behavioral, mood, and physiologic changes. Although the effects of alcohol are proportional to the amount ingested, the destabilization of alcohol and the CNS effects of alcohol differ between people. When alcohol is ingested, about 20% is quickly absorbed through the stomach wall into the bloodstream, and 80% is absorbed more slowly into the bloodstream from the upper digestive tract. When a low dose of alcohol is ingested it produces a lessening of inhibition, sleepiness, relaxation, slurred speech, and loss of coordination. In high doses it may produce profound CNS depression with coma, respiratory arrest, and organ failure.

According to the Centers for Disease Control and Prevention, alcohol abuse is considered the number three cause of preventable death in the United States. Eighteen million Americans have alcohol use disorders but only 7% (per year) receive any treatment. The annual costs of alcohol-related problems in the United States are estimated at $185 billion.

The interplay of numerous biological, psychological, and sociocultural factors appear to be involved in alcohol-related disorders. The human genome is being studied in attempt to identify and define genetic risk factors and understand their interaction with environmental factors. Indeed, a child of one parent with alcohol-related disorder is seven to eight times more likely to become an alcoholic than a child without such a parent. Biological factors may include genetic or biochemical abnormalities, nutritional deficiencies, endocrine imbalances, and allergic responses.

≥ PREVENTION

Teach the pregnant patient that people who were exposed to alcohol prenatally have a higher than average risk for developing an alcohol or substance abuse problem later in life.

Alcohol is the leading cause of death in children younger than age 21. In college-age students, nearly 600,000 are injured annually when under the influence of alcohol, and alcohol abuse is implicated in nearly 100,000 sexual assaults or date rapes. Across the lifespan, alcohol is commonly implicated in both non-fatal and fatal accidents. Children who begin drinking alcohol before age 15 are four times as likely to develop alcohol dependence even if their parents had no parental history of alcohol dependence.

Psychological factors may include self-medicating with alcohol to reduce anxiety or symptoms of mental illness; the desire to avoid responsibility in familial, social, and work relationships; and the need to bolster self-esteem. Alcohol-related disorders are common among individuals who also abuse other drugs. Individuals who are addicted to nicotine and who abuse alcohol aren't as successful at quitting smoking and suffer higher rates of smoking-related illnesses. Further, it's estimated that 90% of people who suffer from cocaine addiction also have alcohol-related disorders.

Sociocultural factors include the availability of alcoholic beverages, group or peer pressure, an excessively stressful lifestyle, and social and familial attitudes that approve of frequent drinking. Research has shown that nearly 80% of adolescents near the end of high school begin to drink. And, nearly 9% of 6th grade students surveyed had consumed a beer in the previous year.

Alcohol-related disorders cuts across all social and economic groups, involves both sexes, and occurs at all stages of the life cycle, beginning as early as elementary school. The focus of research on the cause and treatment of alcohol-related disorders requires a lifespan perspective.

SIGNS AND SYMPTOMS

Because alcohol-related disorders occur across the lifespan, age-specific and sensitive diagnostic assessment tools must be used.

The patient with alcohol dependence may hide or deny his addiction and may temporarily manage to maintain a functional life. Assessing for abuse or dependence can be difficult. Look for these physical and psychosocial symptoms that suggest alcohol-related disorders:

- need for daily or episodic alcohol use to maintain adequate functioning
- inability to discontinue or reduce alcohol intake
- episodes of anesthesia or amnesia (blackouts) during intoxication
- episodes of violence during intoxication
- interference with social and familial relationships

- interference with school or occupational responsibilities
- intake during pregnancy
- malaise, dyspepsia, mood swings, depression, and an increased incidence of infection
- poor personal hygiene
- unexplained injuries, such as burns, fractures, and bruises
- unusually high tolerance of sedatives and opioids
- memory or cognitive impairment (at any age)
- legal problems associated with driving under the influence, property or violent crime, or sexual assault
- abuse of other substances such as cocaine
- mood, anxiety, or personality disorders
- child with fetal alcohol spectrum disorder (FASD)
- multiple minor complaints.

Although each person abusing alcohol may present in a unique way, secretive or manipulative behavior may be a manifestation of the patient's denial of the severity of his addiction. Proactive screening may be necessary to identify alcohol-related disorders in young adult patients because they rarely identify themselves as having alcohol abuse problems. Suspect alcohol-related disorder if the patient uses inordinate amounts of aftershave or mouthwash. When confronted, the patient may deny or rationalize the problem. Or, he may be guarded or hostile in his response and may even sign out of the hospital against medical advice. He also may project his anger or feelings of guilt or inadequacy onto others to avoid confronting his illness. The blood alcohol level in a physically dependent and tolerant drinker may exceed levels that would cause severe dysfunction or death in a nontolerant drinker. For example, a tolerant drinker might have a blood alcohol level of more than 0.5 mg (the usual lethal level) and still be alive, talking, and moving.

After abstinence or reduction of alcohol intake, signs and symptoms of withdrawal—which begin shortly after drinking has stopped and last for 5 to 7 days—may vary. (See *Signs and symptoms of alcohol withdrawal,* page 6.)

The patient initially experiences:
- anorexia, nausea, and diaphoresis
- anxiety with tremor that progresses to severe tremulousness and agitation; possibly hallucinations and violent behavior
- insomnia
- major motor seizures (alcohol withdrawal seizures) during withdrawal.

Suspect alcohol-related disorder in any patient with unexplained seizures.

⚠ ALERT

Remember to consider the possibility of alcohol abuse when evaluating older patients. Research suggests that alcoholism affects 2% to 10% of adults older than age 60. More than half of all elderly hospital admissions are due to alcohol-related problems.

SIGNS AND SYMPTOMS OF ALCOHOL WITHDRAWAL

Alcohol withdrawal signs and symptoms may vary in degree from mild (morning hangover) to severe (alcohol withdrawal delirium). Formerly known as *delirium tremens*, alcohol withdrawal delirium is marked by acute distress following abrupt withdrawal after prolonged or massive use.

Signs and symptoms	Mild	Moderate	Severe
Anxiety	Mild restlessness	Obvious motor restlessness and anxiety	Extreme restlessness and agitation with intense fearfulness
Appetite	Impaired appetite	Marked anorexia	Rejection of all food and fluid except alcohol
Blood pressure	Normal or slightly elevated systolic pressure	Usually elevated systolic pressure	Elevated systolic and diastolic pressures
Confusion	None	Variable	Marked confusion and disorientation
GI symptoms	Nausea	Nausea and vomiting	Dry heaves and vomiting
Hallucinations	None	Vague, transient, visual and auditory hallucinations and illusions (commonly nocturnal)	Visual and occasionally auditory hallucinations, usually of fearful or threatening content; misidentification of people and frightening delusions related to hallucinatory experiences
Seizures	None	Possible	Common
Sleep disturbance	Restless sleep or insomnia	Marked insomnia and nightmares	Total wakefulness
Sweating	Slight	Obvious	Marked hyperhidrosis

COMPLICATIONS

Chronic alcohol abuse is implicated in many physical and psychological complications, including:

- malnutrition
- aggravation of chronic diseases such as hypertension, stroke, and memory loss

- alcoholic liver diseases
- neurotoxicities and brain damage
- cardiac diseases
- immune system changes resulting in diminished disease resistance
- oropharyngeal and GI cancers
- fetal alcohol syndrome
- endocrine system changes (Prenatal alcohol exposure causes changes in the pituitary, adrenal, and hypothalamus glands that result in persistently elevated levels of stress hormones.)
- mood, personality, anxiety, and sleep disorders
- prescription drug interactions that may result in harmful side effects or diminished medication benefit.

Assess for these complications in a patient with suspected alcohol-related disorder. (See *Complications of alcohol use,* page 8.)

DIAGNOSTIC CRITERIA

For characteristic findings in patients with alcoholism, see *Diagnosing substance dependence and related disorders,* page 9.

In addition to client and family assessment, clinical findings may help support the diagnosis of alcohol-related disorder. For example:

- Laboratory tests confirm alcohol use and document recent alcohol ingestion. A blood alcohol level ranging from 0.08% to 0.10% weight/volume (200 mg/dl) is accepted as the level of intoxication, depending on the state or country.
- Blood urea nitrogen level is increased, serum ammonia level is increased, and serum glucose level is decreased in liver disease.
- Liver function studies consistent with liver damage reveal increased levels of serum cholesterol, lactate dehydrogenase, alanine aminotransferase, aspartate aminotransferase, and creatine phosphokinase.
- Elevated serum amylase and lipase levels are consistent with pancreatitis.
- Urine toxicology may reveal other drug use.
- Hematologic studies identify anemia, thrombocytopenia, increased prothrombin time, and increased partial thromboplastin time.
- Liver ultrasound studies can reveal hepatomegaly.
- Cardiac echocardiography may show cardiomyopathy.
- Diagnosis of alcohol-related disorder is confirmed when *Diagnostic and Statistical Manual of Mental Disorders,* Fourth Edition, Text Revision criteria are met.

Researchers are attempting to develop biomarkers to help identify patients with chronic alcohol abuse, alcohol-related tissue injury, and FASD. Current research seeks to identify the pharmacodynamic effects of alcohol, the quantification of and changes in neurotransmitters, and the effects of genetic expression and environmental factors on an individual's potential to develop alcohol-related disorders. In the future, imaging technologies, such as diffusion tensor magnetic resonance imaging, may be useful for identifying

COMPLICATIONS OF ALCOHOL USE

Alcohol can damage body tissues by its direct irritating effects, by changes that take place in the body during its metabolism, by aggravation of existing disease, by accidents occurring during intoxication, and by interactions between the substance and drugs. Such tissue damage can cause these complications:

Cardiopulmonary complications
- Cardiac arrhythmias
- Cardiomyopathy
- Chronic obstructive pulmonary disease
- Essential hypertension
- Increased risk of tuberculosis
- Pneumonia

GI complications
- Chronic diarrhea
- Esophageal cancer
- Esophageal varices
- Esophagitis
- Gastric ulcers
- Gastritis
- GI bleeding
- Malabsorption
- Pancreatitis

Hematologic complications
- Anemia
- Leukopenia
- Reduced number of phagocytes

Hepatic complications
- Alcoholic hepatitis
- Cirrhosis
- Fatty liver

Neurologic complications
- Alcoholic dementia
- Alcoholic hallucinosis
- Alcohol withdrawal delirium
- Korsakoff's syndrome
- Peripheral neuropathy
- Seizure disorders
- Subdural hematoma
- Wernicke's encephalopathy

Psychiatric complications
- Amotivational syndrome
- Depression
- Fetal alcohol syndrome
- Impaired social and occupational functioning
- Multiple substance abuse
- Suicide

Other complications
- Beriberi
- Hypoglycemia
- Infertility
- Leg and foot ulcers
- Impaired respiratory diffusion
- Increased incidence of pulmonary infections
- Myopathies
- Prostatitis
- Sexual performance difficulties

alcohol-induced brain tissue changes.

TREATMENT

Total abstinence from alcohol is the only effective treatment. Supportive programs that offer detoxification, rehabilitation, and aftercare, including continued involvement in Alcoholics Anonymous (AA), may produce good long-term results. For long-term success, the recovering individual must learn to fill the place alcohol once occupied in his life with something constructive.

Supportive counseling or individual, group, or family psychotherapy

DIAGNOSING SUBSTANCE DEPENDENCE AND RELATED DISORDERS

The *Diagnostic and Statistical Manual of Mental Disorders,* Fourth Edition, Text Revision, identifies these diagnostic criteria for substance dependence, abuse, intoxication, and withdrawal.

Substance dependence

A maladaptive pattern of substance use leading to clinically significant impairment or distress, as manifested by three or more of the following, occurring at any time in the same 12-month period:

■ Tolerance, as defined by either of the following: the need for increased amounts of the substance to achieve intoxication or desired effect or a markedly diminished effect with continued use of the same amount of the substance

■ Withdrawal, as manifested by either of the following: the characteristic withdrawal syndrome for the substance, as described by the two criteria above, or the use of the same, or similar, substance to relieve or avoid withdrawal symptoms

■ Inability to moderate usage, e.g., the person commonly takes the substance in larger amounts or over a longer period than was intended

■ Powerful cravings such that the person experiences a persistent desire for—or unsuccessful efforts to cut down or control use of—the substance

■ A lifestyle increasingly oriented around the substance, to the point where the person spends a lot of time in activities needed to obtain the substance, use the substance, or recover from its effects

■ Social withdrawal, e.g., the person abandons or reduces important social, occupational, or recreational activities because of substance use

■ Continued use despite the knowledge that persistent or recurrent physical or psychological problems are likely to have been caused or made worse by the substance

Substance abuse

A maladaptive pattern of substance use leading to clinically significant impairment or distress, as manifested by one or more of the following, occurring within a 12-month period:

■ Recurrent substance use, resulting in a failure to fulfill major role obligations at work, school, or home

■ Recurrent substance use in situations in which using the substance puts the person in physical danger, e.g., while driving a car or operating machinery

■ Recurrent substance-related legal problems

■ Continued substance use despite having persistent or recurrent social or interpersonal problems caused or made worse by the effects of the substance

In addition, the symptoms have never met the criteria for substance dependence for this class of substance.

Substance intoxication

■ Development of a reversible substance-specific syndrome resulting from recent ingestion of, or exposure to, a substance

■ Clinically significant maladaptive behavioral or psychological changes, resulting from the effect of the substance on the central nervous

(continued)

DIAGNOSING SUBSTANCE DEPENDENCE AND RELATED DISORDERS *(continued)*

system and developing during or shortly after use of the substance
■ Symptoms that aren't caused by a general medical condition and aren't better accounted for by another mental disorder

Substance withdrawal
■ Development of a substance-specific syndrome resulting from the cessation or reduction of substance

use that has been heavy and pro-longed
■ Substance-specific syndrome that causes clinically significant distress or impairment in social, occupation-al, or other important areas of func-tioning
■ Symptoms that aren't caused by a general medical condition and aren't better accounted for by another mental disorder

---

may help. Ongoing support groups are helpful. In AA, a self-help group with more than 2 million members worldwide, the alcoholic finds emo-tional support from others with sim-ilar problems. About 40% of AA's members stay sober as long as 5 years, and 30% stay sober longer than 5 years.

⚠ ALERT

Individuals with late-onset problem drinking have fewer alcohol-related health problems and better chances of recovery than early-onset prob-lem drinkers.

Acute intoxication is treated symptomatically by:
● supporting respiration
● preventing aspiration of vomitus
● replacing fluids and giving I.V. glucose to prevent hypoglycemia
● correcting hypothermia or acid-osis
● monitoring for seizure activity or withdrawal
● starting emergency treatment for trauma, infection, or GI bleeding.

Treatment of chronic alcohol abuse requires a varied approach that may include:
● drugs to deter alcohol use and treat effects of withdrawal
● psychotherapy, consisting of be-havior modification techniques, group therapy, and family therapy
● appropriate measures to relieve associated physical problems and psychiatric disorders.

Drugs

Although behavior modification ther-apy has been the cornerstone of treat-ment for alcohol-related disorder, re-searchers are attempting to develop new medications to decrease the symptoms of withdrawal, promote abstinence, and prevent relapse. The primary drugs in use today are:
● Disulfiram (Antabuse) is part of aversion, or deterrent, therapy. A daily oral dose of disulfiram is taken to prevent compulsive drinking.
– It interferes with alcohol metabo-lism and allows toxic levels of

acetaldehyde to accumulate in the patient's blood, producing immediate and potentially fatal distress in the event he consumes alcohol up to 2 weeks after taking it.
– Disulfiram is contraindicated during pregnancy and in the patient with diabetes, heart disease, severe hepatic disease, or any disorder in which such a reaction could be especially dangerous.
● Naltrexone (Revia) is an opiate antagonist that effectively reduces the amount of intake, severity of craving, and relapse incidence.
– It may work by preventing the effects of increased endorphins produced as a product of increased alcohol intake.
● Acamprosate (Campral) is used to maintain abstinence.
– The exact mechanism of action isn't understood, but acamprosate appears to reduce alcohol cravings by regulating neurotransmitter systems that may have been altered by chronic alcohol exposure.
● Benzodiazepines are given to alleviate symptoms of alcohol withdrawal and to prevent withdrawal convulsions.
– They're preferred over other anticonvulsants due to their rapid action.
– They aren't recommended for use during the rehabilitation phase because of their addictive potential.
● Anxiolytics, such as chlordiazepoxide (Librium), are used to treat severe anxiety and to lessen withdrawal symptoms and prevent delirium tremens.

● Vitamin deficiencies are commonly associated with alcohol-related disorders.
– Thiamine (vitamin B_1) is given to decrease ataxia and other symptoms in patients suffering from withdrawal.
– Folic acid is given to help correct anemia related to alcohol abuse.
– Magnesium sulfate is given to patients with a history of seizures to help prevent them and to enhance the body's use of thiamine.
● Antipsychotics control psychotic symptoms and hyperactivity.
● Antiemetics and antidiarrheals help to control nausea and diarrhea related to withdrawal.
– In a manner similar to disulfiram use, another form of aversion therapy attempts to induce aversion by administering alcohol with an emetic.

⚠ ALERT

Because the older patient may be more sensitive to these drugs, withdrawal may take longer (weeks or months) and be more severe than in a younger adult.

SPECIAL CONSIDERATIONS

● During acute intoxication or withdrawal, carefully monitor the patient's mental status, heart rate, breath sounds, blood pressure, and temperature every 30 minutes to 6 hours.
● Assess the patient for signs of inadequate nutrition and dehydration. Start seizure precautions and give drugs prescribed to treat the signs and symptoms of withdrawal in chronic alcohol abuse.

• During withdrawal, orient the patient to reality because he may have hallucinations and may try to harm himself or others. Maintain a calm environment, minimizing noise and shadows to reduce the incidence of delusions and hallucinations. Avoid restraining the patient unless necessary to protect him or others.

• Approach the patient in a non-threatening way. Limit sustained eye contact. Even if he is verbally abusive, listen attentively and respond with empathy. Explain all procedures.

• Monitor the patient for signs of depression or impending suicide.

• In chronic alcohol-related disorder, help the patient accept his drinking problem and the necessity for abstinence. Confront him about his behavior, urging him to examine his actions more realistically.

• If the patient is taking disulfiram (or has taken it within the past 2 weeks), warn him of the effects of alcohol ingestion, which may last from 30 minutes to 3 hours or longer. The reaction includes nausea, vomiting, facial flushing, headache, shortness of breath, red eyes, blurred vision, sweating, tachycardia, hypotension, and fainting. Emphasize that even a small amount of alcohol will induce this adverse reaction and that the longer he takes the drug, the greater his sensitivity to alcohol will be. Even medicinal sources of alcohol, such as mouthwash, cough syrups, liquid vitamins, and cold remedies, must be avoided.

• Refer the patient to AA and offer to arrange a visit from an AA member. Stress the effectiveness of this organization.

• For the individual who has lost all contact with his family and friends and who has a long history of unemployment, trouble with the law, or other problems associated with alcohol abuse, rehabilitation may involve job training, sheltered workshops, halfway houses, and other supervised facilities.

• Refer the spouse of an alcoholic to Al-Anon and children of an alcoholic to Alateen. By participating in these self-help groups, family members learn to relinquish responsibility for the individual's drinking. Point out that family involvement in rehabilitation can reduce family tensions.

• Refer adult children of an alcoholic to the National Association for Children of Alcoholics.

Anorexia nervosa

The key feature of anorexia nervosa is self-imposed starvation, resulting from a distorted body image and an intense, irrational fear of gaining weight, even when the patient is obviously emaciated. Individuals with anorexia may severely restrict their food intake or engage in regular binge-eating or purging behaviors such as self-induced vomiting or misuse of laxatives. A patient with anorexia is at least 15% below expected body weight, is preoccupied with body size, describes him or herself as "fat," and commonly expresses dissatisfaction with a particular aspect of her physical appearance. Although the term anorexia suggests that the patient's weight loss is associated with a loss of appetite, this is rarely the case.

CAUSES AND INCIDENCE

No causes of anorexia nervosa have been identified; however, genetic, social, and psychological factors have been implicated. Researchers in neuroendocrinology continue to seek a physiologic cause, but have found nothing definitive. Clearly, social attitudes that equate slimness with beauty play some role in provoking this disorder and family factors are also implicated. Most theorists believe that refusing to eat is a subconscious effort to exert personal control over one's life. Anorexia nervosa has been associated with other psychiatric disorders, such as obsessive-compulsive disorder (OCD), depression, and anxiety.

Anorexia occurs in 5% to 10% of the population; about 95% of those affected are women. This disorder occurs primarily in adolescents and young adults but may also affect older adults or even children. It is estimated that about 1 million boys and men suffer from either anorexia nervosa or bulimia. The prognosis for the disease varies but improves if the patient is diagnosed early or if help is sought voluntarily. Mortality ranges from 5% to 15%—the highest mortality associated with a psychiatric disturbance. Some studies report that people with anorexia are up to 10 times as likely to die from the disorder when compared to people without the disorder. One-third of these deaths can be attributed to suicide.

SIGNS AND SYMPTOMS

The patient's history usually reveals a 25% or greater weight loss for no organic reason, coupled with a morbid dread of being fat, a compulsion to be thin, and a distorted body image. Many patients tend to be angry and ritualistic with low self-esteem and perfectionism. Other signs of anorexia nervosa include:

- emaciated appearance, with skeletal muscle atrophy, loss of fatty tissue, and atrophy of breast tissue
- wearing of over-sized clothing to disguise body size
- severe lethargy and fatigue or hyperactivity with excessive exercising
- cold intolerance
- expression of morbid fear of gaining weight and an obsession with physical appearance (Paradoxically, the individual may also be obsessed with food, preparing elaborate meals for others.)
- sallow skin
- lanugo on the face and body
- dry brittle nails and hair
- calluses on the knuckles and abrasions and scars on the dorsum of the hand resulting from tooth injury during self-induced vomiting
- painless salivary gland enlargement and bowel distention on palpation
- slowed reflexes on percussion
- sleep alterations
- social regression, including poor sexual adjustment and fear of failure

COMPLICATIONS OF ANOREXIA NERVOSA

Serious medical complications can result from the malnutrition, dehydration, and electrolyte imbalances caused by prolonged starvation, frequent vomiting, or laxative abuse that's typical in anorexia nervosa.

Malnutrition and related problems

Malnutrition may cause hypoalbuminemia and subsequent edema or hypokalemia, leading to ventricular arrhythmias and renal failure.

Poor nutrition and dehydration, coupled with laxative abuse, produce changes in the bowel similar to those in chronic inflammatory bowel disease. Frequent vomiting can cause esophageal erosion, ulcers, tears, and bleeding as well as tooth and gum erosion and dental caries.

Cardiovascular consequences

Cardiovascular complications, which can be life-threatening, include decreased left ventricular muscle mass, chamber size, and myocardial oxygen uptake; reduced cardiac output; hypotension; bradycardia; electrocardiographic changes, such as a nonspecific ST interval, T-wave changes, and a prolonged PR interval; heart failure; and sudden death, possibly caused by ventricular arrhythmias.

Infection and amenorrhea

Anorexia nervosa may increase the patient's susceptibility to infection.

In addition, amenorrhea, which may occur when the patient loses about 25% of her normal body weight, usually is associated with anemia. Possible complications of prolonged amenorrhea include estrogen deficiency (increasing the risk of calcium deficiency and osteoporosis) and infertility. Menses usually return to normal when the patient weighs at least 95% of her normal weight.

• depression, OCD, and anxiety
• feelings of despair, hopelessness, and worthlessness as well as suicidal thoughts.

COMPLICATIONS

(See *Complications of anorexia nervosa*.)

DIAGNOSTIC CRITERIA

For the diagnostic criteria in patients with this condition, see *Diagnosing anorexia nervosa*.

Laboratory tests help to identify various disorders and deficiencies and help to rule out endocrine, metabolic, and central nervous system abnormalities; cancer; malabsorption syndromes; and other disorders that cause physical wasting.

Abnormal findings that may accompany a weight loss exceeding 30% of normal body weight include:

• low hemoglobin level, platelet count, and white blood cell count
• prolonged bleeding time caused by thrombocytopenia
• decreased erythrocyte sedimentation rate

• decreased levels of serum creatinine, blood urea nitrogen, uric acid, cholesterol, total protein, albumin, sodium, potassium, chloride, calcium, and fasting blood glucose (resulting from malnutrition)

• elevated levels of alanine aminotransferase and aspartate aminotransferase in severe starvation states

• elevated serum amylase levels when pancreatitis isn't present

• decreased levels of serum luteinizing hormone and follicle-stimulating hormone in females

• decreased triiodothyronine levels resulting from a lower basal metabolic rate

• dilute urine caused by the kidneys' impaired ability to concentrate urine

• nonspecific ST interval, prolonged PR interval, and T-wave changes on the electrocardiogram. Ventricular arrhythmias may also be present.

TREATMENT

Appropriate treatment aims to promote weight gain or control the patient's compulsive binge eating and purging. Malnutrition and the underlying psychological dysfunction must be corrected. Hospitalization in a medical, psychiatric, or specialized unit may be needed to improve the patient's precarious physical condition. All forms of psychotherapy, from psychoanalysis to hypnotherapy, have been used in treating anorexia nervosa, with varying success. To be successful, psycho-

---

DIAGNOSING ANOREXIA NERVOSA

A diagnosis of anorexia nervosa is made when the patient meets the following criteria put forth in the *Diagnostic and Statistical Manual of Mental Disorders,* Fourth Edition, Text Revision:

■ The patient refuses to maintain body weight over a minimal normal weight for age and height (for instance, weight loss leading to maintenance of body weight 15% below that expected) or fails to achieve expected weight gain during a growth period, leading to body weight 15% below that expected.

■ The patient experiences intense fear of gaining weight or becoming fat, despite her underweight status.

■ The patient has a distorted perception of body weight, size, or shape (that is, the person claims to feel fat even when emaciated or believes that one body area is too fat even when it's obviously underweight).

■ The patient experiences amenorrhea for at least three consecutive menstrual cycles when otherwise expected to occur.

---

therapy should address the underlying problems of low self-esteem, guilt, anxiety, feelings of hopelessness and helplessness, and depression. The hospital stay may be as brief as 2 weeks or may stretch from a few months to 2 years or longer. Even with treatment, only half of the individuals diagnosed with anorexia or bulimia will fully recover. Team approaches to care include:

- aggressive medical management with curtailed activity, increased oral intake with liquid supplementation, enteral hyperalimentation, and vitamin and mineral supplementation
- nutritional counseling
- individual, group, or family psychotherapy
- behavior modification therapy.

Drugs

- Antidepressants, such as fluoxetine (Prozac), sertraline (Zoloft), and paroxetine (Paxil), are approved to treat depression and OCD. They may be prescribed for individuals who have symptoms of depression and obsession with weight. Individuals may respond better once they have reached an acceptable weight because people with low weight may suffer more side effects. Studies on the use of antidepressants have demonstrated limited benefits and have not prevented relapses in patients once normal weight has been achieved.

⊵ PREVENTION

During the first 4 weeks of therapy with selective serotonin reuptake inhibitors, closely monitor children and adolescents for signs of increasing depression or suicidal thoughts.

- Anxiolytics, such as alprazolam (Xanax), a benzodiazepine, may be prescribed to treat anxiety in the short term. The patient must be carefully monitored because the potential for addiction is high. For this reason, the drug shouldn't be prescribed if the patient has a history of substance abuse.

- Vitamin and minerals may be prescribed to correct deficiencies caused by inadequate nutritional intake.

SPECIAL CONSIDERATIONS

- During hospitalization, regularly monitor the patient's vital signs, nutritional status, and intake and output.
- Weigh the patient daily—before breakfast if possible. Varying the weighing routine may help diminish anxiety associated with being weighed. Keep in mind that weight should increase from morning to night. Monitor the patient for excessive drinking of liquids prior to being weighed and weigh the patient in the same clothes each time.
- Help the patient establish a target weight and support her efforts to achieve this goal.
- Negotiate an adequate food intake with the patient. Make sure the patient understands the need to comply with this contract and the consequences for not complying.
- Frequently offer small portions of food or drink if the patient wants them. Allow the patient to maintain control over the types and amounts of food eaten, if possible.

⚠ ALERT

Maintain one-on-one supervision of the patient during meals and for 1 hour afterward to ensure compliance with the dietary treatment program. For the hospitalized patient with anorexia, food is considered a medication.

• During an acute anorexic episode, nutritionally complete liquids are more acceptable than solid food because they eliminate the need to choose between foods—something the patient with anorexia may find difficult.

• Teach the patient how to keep a food journal, including the types of food eaten, eating frequency, and feelings associated with eating and exercise.

• Advise family members to avoid discussing food with the patient.

• If tube feedings or other special feeding measures become necessary, fully explain these measures to the patient and be ready to discuss any fears or reluctance; limit the discussion about food itself.

• Expect a weight gain of about 1 lb (0.5 kg) per week.

• If edema or bloating occurs after the patient has returned to normal eating behavior, provide reassurance that this phenomenon is temporary. The patient may fear that she is becoming fat and stop complying with the plan of treatment.

• Encourage the patient to recognize and express feelings freely. The individual may learn that expressing true feelings won't result in losing control or love.

• If a patient receiving outpatient treatment must be hospitalized, maintain contact with the treatment team to facilitate a smooth return to the outpatient setting.

⚠ ALERT

Remember that the patient with anorexia uses exercise, preoccupation with food, ritualism, manipulation, and lying as mechanisms to preserve control.

• The patient and family who need additional information should be referred to the National Association for Anorexia Nervosa and Associated Eating Disorders, a national information and support organization. This organization will provide information about anorexia, may help convince them that they need help, and help them find a psychotherapist or practitioner who is experienced in treating this disorder.

Asperger's disorder

Asperger's disorder is a condition whose primary characteristics are social insensitivity and restricted, repetitive, narrow interests and patterns of behavior. Asperger's disorder causes diminished social and occupational functioning. A lack of empathy and motor clumsiness are also frequently noted. The patient with Asperger's disorder scores within the normal range in intelligence testing and doesn't demonstrate cognitive or language developmental delays.

Asperger's disorder was first described in 1944; however, it wasn't listed in the *Diagnostic and Statistical Manual of Mental Disorders,* Fourth Edition, until 1994. It's listed as a type of pervasive developmental disorder in the current *Diagnostic and Statistical Manual of Mental Disorders,* Fourth Edition, Text Revision (*DSM-IV-TR*). Some professionals consider Asperger's disorder to be identical to higher functioning autism or autism without mental retardation, whereas others see Asperger's disorder as a separate and distinct entity.

CAUSES AND INCIDENCE

There is no clear consensus on the cause of Asperger's disorder. Research continues to focus on biological factors such as brain damage, biochemical abnormalities, genetic factors, and interactions among these factors that may influence the development of Asperger's disorder. Using brain imaging, researchers suggest that there may be differences in the cerebrum, cerebellar, and limbic areas in patients with the disorder. The neuronal theory suggests that there are connection problems within the neuronal networks that link the cerebral areas. It's theorized that there may be more than 20 genes involved with autism spectrum disorders. Although some research suggests that up to 33% of patients with Asperger's also have a first-degree relative with "social difficulties" (suggesting inherited traits), no consistent abnormal genes or chromosomes have been identified. Estimating the actual number of individuals with Asperger's is challenging as individuals may be diagnosed at different ages and usually not until they attend school. The Centers for Disease Control and Prevention estimates that the number of individuals with autism spectrum disorders ranges from 1:150 to 1:166. In addition, males with Asperger's disorder outnumber females by about 4:1.

SIGNS AND SYMPTOMS

Individuals with Asperger's disorder have serious problems with social and communication skills. Intelligence is typically in the normal to superior range and most children are in the mainstream in school, commonly with additional help. In the occupational realm, individuals excel in fields (such as mathematics and computer science) that aren't dependent on social interaction. Individuals with Asperger's disorder desire to fit in socially and make friends but often have great difficulty making social connections. As these individuals approach adolescence, they may be particularly vulnerable to developing anxiety and depression. Tourette's syndrome and obsessive-compulsive disorder (OCD) may also be noted, particularly in males.

Individuals with Asperger's disorder may have some or all of the following characteristics:
- shows no delay in language development, but may have impaired speech and communication skills
- commonly has an extremely formal speech style
- demonstrates literal language interpretation with inability to understand implied meanings

- exhibits early reading ability with large vocabulary and excellent rote memory
- doesn't understand nonverbal social cues such as facial expressions
- has difficulty understanding other people's feelings
- has great difficulty making friends and interacting with peers
- desires adherence to routines
- exhibits preoccupation with one subject
- displays clumsiness
- exhibits heightened sensitivity to the environment (loud noises, smells, clothing fit, etc.).

COMPLICATIONS

- Learning problems caused by difficulties with social integration
- Occupational problems caused by difficulties with social integration
- Depression
- Anxiety
- OCD
- Tourette's syndrome

DIAGNOSTIC CRITERIA

Neuropsychological testing using tests and scales such as:
- Wisconsin Card Sorting test
- Trail Making Test
- Stanford-Binet scale
– Speech testing to identify problems and target interventions
– Audiography testing to exclude auditory deficits.

A diagnosis is made if the patient's symptoms match those in the *DSM-IV-TR*. (See *Diagnosing Asperger's disorder,* page 20.)

TREATMENT

Because Asperger's disorder is a life-long condition, therapy centers on controlling symptoms, improving social skills, and providing educational opportunities and supportive care for the individual and his family.

Because most children with Asperger's disorder are in regular classes in school, special help and coaching are usually needed to help the child adapt to these settings. For example, occupational or physical therapy may improve functioning in group situations and aid in motor coordination. Behavioral therapy may also be useful in some cases. Speech therapy may help improve irregularities in volume, rhythm, or tone. In addition, social skills training and cognitive orientation for daily occupational performance are examples of newer training programs offering potential future benefits.

Family members will also benefit from educational programs or sessions that address information on the disorder, treatment goals for the patient, and psychoeducational material.

Drugs

There are currently no medications to treat the underlying primary characteristics of Asperger's disorder; rather, medication therapy is usually used to control symptoms.
- Central nervous system stimulants, such as methylphenidate (Ritalin) and dextroamphetamine-methamphetamine (Adderall), help

DIAGNOSING ASPERGER'S DISORDER

The following criteria described in the *Diagnostic and Statistical Manual of Mental Disorders,* Fourth Edition, Text Revision, are used to diagnose a person with Asperger's disorder.

■ Impairment in social interaction, including (minimally) two of the following:
– impairment in the use of multiple nonverbal behaviors
– failure to develop peer relations appropriate to developmental level
– lack of sharing experiences spontaneously
– lack of social or emotional reciprocity.

■ Restricted repetitive and stereotyped patterns of behavior, interests, and activities, including (minimally) one of the following:
– preoccupation with one or more stereotyped and restricted patterns of interest that's abnormal either in intensity or focus
– inflexible adherence to specific, nonfunctional routines or rituals
– repetitive motor mannerisms or whole-body movements
– persistent preoccupation with parts of objects.

■ Significant impairment in social, occupational, or other important areas of functioning

■ No clinically significant delay in language or cognitive development

■ No clinically significant delay in the development of age-appropriate self-help skills, adaptive behavior (except in social interaction), and curiosity about the environment (in childhood)

■ Criteria not fitting another specific pervasive developmental disorder or schizophrenia

to control symptoms of hyperactivity and impulsiveness.

● Antipsychotics, such as risperidone (Risperdal), olanzapine (Zyprexa), and haloperidol (Haldol), help to decrease irritability and aggression.

● Antidepressants, such as fluoxetine (Prozac), sertraline (Zoloft), and paroxetine (Paxil), help to treat depression and OCD. Such selective serotonin reuptake inhibitors as fluoxetine act on the brain to help balance levels of serotonin. Tricyclic antidepressants, such as clomipramine (Anafranil), help to balance serotonin and norepinephrine and are used to treat anxiety and depression.

⊠ PREVENTION
Closely monitor patients taking antidepressants for suicidal thoughts, especially during the first 4 weeks of starting therapy.

SPECIAL CONSIDERATIONS
● Provide structure and keep to a routine as much as possible.

● Minimize separations from family members and friends as much as possible.

● Keep any instructions simple and explicit.

● Don't expect nonverbal communication to be perceived and understood.

- Encourage the child's family to work with the school system and individual teachers to provide appropriate learning opportunities.
- Refer the patient and family to professionals who specialize in pervasive developmental disorders.
- Decrease environmental stimuli to which the individual is sensitive. For example, wearing sunglasses and avoiding intense light may help children with Asperger's disorder who exhibit photosensitivity. Earplugs may help those who are sensitive to sounds.
- Assistive technology, such a laptop computer, may help those who have problems with fine motor coordination and handwriting.

Attention deficit hyperactivity disorder

The patient with attention deficit hyperactivity disorder (ADHD) has difficulty focusing his attention and displays impulsiveness and hyperactivity. Although the disorder is present at birth, diagnosis before age 4 or 5 is difficult unless the child shows severe symptoms. Occasionally, the patient isn't diagnosed until adulthood; however, in order to meet criteria, onset must be in childhood and he must have persistent, recurrent symptoms.

CAUSES AND INCIDENCE

ADHD is thought to be a physiologic brain disorder with a familial tendency. Some studies show that when a child has been diagnosed with ADHD, up to 25% of his close relatives also have ADHD. Other studies indicate that it may result from disturbances in neurotransmitter levels in the brain caused by reduced blood flow in the striated area of the brain. Environmental studies show a positive correlation between maternal use of cigarettes and alcohol and the development of ADHD. Children exposed to lead also have a higher incidence of ADHD. ADHD affects 3% to 5% of school-age children and is three times more common in boys than in girls. Of the children diagnosed with ADHD, 30% to 70% continue to exhibit symptoms into adulthood.

SIGNS AND SYMPTOMS

The principal sign of ADHD is persistent patterns of inattention hyperactivity that is present over a long period, in at least two settings (such as school and home), and is accompanied by easy distractibility or hyperactivity with impulsivity. The patient typically demonstrates average to high intelligence. The patient may also exhibit:

- emotional lability
- irritability
- disorganization
- inability to concentrate and complete tasks
- inability to remain seated or wait in line
- frequent daydreaming
- attention to irrelevant thoughts, sounds, or sights.

The patient may have an attention deficit without hyperactivity; if so, he is less likely to be diagnosed and treated. His disorganization becomes apparent as he has difficulty meeting deadlines and keeping track of school or work tools and materials.

COMPLICATIONS

• Emotional problems, such as anxiety and depression
• Social complications, such as school, work, and interpersonal relationship problems
• Poor nutrition
• Higher incidence of trauma-related injuries

DIAGNOSTIC CRITERIA

The child is usually referred for evaluation by the school. (See *Diagnosing attention deficit hyperactivity disorder*.)

A diagnosis of ADHD requires:
• obtaining data from several sources, including the parents, teachers, and the child himself
• completing psychological, medical, and neurologic evaluations to rule out other problems
• evaluating hearing and vision
• evaluating speech and language
• performing a psychiatric evaluation to assess intellect, academic achievement, presence of emotional problems, and learning disorders
• performing professional testing to measure impulsiveness, attention, and the ability to sustain a task.

The combined findings portray a clear picture of the disorder and the areas of support the child will need.

TREATMENT

Education is the first step in effective treatment. The entire treatment team (which ideally includes parents, teachers, and therapists as well as the patient and the practitioner) must understand the disorder and its effect on the patient's functioning.

Treatment may consist of:
• behavior modification
• coaching
• use of planning and organizing systems
• supportive psychotherapy to help the patient cope with the disorder.

Drugs

The patient may benefit from medication to relieve symptoms. Ideally, the treatment team identifies the symptoms to be managed, selects appropriate medication, and then tracks the patient's symptoms carefully to determine the drug's effectiveness. Eighty percent of the children diagnosed with ADHD need to continue medication treatment into their teens and 50% need medication into adulthood. The drugs most commonly used are:
• Central nervous system (CNS) stimulants help control the symptoms of inattention and hyperactivity. CNS stimulants, such as methylphenidate (Ritalin) and dextroamphetamine-amphetamine (Adderall), act to decrease dopamine levels in the brain. There has been no evidence to suggest that these drugs cause dependence in children. Long-term studies show

DIAGNOSING ATTENTION DEFICIT HYPERACTIVITY DISORDER

The *Diagnostic and Statistical Manual of Mental Disorders,* Fourth Edition, Text Revision, groups certain signs and symptoms into inattention and hyperactivity-impulsivity categories. The diagnosis of attention deficit hyperactivity disorder is based on the person demonstrating at least six signs or symptoms from the inattention group or at least six from the hyperactivity-impulsivity group. They must have persisted for at least 6 months to a degree that's maladaptive and inconsistent with the person's developmental level.

Symptoms of inattention

The person manifesting *inattention:*
- often fails to give close attention to details or makes careless mistakes in schoolwork, work, or other activities
- often has difficulty sustaining attention in tasks or play activities
- often doesn't seem to listen when spoken to directly
- often doesn't follow through on instructions and fails to finish schoolwork, chores, or duties in the workplace (not because of oppositional behavior or failure to understand instructions)
- often has difficulty organizing tasks and activities
- often avoids, dislikes, or is reluctant to engage in tasks that require sustained mental effort (such as schoolwork or homework)
- often loses things needed for tasks or activities (for example, toys, school assignments, pencils, books, or tools)
- often becomes distracted by extraneous stimuli

- often demonstrates forgetfulness in daily activities.

Symptoms of hyperactivity

The person manifesting *hyperactivity:*
- often fidgets with hands or feet or squirms in his seat
- often leaves his seat in the classroom or in other situations in which remaining seated is expected
- often runs about or climbs excessively in situations in which remaining seated is expected
- often has difficulty playing or engaging in leisure activities quietly
- often is characterized as "on the go" or acts as if "driven by a motor"
- often talks excessively.

Symptoms of impulsivity

The person manifesting *impulsivity:*
- often blurts out answers before questions have been completed
- often has difficulty awaiting his turn
- often interrupts or intrudes on others.

Additional features

- Some symptoms that cause impairment are evident before age 7.
- Some impairment from the symptoms is present in two or more settings.
- Clinically significant impairment in social, academic, or occupational functioning must be clearly evident.
- The symptoms don't occur exclusively during the course of a pervasive developmental disorder, schizophrenia, or another psychotic disorder and aren't better accounted for by another mental disorder.

that adolescents who continue their medication through their teen years have a lower-than-average incidence of substance abuse.

● Antidepressants help control symptoms of inattention and hyperactivity along with anxiety and depression. Venlafaxine (Effexor) acts to increase norepinephrine in the brain, and bupropion (Wellbutrin) may act to block serotonin and to decrease dopamine. Older tricyclic antidepressants, such as amitriptyline, have affects on both dopamine and norepinephrine. Children who can't tolerate stimulants are often prescribed antidepressants.

SPECIAL CONSIDERATIONS

● Work with professional staff to help the patient and his parents develop external structure and controls.

● Help the patient and family set realistic expectations and limits because the patient with ADHD is easily frustrated (which leads to decreased self-control).

● Provide a calm and consistent environment.

● Teach the patient and family to breakdown tasks into smaller, more manageable steps.

● Teach the parents that physical problems, such as hunger and thirst, may trigger undesirable behavior.

● Teach the family to keep instructions short and simple.

● Tell the family to provide praise, rewards, and positive feedback whenever possible.

Autistic disorder

A severe, pervasive developmental disorder, autistic disorder is marked by unresponsiveness to social contact, deficits in language development, ritualistic and compulsive behaviors, restricted capacity for developmentally appropriate activities and interests, and bizarre responses to the environment. Autistic disorder may be complicated by epileptic seizures, depression and, during periods of stress, catatonic phenomena. Autism becomes apparent before the child reaches age 36 months but, in some children, the actual onset is difficult to determine. According to the National Institute of Mental Health, about 50% of children with autism aren't diagnosed before kindergarten age. (See *Other pervasive developmental disorders.*)

The prognosis for autistic disorder is poor; most patients require a structured environment throughout life.

CAUSES AND INCIDENCE

Studies by the Centers for Disease Control and Prevention reveal that the incidence of autism in the states surveyed is about 1 in 150 8-year-old children. The causes of autistic disorder remain unclear, but researchers are looking at neurobiology and genetic and environmental influences. Magnetic resonance imaging and post-mortem studies demonstrate significant brain changes in people with autism. Some neuroimaging studies are able to locate abnormal brain growth in the first few months of an infant's life. Studies on the families of autistic individuals and twins suggest a genetic predisposition to developing autism. Fragile X syndrome, an inherited disease and the most common cause of mental retardation, is strongly linked to autism. Children with tuberous sclerosis, another inherited disease that causes benign brain and organ tumors, is also strongly associated with autism.

Some autistic children show abnormal but nonspecific EEG findings that suggest brain dysfunction, possibly resulting from trauma, disease, or a structural abnormality. Many children have some degree of mental impairment and may score well in some areas but very poorly in others. Studies have also established a link with abnormalities in neurotransmitters, including (in some cases) increased dopamine and increased serotonin.

SIGNS AND SYMPTOMS

Characteristics of autism include:
• decreased responsiveness to people (Infants with this disorder won't cuddle; they avoid eye contact and are indifferent to affection and physical contact. Parents may report that the child becomes rigid or flaccid when held, cries when touched, and shows little or no interest in human contact.)
• delayed or absent smiling response
• severe language impairment or loss of language by age 3
• lack of imaginative play

OTHER PERVASIVE DEVELOPMENTAL DISORDERS

Although autistic disorder is the most severe and most typical of the pervasive developmental disorders, recent evidence points to other similar disorders in this class.

For example, the *Diagnostic and Statistical Manual of Mental Disorders,* Fourth Edition, Text Revision category *pervasive developmental disorder not otherwise specified* refers to those patients who don't meet the criteria for autistic disorder but who *do* exhibit impaired development of reciprocal social interaction and of verbal and nonverbal communication skills.

Some patients with this diagnosis exhibit a markedly restricted repertoire of activities and interests, but others don't. Research suggests that these disorders are more common than autistic disorder, occurring in 6 to 10 of every 10,000 children.

• poor eye contact
• inability to play with toys or abnormal attachment to objects
• appearance of being hearing impaired
• lack of insight into other people's emotions
• difficulty regulating emotions (He may have outbursts, cry without tears, and demonstrate self-destructive behavior such as hand biting, eye gouging, hair pulling, or head banging when overwhelmed.)

- disturbed sleeping and eating patterns
- repetitive behaviors such as arm flapping or rocking
- obsessive interest in objects such as vacuum cleaners or numbers
- extreme sensitivity to sound, tastes, touch, or other sensory stimulation.

COMPLICATIONS

- About 1 in 4 children with autism develop seizures.
- There are significant social, emotional, and economic stressors for the family related to caring for the autistic individual. The cost of autism to society is estimated at $35 billion per year.

DIAGNOSTIC CRITERIA

For characteristic findings in patients with this condition, see *Diagnosing autistic disorder*.

Diagnosing autism requires a team approach in order to rule out medical, neurologic, psychiatric problems that impact the diagnosis. Identifying autism consists of:
- obtaining data from several sources, including the parents, caregivers, and the child himself
- performing a complete psychological, medical, and neurologic evaluation to rule out additional problems
- evaluating hearing and vision
- evaluating speech and language
- performing a psychiatric evaluation to assess intellect, academic achievement, presence of emotional problems, and learning disorders
- obtaining professional testing to measure impulsiveness, attention, and the ability to sustain a task.

TREATMENT

The most successful treatment for autism consists of early intensive interventions (as soon as the diagnosis is obtained) that focus on encouraging social adjustment, reducing self-injurious behavior, promoting speech development, and providing education. Treatment may consist of:
- home care to assist with the child's physical and behavioral management
- applied behavioral techniques to decrease inappropriate behavior and improve communication, learning, and social behavior
- special education programs
- family counseling.

Drugs

No drug has been shown to successfully treat autistic disorder, but drug therapy may help to manage behavioral symptoms and decrease seizure activity. Some drugs are prescribed "off-label" (not approved by the Food & Drug Administration [FDA] for use in children) because they have shown effectiveness in treating behavioral problems associated with other disorders. Drugs commonly prescribed for autistic individuals may include:
- older antipsychotics, such as haloperidol (Haldol), which reduce the activity of dopamine, thereby alleviating such symptoms as aggression
- newer antipsychotics, such as risperidone (Risperdal) and olanzapine (Zyprexa), which reduce severe

DIAGNOSING AUTISTIC DISORDER

Autism is diagnosed when the patient meets the criteria in the *Diagnostic and Statistical Manual of Mental Disorders,* Fourth Edition, Text Revision. At least six characteristics from the following three categories must be present, including at least two from the social interaction category and one each from the communication and patterns categories.

Social interaction
Impairment in social interaction, as shown by at least two of the following:
■ marked impairment in the use of multiple nonverbal behaviors, such as eye-to-eye gaze, facial expression, body postures, and gestures to regulate social interaction
■ failure to develop peer relationships appropriate to developmental level
■ no spontaneous sharing of enjoyment, interests, or achievements with others
■ lack of social or emotional reciprocity
■ gross impairment in ability to make peer friendships.

Communication
Impairment in communication, as shown by at least one of the following:
■ delay in, or total lack of, spoken language development

■ in individuals with adequate speech, marked impairment in initiating or sustaining a conversation with others
■ stereotyped and repetitive use of language or idiosyncratic language
■ lack of varied, spontaneous make-believe play or social imitative play appropriate to developmental level.

Patterns
Restricted, repetitive, and stereotyped patterns of behavior, interests, and activities, as manifested by at least one of the following:
■ encompassing preoccupation with one or more stereotyped and restricted patterns of interest that's abnormal either in intensity or focus
■ apparently inflexible adherence to specific nonfunctional routines or rituals
■ stereotyped and repetitive motor mannerisms
■ persistent preoccupation with parts of objects.

Additional criteria
Delays or abnormal functioning in at least one of the following before age 3:
■ social interaction
■ language as used in social communication
■ symbolic or imaginative play
■ disturbance that isn't better accounted for by Rett's disorder or childhood disintegrative disorder.

behavior problems (More long-term studies are needed to look at the long-term effects of treatment.)
• antidepressants, such as fluoxetine (Prozac), which is FDA-approved

for children (age 7 and older) to treat depression and obsessive-compulsive disorder
• antidepressants, such as fluvoxamine (Luvox) and sertraline

(Zoloft), which reduce repetitive behavior and improve social contact

• stimulants, such as methyl-phenidate (Ritalin) (Methylphenidate has been effective at decreasing impulsivity and hyperactivity in attention deficit hyperactivity disorder.)

• anxiolytics, such as diazepam (Valium) and lorazepam (Ativan), which treat behavioral symptoms (Safe use in children hasn't been established, however.)

• anticonvulsants, such as carbamazepine (Tegretol), topiramate (Topamax), and valproic acid (Depakene), which decrease seizure activity.

SPECIAL CONSIDERATIONS
⚠ ALERT

Autistic individuals respond best to regular, predictable routines. Carefully preparing children for changes in routine can help to reduce outbursts and undesirable behavior.

• Identify positive ways for the child to channel his energy.

• Provide positive reinforcement for good behavior.

• Instruct the family on ways to make the home environment safer, such as installing locking gates, cabinet locks, and outlet covers.

• Provide emotional support to the parents, and refer them to the Autism Society of America.

Bipolar disorders

Marked by severe pathologic mood swings from hyperactivity and euphoria to sadness and depression, bipolar disorders involve various symptom combinations. Type I bipolar disorder is characterized by alternating episodes of mania and depression, whereas type II is characterized by recurrent depressive episodes and occasional mild manic (hypomanic) episodes. In some patients, bipolar disorder assumes a seasonal pattern, marked by a cyclic relation between the onset of the mood episode and a particular 60-day period of the year.

CAUSES AND INCIDENCE

The cause of bipolar disorder is unclear, but hereditary, biological, and psychological factors may play a part. For example, the incidence of bipolar disorder among relatives of affected patients is higher than in the general population and highest among maternal relatives. The closer the relationship, the greater the susceptibility. Children with one affected parent have a 25% chance of developing bipolar disorder; children with two affected parents, a 50% chance. The incidence of this illness in siblings is 20% to 25%; in identical twins, the incidence is 66% to 96%.

Although certain biochemical changes accompany mood swings, it isn't clear whether these changes cause the mood swings or result from them. In mania and depression, intracellular sodium concentration increases during illness and returns to normal with recovery.

Patients with mood disorders have a defect in the way the brain handles certain neurotransmitters—chemical messengers that shuttle nerve impulses between neurons. Low levels of the chemicals dopamine and norepinephrine, for example, have been linked to depression, whereas excessively high levels of these chemicals are associated with mania.

Changes in the concentration of acetylcholine and serotonin may also play a role. Although neurobiologists have yet to prove that these chemical shifts cause bipolar disorder, it's widely assumed that most antidepressant medications work by modifying these neurotransmitter systems.

New data suggest that changes in the circadian rhythms that control hormone secretion, body temperature, and appetite may contribute to the symptoms of bipolar disorder.

Emotional or physical trauma, such as bereavement, disruption of an important relationship, or a serious accidental injury, may precede the onset of bipolar disorder; however, bipolar disorder commonly appears without identifiable predisposing factors.

Manic episodes may follow a stressful event, but they're also associated with antidepressant therapy and childbirth. Major depressive episodes may be caused by chronic physical illness, psychoactive drug dependence, psychosocial stressors, and childbirth. Other familial influences, especially the early loss of a parent, parental depression, incest, or abuse, may predispose a person to depressive illness. (See *Cyclothymic disorder.*)

The American Psychiatric Association estimates that 0.4% to 1.2% of adults experience bipolar disorder. This disorder affects women and men equally and is more common in higher socioeconomic groups. It can begin any time after adolescence, but onset usually occurs between ages 20 and 35; about 35% of patients experience onset between ages 35 and 60. Before the onset of overt symptoms, many patients with bipolar disorder have an energetic and outgoing personality with a history of wide mood swings.

Bipolar disorder recurs in 80% of patients; as they grow older, the episodes recur more frequently and last longer.

SIGNS AND SYMPTOMS

Signs and symptoms vary widely, depending on whether the patient is

---

CYCLOTHYMIC DISORDER

A chronic mood disturbance of at least 2 years' duration, cyclothymic disorder involves numerous episodes of hypomania or depression that aren't of sufficient severity or duration to qualify as a major depressive episode or a bipolar disorder.

Cyclothymic disorder commonly starts in adolescence or early adulthood. Beginning insidiously, this disorder leads to persistent social and occupational dysfunction.

Signs and symptoms
In the hypomanic phase, the patient may experience insomnia; hyperactivity; inflated self-esteem; increased productivity and creativity; over involvement in pleasurable activities, including an increased sexual drive; physical restlessness; and rapid speech. Depressive symptoms may include insomnia, feelings of inadequacy, decreased productivity, social withdrawal, loss of libido, loss of interest in pleasurable activities, lethargy, slow speech, and crying.

Diagnosis
Many medical disorders (for example, Cushing's syndrome, stroke, brain tumors, and head trauma) and drug overdose can produce a similar pattern of mood alteration. These organic causes must be ruled out before making a diagnosis of cyclothymic disorder.

experiencing a manic or a depressive episode. The manic patient:
- typically appears grandiose, euphoric, expansive, or irritable with little control over his activities and responses
- may appear hyperactive or describe excessive behavior, including elaborate plans for numerous social events, efforts to renew old acquaintances by telephoning friends at all hours of the night, buying sprees, or promiscuous sexual activity
- may have a bizarre quality, such as dressing in colorful or strange garments, wearing excessive makeup, or giving advice to passing strangers
- commonly expresses an inflated sense of self-esteem, ranging from uncritical self-confidence to marked grandiosity, which may be delusional
- may have accelerated and pressured speech, frequent changes of topic, and flight of ideas
- is easily distracted and responds rapidly to external stimuli, such as background noise or a ringing telephone
- may have signs of malnutrition and poor personal hygiene
- may report sleeping and eating less as well as being more physically active than usual.

Hypomania, more common than acute mania, can be recognized during the assessment interview by three classic symptoms:
- euphoric but unstable mood
- pressured speech
- increased motor activity.

The hypomanic patient:
- may appear elated, hyperactive, easily distracted

- is talkative, irritable, impatient, impulsive, and full of energy
- seldom exhibits flight of ideas. (Delusions and other symptoms of psychotic intensity are never present.)

The patient who experiences a depressive episode may speak and respond slowly but is not usually disoriented or intellectually impaired. His growing sadness, guilt, negativity, and fatigue place extraordinary burdens on his family. He may report:
- loss of self-esteem
- overwhelming inertia
- difficulty concentrating
- social withdrawal
- feelings of hopelessness, apathy, or self-reproach
- feelings of being wicked and that he deserves to be punished.

Physical examination of the patient with a depressive episode may reveal:
- reduced psychomotor activity
- lethargy
- low muscle tonus
- weight loss
- slowed gait
- constipation
- sleep disturbances (falling asleep, staying asleep, or early morning awakening)
- sexual dysfunction
- headaches, chest pains, and heaviness in the limbs.

Typically, symptoms are worse in the morning and gradually subside as the day progresses.

The patient's concerns about his health may become hypochondriacal, such that he may worry excessively about having cancer or some other serious illness. In an elderly patient, physical symptoms may be the only clues to depression.

≥ PREVENTION

Suicide is an ever-present risk, especially as the depression begins to lift. At that point, a rising energy level may strengthen the patient's resolve to carry out suicidal plans. The suicidal patient may also harbor homicidal ideas—for example, thinking of killing his family either in anger or to spare them pain and disgrace.

COMPLICATIONS

- This illness is associated with a significant mortality; 20% of patients commit suicide, many just as the depression lifts.

≥ PREVENTION

Suicidal behavior is linked to increases in impulsivity and to alcohol abuse in patients with bipolar disorder.

- There are significant economic and social stresses associated with bipolar disorder. For example, families may suffer economic hardship if an individual's mania is associated with unchecked spending.
- Studies show that the prevalence of cardiovascular disease risk factors (smoking, obesity, hypertension, dyslipidemia, and type 2 diabetes) is twice as high among individuals with bipolar disorder than in the general population.

≥ PREVENTION

Strategies to reduce the risk of developing cardiovascular disease need to be developed and implemented.

DIAGNOSTIC CRITERIA

For characteristic findings in patients with this condition, see *Diagnosing bipolar disorders,* page 33.

Diagnosing bipolar disorder requires a team approach in order to rule out medical, neurologic, and psychiatric problems that impact the diagnosis. In addition to physical and psychological examinations the patient may require:

- hematologic, endocrine, and other laboratory tests to rule out medical causes of mood changes, such as hypothyroidism, hyperthyroidism, uremia, or psychoactive substance abuse
- neurologic evaluation and imaging studies to rule out disturbances, such as cerebral arteriosclerosis, parkinsonism, psychoactive drug abuse, brain tumor, and uremia
- review of the medications prescribed for other disorders, which may indicate the possibility of drug-induced depression or mania.

TREATMENT

Treatment for bipolar disorder commonly consists of:

- drug therapy prescribed by a psychiatrist
- psychotherapy, which provides support and guidance
- cognitive behavioral therapy, which helps patient change negative thought patterns
- family therapy

DIAGNOSING BIPOLAR DISORDERS

The diagnosis of a bipolar disorder is confirmed when the patient meets the criteria documented in the *Diagnostic and Statistical Manual of Mental Disorders,* Fourth Edition, Text Revision.

For a manic episode

■ A distinct period of abnormally and persistently elevated, expansive, or irritable mood lasting at least 1 week (or any duration if hospitalization is needed).

■ During the mood disturbance period, at least three of the following symptoms must have persisted (four, if the mood is only irritable) and have been present to a significant degree:
– inflated self-esteem or grandiosity
– decreased need for sleep
– more talkative than usual or pressured to keep talking
– flight of ideas or subjective experience that thoughts are racing
– distractibility
– increased goal-directed activity or psychomotor agitation
– excessive involvement in pleasurable activities that have a high potential for painful consequences.

■ The symptoms don't meet the criteria for a mixed episode.

■ The mood disturbance is sufficiently severe to cause one of the following to occur:
– marked impairment in occupational functioning or in usual social activities or relationships with others
– hospitalization to prevent harm to self or others
– evidence of psychotic features.

■ The symptoms aren't due to the direct physiologic effects of a substance or a general medical condition.

For a hypomanic episode

■ A distinct period of abnormally and persistently elevated, expansive, or irritable mood lasting at least 4 days that's clearly different from the usual nondepressed mood.

■ During the mood disturbance period, at least three of the following symptoms must have persisted (four, if the mood is only irritable) and have been present to a significant degree:
– inflated self-esteem or grandiosity
– decreased need for sleep
– more talkative than usual or pressured to keep talking
– flight of ideas or subjective experience that thoughts are racing
– distractibility
– increased goal-directed activity or psychomotor agitation
– excessive involvement in pleasurable activities that have a high potential for painful consequences.

■ The episode is associated with an unequivocal change in functioning that's uncharacteristic of the person when not symptomatic.

■ Others can recognize the disturbance in mood and the change in functioning.

■ The episode isn't severe enough to markedly impair social or occupational functioning or to necessitate hospitalization to prevent harm to self or others. No psychotic features are evident.

■ The symptoms aren't caused by the direct physiologic effects of a substance or a general medical condition.

(*continued*)

DIAGNOSING BIPOLAR DISORDERS *(continued)*

For a bipolar I single manic episode

- The presence of only one manic episode and no past major depressive episodes.
- The manic episode isn't better accounted for by schizoaffective disorder and isn't superimposed on schizophrenia, schizophreniform disorder, delusional disorder, or psychotic disorder not otherwise specified.

For a bipolar I disorder, most recent episode hypomanic

- The person is currently (or was most recently) in a hypomanic episode.
- The person previously had at least one manic episode or mixed episode.
- The mood symptoms cause clinically significant distress or impairment in social, occupational, or other important areas of functioning.
- The first two exacerbations of the mood episode (above) aren't better accounted for by schizoaffective disorder and aren't superimposed on schizophrenia, schizophreniform disorder, delusional disorder, or psychotic disorder not otherwise specified.

For a bipolar I disorder, most recent episode manic

- The person is currently (or was most recently) in a manic episode.
- The person previously had at least one major depressive episode, manic episode, or mixed episode.
- The first two exacerbations of mood episode (above) aren't better accounted for by schizoaffective disorder and aren't superimposed on schizophrenia, schizophreniform

disorder, delusional disorder, or psychotic disorder not otherwise specified.

For a bipolar I disorder, most recent episode mixed

- The person is currently (or was most recently) in a mixed episode.
- The person previously had at least one major depressive episode, manic episode, or mixed episode.
- The first two exacerbations of mood episode (above) aren't better accounted for by schizoaffective disorder and aren't superimposed on schizophrenia, schizophreniform disorder, delusional disorder, or psychotic disorder not otherwise specified.

For a bipolar I disorder, most recent episode depressed

- The person is currently (or was most recently) in a major depressive episode.
- The person previously had at least one manic episode or mixed episode.
- The first two exacerbations of mood episode (above) aren't better accounted for by schizoaffective disorder and aren't superimposed on schizophrenia, schizophreniform disorder, delusional disorder, or psychotic disorder not otherwise specified.

For a bipolar I disorder, most recent episode unspecified

- Criteria, except for duration, are currently (or most recently) met for a manic, hypomanic, mixed, or major depressive episode.
- The person previously had at least one manic episode or mixed episode.

DIAGNOSING BIPOLAR DISORDERS *(continued)*

- The mood symptoms cause clinically significant distress or impairment in social, occupational, or other important areas of functioning.
- The first two exacerbations of mood episode (above) aren't better accounted for by schizoaffective disorder and aren't superimposed on schizophrenia, schizophreniform disorder, delusional disorder, or psychotic disorder not otherwise specified.
- The first two exacerbations of mood episode (above) aren't caused by the direct physiologic effects of a substance or a general medical condition.

For a bipolar II disorder
- The presence (or history) of one or more major depressive episodes.

- The presence (or history) of at least one hypomanic episode.
- The patient has never had a manic episode or a mixed episode.
- The first two exacerbations of mood episode (above) aren't better accounted for by schizoaffective disorder and aren't superimposed on schizophrenia, schizophreniform disorder, delusional disorder, or psychotic disorder not otherwise specified.
- The symptoms cause clinically significant distress or impairment in social, occupational, or other important areas of functioning.

- psychoeducational therapy, which educates the individual and family about the disorder and treatments in order to prevent relapse
- electroconvulsive therapy (rarely) when the disorder is refractory to other interventions.

Drugs
- Lithium (Eskalith) stabilizes mood and prevents relapse and rapid cycling. Therapeutic blood levels must be maintained for 7 to 10 days before the drug's beneficial effects appear. Long-term use of lithium may affect thyroid function.

⚠ ALERT
Lithium has a narrow therapeutic range; so, treatment must be started cautiously and the dosage must be adjusted slowly. Teach the patient and his family to immediately notify the practitioner if signs or symptoms of toxicity, such as diarrhea, abdominal cramps, vomiting, unsteadiness, drowsiness, muscle weakness, polyuria, and tremors, occur.

- Anticonvulsants stabilize mood and are useful in difficult-to-treat episodes. Valproate (Depakote), carbamazepine (Tegretol), and others may be combined with each other or with lithium to achieve maximum effects.

⚠ ALERT
Young women taking valproate should be monitored carefully. Some research suggests that use of valproate in women younger than age 20 may lead to abnormal hormone levels and polycystic ovary syndrome.

• Antipsychotics may help to relieve symptoms of psychotic depression. Olanzapine (Zyprexa) is approved by the Food and Drug Administration to treat acute mania.

⚠ ALERT

Research suggests that antidepressant drug therapy may cause rapid mood cycling in some patients.

SPECIAL CONSIDERATIONS
For the manic patient

• Remember the manic patient's physical needs. Encourage him to eat. Offer small, frequent meals. Alter the diet so that it's high in calories, carbohydrates, and liquids.

• As the patient's symptoms subside, encourage him to assume responsibility for personal care.

• Provide emotional support, maintain a calm environment, and set realistic goals for behavior.

• Provide diversionary activities suited to a short attention span.

• Encourage the patient to keep a daily mood diary to identify patterns and recognize symptoms associated with relapse.

• When necessary, reorient the patient to reality.

• Set limits in a calm, clear, and self-confident manner for the manic patient's demanding, hyperactive, manipulative, and acting-out behaviors.

• Listen to requests attentively and with a neutral attitude. Avoid power struggles if a patient tries to put you on the spot for an immediate answer.

• Encourage solitary activities such as writing out one's thoughts.

• Collaborate with other staff members to provide a consistent response to the patient's manipulative or acting-out behaviors.

• Watch for early signs of frustration (when the patient's anger may escalate from verbal threats to hitting an object). Tell the patient firmly that threats and hitting are unacceptable. Explain that these behaviors show that he needs help to control his behavior. Inform him that the staff will help him move to a quiet area to help him control his behavior so he won't hurt himself or others. Staff members who have practiced as a team can work effectively to prevent acting-out behavior or to remove and confine a patient.

⚠ ALERT

Tell the staff promptly when acting-out behavior escalates. It's safer to have help available before you need it than to try controlling an anxious or frightened patient by yourself.

• After the incident is over and the patient is calm and in control, discuss his feelings with him and offer suggestions on how to prevent a recurrence.

For the depressed patient

• The depressed patient needs ongoing positive reinforcement to improve his self-esteem.

• Provide a structured routine, including activities to boost his self-confidence and promote interaction with others (for instance, group therapy).

• Encourage the patient to talk or to write down his feelings if he's having trouble expressing them.

• To prevent possible self-injury or suicide, remove harmful objects (such as glass, belts, rope, or bobby pins) from the patient's environment, observe him closely, and strictly supervise his medications. Institute suicide precautions, when necessary, as dictated by facility policy.

• Provide for the patient's physical needs. If he's too depressed to take care of himself, help him with personal hygiene measures. Encourage him to eat, or feed him if necessary. If he's constipated, add high-fiber foods to his diet; offer small, frequent meals; and encourage physical activity.

• Help the patient establish good sleep hygiene measures to improve sleep.

• For additional support and guidance refer the patient and family to the National Depressive and Manic Depressive Association and the National Alliance for the Mentally Ill.

Body dysmorphic disorder

In body dysmorphic disorder (BDD), the patient is preoccupied with an imagined or slight defect in physical appearance. The perceived flaw may involve one or several body parts. He may think he's hideous or grotesque even though others reassure him that he looks fine. The patient with this disorder thinks about the defect for at least 1 hour each day and the intense preoccupation may consume many hours each day. It's frequently associated with other disorders, such as depression, social phobias, and obsessive-compulsive and substance abuse disorders.

CAUSES AND INCIDENCE

No one cause for BDD has been identified, although several theories are being explored. The neurobiological theory holds that some individuals may have a genetic predisposition to psychiatric disorders, making them more likely to develop BDD. It may also be associated with lower brain levels of serotonin or other neurotransmitters.

The psychological theory holds that low self-esteem and a tendency to judge oneself almost exclusively by appearance may contribute to BDD. These patients may be perfectionists who strive for an impossible ideal. In such patients, heightened perception about appearance causes increasing focus on every imperfection or slight abnormality. Certain stresses or life events, especially during adolescence, may precipitate the onset of the disorder. Children of parents who are highly critical of their children's appearance are more likely to develop BDD as adolescents.

In the United States, BDD is estimated to occur in 1% to 3% of the general population. Although the gender ratio is unclear, it does affect both males and females. The incidence may be underestimated because it's frequently undiagnosed unless the patient seeks help for another psychiatric problem such as depression. Some studies estimate that of all individuals who seek dermatologic or cosmetic surgery, the incidence of BDD is between 6% and 15%. BDD is a chronic condition with a varying course that usually begins during the late teens and persists into adulthood. The average age of onset is 17.

SIGNS AND SYMPTOMS

BDD may be suspected in the patient who reports or exhibits any of these behaviors:

- commonly checks reflection in the mirror or avoids mirrors
- frequently compares appearance against that of other people
- frequently examines the appearance of other people
- tries to camouflage the perceived defect with clothing, makeup, or a hat or by changing posture
- seeks corrective treatment, such as surgery or dermatologic therapy, to eradicate the perceived defect, even though practitioners, family members, and friends think such measures are unnecessary
- constantly seeks reassurance from others about the perceived flaw or, conversely, tries to convince others of its repulsiveness
- performs long grooming rituals, such as repeatedly combing or cutting the hair or applying makeup or cover-up creams
- picks at the skin or squeezes pimples or blackheads for hours
- frequently touches the perceived problem area

- frequently measures the body part he considers repulsive
- feels anxious and extremely self-conscious
- feels such acute distress over his appearance that he is functionally impaired
- avoids social situations where the perceived defect may be exposed
- has difficulty maintaining relationships with peers, family, and spouse
- performs poorly in school or work or may not be able to work
- has low self-esteem
- expresses suicidal ideation.

⊗ PREVENTION

Assess all individuals with BDD for suicidal ideation. Some studies of individuals with BDD show that up to 30% had made at least one suicide attempt.

COMPLICATIONS

Complications from BDD include:

- varying degrees of functional impairment, some so severe that the individual avoids all social interaction
- self-destructive behavior that may consist of performing self surgery (such as attempted liposuction) or using sandpaper on the skin to remove lesions.

DIAGNOSTIC CRITERIA

BDD shares many of the same symptoms and signs as other psychological illnesses, especially obsessive-compulsive disorder. To assess the severity, testing may include diagnostic instruments such as the Yale-Brown Obsessive-Compulsive Scale modified for BDD or various others.

The diagnosis of BDD is confirmed when the patient meets criteria from the *Diagnostic and Statistical Manual of Mental Disorders,* Fourth Edition, Text Revision. Criteria include the following:

• The patient is preoccupied with an imagined defect in appearance. If a slight physical abnormality actually is present, concern over it is markedly excessive.

• The preoccupation causes clinically significant distress or impairment in social, occupational, or other important areas of functioning.

• The preoccupation isn't better explained by another mental disorder such as anorexia nervosa.

TREATMENT

Successful treatments include both psychotherapy and the use of drugs such as selective serotonin reuptake inhibitors (SSRIs).

The goals of treatment for the patient include enhancement of his self-esteem, reduced preoccupation with the perceived flaw, and elimination of the harmful effects of compulsive behaviors. The patient also needs to improve functional and social interaction as well as express (and cope with) feelings of anxiety without resorting to excessive behaviors.

Cognitive-behavioral therapy with cognitive restructuring and group therapies have consistently proven helpful. Behavioral methods,

including aversion therapy, thought-stopping, and flooding (also called *implosion therapy*), have also proven effective.

Drugs

• SSRIs, such as fluoxetine (Prozac), fluvoxamine (Luvox), and paroxetine (Paxil), have demonstrated favorable responses in reducing BDD-associated obsessive-compulsive behavior, anxiety, and depression. Individuals taking SSRIs for BDD may require higher doses than individuals being treated for depression alone.

SPECIAL CONSIDERATIONS

• Provide an accepting, nonjudgmental atmosphere when caring for the patient.

• If the patient becomes involved in ritualistic thoughts and behaviors to the point of self-neglect, provide for basic needs, such as rest, nutrition, and grooming. Don't block ritualistic behavior, but attempt to set limits with the patient.

• Help the patient explore feelings associated with the behavior.

• Engage the patient in activities that create positive accomplishments and raise self-esteem and confidence.

• Suggest active diversions to divert the patient's attention away from unwanted thoughts.

• Encourage the patient to use appropriate techniques to relieve stress, loneliness, and isolation.

• Monitor drug therapy for effectiveness and adverse effects.

Bulimia nervosa

The essential features of bulimia nervosa include eating binges followed by feelings of guilt, humiliation, and self-deprecation. These feelings cause the patient to engage in self-induced vomiting, use laxatives or diuretics, follow a strict diet, or fast to overcome the effects of the binges. These episodes must occur at least twice a week for 3 months. Unless the patient spends an excessive amount of time bingeing and purging, bulimia nervosa seldom is incapacitating. However, electrolyte imbalances (metabolic alkalosis, hypochloremia, and hypokalemia) and dehydration can occur, increasing the risk of life-threatening physical complications.

CAUSES AND INCIDENCE

The cause of bulimia nervosa is unknown, but psychosocial factors are thought to contribute. These factors include family disturbance or conflict, sexual abuse, maladaptive learned behavior, struggle for control or self-identity, cultural overemphasis on physical appearance, and parental obesity. Bulimia nervosa is associated with depression, anxiety, phobias, and obsessive-compulsive disorder.

Eating disorders are most prevalent in affluent cultural groups and are essentially unknown in cultural groups where poverty and malnutrition are prevalent. In developing countries, almost no cases of eating disorders have been recognized.

Cultural forces that influence body image are major factors in the development of eating disorders. In most cultures in the United States, thinness is valued and being overweight is frowned upon. However, media messages are mixed. Indeed, one may see a commercial for fast food, immediately followed by a commercial for a weight-loss program. Young girls are especially at risk for these mixed messages, although boys may be influenced as well. Further, certain sports or activities, such as ballet, wrestling, and gymnastics, may encourage potentially unhealthy weight loss.

Bulimia nervosa usually begins in adolescence or early adulthood and can occur simultaneously with anorexia nervosa. It affects nine women for every man. Nearly 2% of adult women meet the diagnostic criteria for bulimia nervosa; 5% to 15% have some symptoms of the disorder.

SIGNS AND SYMPTOMS

The history of a patient with bulimia nervosa is characterized by episodes of binge eating that may occur up to several times per day. A binge is usually defined as consuming an excess amount of food over a discrete period of time (usually less than 2 hours). The patient commonly reports a loss of control over the bingeing episode, during which she continues eating until abdominal pain, sleep, or the presence of another person interrupts it. The preferred food is usually sweet, soft, and high in calories and carbohydrate content.

The patient with bulimia may:
- appear thin or of normal weight, but have wide fluctuations in weight (Patients are never as thin as those suffering from anorexia nervosa.)
- use purging behaviors, such as self-induced vomiting, diuretics, and laxatives, to compensate for bingeing behavior
- exercise excessively to lose weight
- use stimulant substances to lose weight
- feel guilty and ashamed and attempt to hide bingeing and purging behavior
- ritualize eating behavior
- complain of abdominal and epigastric pain caused by acute gastric dilation.

About 80% to 90% of patients suffering from bulimia nervosa use self-induced vomiting to compensate for bingeing behavior. This may occur several times a day or several times a week. Signs of repetitive vomiting include:
- discolored tooth enamel
- painless swelling of the salivary glands
- hoarseness, throat irritation, or lacerations
- calluses on the knuckles or abrasions and scars on the dorsum of the hand, resulting from tooth injury from attempts to induce vomiting
- frequent use of ipecac to induce vomiting.

A patient with bulimia nervosa is commonly perceived by others as a "perfect" student, mother, or career

woman; an adolescent may be distinguished for participation in competitive activities such as sports. However, the patient's psychosocial history may reveal an exaggerated sense of guilt, symptoms of depression, childhood trauma (especially sexual abuse), parental obesity, or a history of unsatisfactory sexual relationships. Overt clues to this disorder also include hyperactivity, frequent weighing, and a distorted body image. (See *Characteristics of patients with bulimia,* page 42.)

COMPLICATIONS

Complications from purging can be severe and even life-threatening. They may include:
- gastric rupture from binge eating
- erosion of tooth enamel, dental caries, and gingivitis from vomiting
- esophageal inflammation and tears from vomiting
- heart failure from ipecac toxicity
- dehydration
- electrolyte imbalances, such as metabolic alkalosis, hypochloremia, and hypokalemia that may lead to cardiac arrhythmias and sudden death
- chronic constipation from excessive laxative use
- metabolic acidosis from laxative abuse.

⊠ PREVENTION

Assess all individuals with eating disorders about suicidal thoughts as they may have a 10% to 30% risk of attempting suicide at least once. The incidence of attempted suicide increases if the patient has a personality disorder, a history of substance

CHARACTERISTICS OF PATIENTS WITH BULIMIA

Recognizing patients with bulimia isn't always easy. Unlike patients with anorexia, patients with bulimia don't deny that their eating habits are abnormal, but they commonly conceal their behavior out of shame. If you suspect bulimia nervosa, watch for these features:

- difficulty with impulse control
- chronic depression
- exaggerated sense of guilt
- low tolerance for frustration
- recurrent anxiety
- feelings of alienation
- self-consciousness
- difficulty expressing feelings such as anger
- impaired social or occupational adjustment.

- Baseline electrocardiogram detects cardiac arrhythmias.
- Serum glucose levels may reveal hypoglycemia.

TREATMENT

Treatment of bulimia nervosa may continue for several years. Interrelated physical and psychological symptoms must be treated simultaneously. Merely promoting weight gain isn't sufficient to guarantee long-term recovery. A patient whose physical status is severely compromised by inadequate or chaotic eating patterns is difficult to engage in the psychotherapeutic process.

abuse, or a childhood history of sexual or physical abuse.

DIAGNOSTIC CRITERIA

For characteristic findings of bulimia nervosa, see *Diagnosing bulimia nervosa*.

Additional diagnostic tools include the following:

- Beck Depression Inventory helps to identify coexisting depression.
- Laboratory tests help to determine the presence and severity of complications. Abnormal serum electrolyte studies may show elevated bicarbonate, decreased potassium, and decreased sodium levels and abnormal pH.

DIAGNOSING BULIMIA NERVOSA

The diagnosis of bulimia is made when the patient meets criteria put forth in the *Diagnostic and Statistical Manual of Mental Disorders*, Fourth Edition, Text Revision. Both of the behaviors listed below must occur at least twice per week for 3 months:

- recurrent episodes of binge eating (rapid consumption of a large amount of food in a discrete period and a feeling of lack of control over eating behavior during the eating binges)
- recurrent inappropriate compensatory behavior to prevent weight gain (self-induced vomiting; misuse of laxatives, diuretics, enemas, or other medications; fasting; excessive exercise).

Treating bulimia may require inpatient hospitalization although outpatient treatment is more common. Psychotherapy is commonly used to treat bulimia nervosa and includes cognitive behavioral, individual, family, and group therapies. With adolescents, studies have shown that family-based therapy is more effective than individual-based therapy. The patient may also benefit from participation in self-help groups, such as Overeaters Anonymous, or in a drug rehabilitation program if she has a concurrent substance abuse problem. The patient may also benefit from nutritional counseling.

The goals of psychotherapy include:

• interrupting the binge-purge cycle and helping the patient regain control over her eating behavior

• strategies to help the patient address the eating disorder as a symptom of unresolved conflict

• helping the patient understand the basis of her behavior and teaching her self-control strategies.

Drugs

• Fluoxetine (Prozac) is the only drug approved by the Food and Drug Administration to treat bulimia. It may be especially beneficial for those patients who are also suffering from anxiety and depression. Fluoxetine has been shown to decrease the frequency of bingeing/purging behaviors and to help improve the patient's attitude toward eating. Studies have also shown that patients are less likely to relapse.

⊵ PREVENTION

Closely monitor children and adolescents for signs of increasing depression or suicidal thoughts especially during the first 4 weeks of starting therapy with selective serotonin reuptake inhibitors.

SPECIAL CONSIDERATIONS

• Supervise the patient during mealtimes and for a specified period after meals (usually 1 hour). Set a time limit for each meal. Provide a pleasant, relaxed environment for eating.

• Use behavior modification techniques, and reward the patient for satisfactory weight gain.

• Outline the risks of laxative, emetic, and diuretic abuse for the patient.

• Establish a contract with the patient, specifying the amount and type of food to be eaten at each meal.

• Teach the patient how to keep a food journal to monitor treatment progress.

• Encourage her to recognize and express her feelings about her eating behavior.

• Maintain an accepting and nonjudgmental attitude.

• Encourage the patient to talk about stressful issues, such as achievement, independence, socialization, sexuality, family problems, and control.

- Provide assertiveness training to help the patient gain control over her behavior and achieve a realistic and positive self-image.
- Identify the patient's elimination patterns.
- Assess her suicide potential.

- Refer the patient and her family to the National Association of Anorexia Nervosa and Associated Disorders and the National Eating Disorders Association for additional information and support.

Conduct disorder

Aggressive behavior is the hallmark of conduct disorder. A child with this disorder fights, bullies, intimidates, and assaults others physically or sexually and is truant from school at an early age. Typically, the patient has poor relationships with peers and adults and violates others' rights and society's rules. Conduct disorder evolves slowly over time until a consistent pattern of behavior is established.

CAUSES AND INCIDENCE

Factors that influence the development of conduct disorder include biological factors (including genetic factors), brain trauma, child abuse and other childhood traumas, failure in school, and psychosocial components. Children of a parent who has antisocial personality disorder have an increased risk of developing conduct disorder. Siblings of individuals with conduct disorder also have an increased risk of developing the disorder.

Studies of the neurobiology of the disorder have linked it to underarousal of the autonomic nervous system and impaired functioning of the nonadrenergic system. Researchers have demonstrated that the brains of patients with severe conduct disorder and who demonstrate callous behavior show less activity in the amygdala region—an area of the brain that typically responds to situations that would elicit empathy. Social risk factors that may predispose a child to conduct disorder include socioeconomic deprivation; harsh, punitive parenting with verbal or physical aggression; separation from parents; early institutionalization; family neglect, parental psychiatric illness, substance abuse, or marital discord; and large family size, crowding, and divorce with persistent hostility between the parents. Roughly 30% to 50% of clinical populations with conduct disorder also have attention deficit hyperactivity disorder (ADHD).

The prevalence of conduct disorder among people ages 9 to 17 is about 1% to 4%. An estimated 6% to 16% of boys and 2% to 9% of girls younger than age 18 have the disorder. Studies of youths show that up to 40% of those detained in juvenile detention centers have disruptive behavior disorders. The prognosis is worse in children with an earlier onset; these children are more likely to develop antisocial personality disorder as adults.

SIGNS AND SYMPTOMS

The individual with conduct disorder may exhibit:

- aggressive behavior with family members and peers
- cruelty to animals
- sexually abusive behavior
- sexually precocious behavior and prostitution
- lying
- cheating in school
- truancy
- substance abuse
- criminal behavior such as property destruction or stealing.

COMPLICATIONS

- Poor performance in school
- Societal costs caused by delinquency and crime
- Occupational difficulties
- Legal problems
- Physical injuries from fighting
- Sexually transmitted diseases
- Unplanned pregnancy
- Higher incidence of other psychosocial disorders, such as ADHD, oppositional-defiance disorder, mood disorders, anxiety disorders, depression, and learning disabilities

DIAGNOSTIC CRITERIA

Medical and psychiatric evaluations, feedback from parents, a school consultant's recommendations, case manager plan, and reports from a probation officer can assist in a team approach to diagnosis. Some of the assessment tools include:

- Rating of Aggression Against People and/or Property Scale
- Nisonger Child Behavior Rating Form
- Conners Parent Rating Scale.

The diagnosis is made when the patient meets the criteria in the *Diagnostic and Statistical Manual of Mental Disorders,* Fourth Edition, Text Revision. (See *Diagnosing conduct disorder.*)

TREATMENT

Treatment focuses on coordinating the child's psychological, physiologic, and educational needs. Studies have shown that multifaceted psychosocial treatments coupled with early intervention have demonstrated the most effectiveness. A structured living environment with consistent rules and consequences can help reduce many symptoms. Parents need to be taught consistent parenting and how to deal with the child's demands, and to set realistic goals for his behavior. Juvenile justice interventions may also be necessary to monitor and help control the individual's behavior.

Drugs

Medication can be useful as an adjunct to treatment. Drugs that have been useful in managing behavior include:

- Antipsychotics, such as risperdone (Risperdal), quetiapine (Seroquel), and others, have been shown to be useful in reducing overt aggression.
- Anticonvulsants, such as carbamazepine (Tegretol), have been used

DIAGNOSING CONDUCT DISORDER

A patient with conduct disorder must meet at least three of the criteria from any of the categories below; these criteria must have been noted within the year before the time of examination, and at least one criterion must have been present within the past 6 months.

Aggression to people and animals
- Bullies, threatens, or intimidates others
- Commonly starts physical fights
- Has used a weapon that can cause serious physical harm to others
- Has been physically cruel to people
- Has stolen while confronting a victim
- Has forced someone into sexual activity

Destruction of property
- Deliberately sets fire with the intention of causing serious damage
- Deliberately destroys others' property

Deceitfulness
- Has broken into someone else's house, car, or building
- Commonly lies to obtain goods or favors or to avoid obligations
- Has stolen items of nontrivial value without confronting a victim

Serious violations of rules
- Often stays out at night despite parental prohibitions, starting before age 13
- Has run away from home overnight at least twice while living in the parents' or surrogate parents' home
- Commonly skips school, beginning before age 13

Additional criteria
- The behavior disturbance must cause clinically significant impairment in social, academic, or occupational functioning.
- The patient is age 18 or older and doesn't meet the criteria for antisocial personality disorder.

Other features
- The disorder is considered mild if the person exhibits few if any conduct problems beyond those required to make the diagnosis and if the conduct problems cause only minor harm to others.
- The disorder is considered moderate if the conduct problems and their effects on others fall somewhere in between mild and severe.
- The disorder is considered severe if the person has many conduct problems beyond those needed to make the diagnosis, or, if the conduct problems cause considerable harm to others.

to treat nonspecific aggressive behavior.

- Mood regulators, such as lithium (Eskalith), have been shown to reduce aggressive behavior in some patients.

In patients who also have ADHD, the following may also be prescribed:
- Central nervous system (CNS) stimulants help control the symptoms of inattention and hyperactivity caused by ADHD.

Methylphenidate (Ritalin) and dex-troamphetamine-amphetamine (Adderall) act to decrease dopamine levels in the brain.

• Antidepressants help control symptoms of inattention and hyperactivity along with anxiety and depression. Venlafaxine (Effexor) acts to increase norepinephrine in the brain and bupropion (Wellbutrin) may act to block serotonin and to decrease dopamine. Older tricyclic antidepressants, such as amitriptyline, have effects on both dopamine and norepinephrine. Children who can't tolerate stimulants are often prescribed antidepressants.

SPECIAL CONSIDERATIONS

• Work to establish a trusting relationship with the child.

• Provide clear behavioral guidelines, including consequences for disruptive and manipulative behavior.

• Teach the child to express anger appropriately through constructive methods to release negative feelings and frustrations.

• Teach the child effective coping, social, and problem-solving skills, and have him demonstrate them in return.

• Help the child accept responsibility for behavior rather than blaming others, becoming defensive, and wanting revenge.

• Use role-playing to help the child practice handling stress and gain skill and confidence in managing difficult situations.

• Support the parents in setting firm, appropriate limits for the child.

Conversion disorder

A conversion disorder allows a patient to express a psychological conflict as physical symptoms—for example, by paralysis, blindness, inability to swallow, or even seizures. Unlike factitious disorders or malingering, conversion disorder results in an involuntary loss of physical function. The problem impairs the patient's functioning in important ways; however, laboratory tests and diagnostic procedures fail to disclose an organic cause and the patient may exhibit a lack of concern about her condition. The conversion symptom itself isn't life threatening and usually has a short duration, generally less than 2 weeks in hospitalized patients.

CAUSES AND INCIDENCE

The patient suddenly develops the conversion symptom soon after experiencing a traumatic conflict or stressful event. Two theories may explain why this occurs. According to the first, the patient achieves a "primary gain" when the symptom keeps a psychological conflict out of conscious awareness. For example, a person may experience blindness after witnessing a violent crime. In this case, the anxiety related to witnessing a violent crime is converted into a physical symptom.

The second theory suggests that the patient achieves "secondary gain" from the symptom by avoiding a traumatic activity. For example, a soldier may develop a "paralyzed" hand that prevents him from entering into combat.

An uncommon disorder, it can occur in either sex at any age but most commonly occurs between ages 10 and 35. More women than men are affected. Careful assessment is needed because it's estimated that approximately 4% of patients falsely diagnosed with conversion disorder are later found to have a neurologic disease.

Patients have a higher incidence of developing conversion disorder if:
• they have a family member with a history of conversion disorder
• they suffer from depression or anxiety
• they have been diagnosed with schizophrenia
• the patient is a child who has a parent who is very ill.

⚠ ALERT

Physical or sexual abuse is linked to the development of conversion disorder in children.

SIGNS AND SYMPTOMS

The history of a patient with conversion disorder reveals the sudden onset of a single, debilitating sign or symptom that prevents normal functioning of the affected body part. Common symptoms include:
• weakness, paralysis, or loss of sensation in one body part

• pseudoseizures
• loss of special sense, such as vision or hearing
• aphonia
• dysphagia
• urine retention
• gait disturbance and inability to stand.

Other common findings include:
• psychologically stressful event that recently preceded the development of the symptom
• lack of concern about the condition
• physical assessment findings that are inconsistent with the primary symptom. (For instance, tendon reflexes may be normal in a "paralyzed" part of the body and loss of motor function fails to follow anatomic patterns of nerve innervation. Pupillary responses and evoked potentials are normal in a patient who reports blindness.)

COMPLICATIONS

• Muscle wasting caused by paralysis or limb disuse
• Depression
• Development of another mental illness, such as somatization disorder, anxiety, or panic disorder

DIAGNOSTIC CRITERIA

For characteristic findings in patients with this condition, see *Diagnosing conversion disorder,* page 50.

A thorough physical evaluation must rule out a physical cause, especially diseases that typically produce vague, intermittent physical

DIAGNOSING CONVERSION DISORDER

The diagnosis of conversion disorder is based on the following criteria put forth in the *Diagnostic and Statistical Manual of Mental Disorders*, Fourth Edition, Text Revision:

- The person has one or more symptoms or deficits affecting voluntary motor or sensory function that suggest a neurologic or other general medical condition.
- The person exhibits psychological factors judged to be associated with the symptom or deficit because conflicts or other stressors preceded the symptom's or deficit's manifestation.
- The person's symptom or deficit isn't intentionally produced or feigned.
- The person's symptom or deficit can't, after appropriate investigation, be fully explained by a general medical condition, by the direct effects of a substance, or as a culturally sanctioned behavior or experience.
- The person's symptom or deficit warrants medical evaluation, causes clinically significant distress, or impairs social, occupational, or other important areas of functioning.
- The person's symptom or deficit isn't limited to pain or sexual dysfunction, doesn't occur exclusively during the course of somatization disorder, and isn't better accounted for by another mental disorder.

symptoms, such as multiple sclerosis, myasthenia gravis, or systemic lupus erythematosus.

Diagnostic testing to exclude organic disease may consist of the following:

- computed tomography or magnetic resonance imaging to rule out lesions of the spinal cord and brain
- chest radiography to exclude malignancy
- laboratory tests to exclude the presence of toxins, drugs, systemic infection, electrolyte disturbances, renal failure, hypoglycemia, or hyperglycemia.

TREATMENT

Treatment consists of helping the patient recognize and cope with the underlying stressful event or conflict that preceded the disorder and the anxiety and depression that commonly results.

- Psychotherapy
- Family therapy
- Behavior modification
- Hypnosis
- Biofeedback training
- Physical therapy

Drugs

- Anxiolytics (benzodiazepines), such as alprazolam (Xanax), may be prescribed to treat anxiety in the short term. The patient must be carefully monitored because the potential for addiction is high. For this reason, they shouldn't be prescribed if the patient has a history of substance abuse.
- Antidepressants are commonly prescribed to treat depression.

Selective serotonin reuptake inhibitors act on the brain to help balance levels of serotonin. Tricyclic antidepressants and monoamine oxidase inhibitors (MAOIs) help to balance serotonin and norepinephrine. Other drugs may act to balance a combination of dopamine, norepinephrine, serotonin, and other chemicals.

⊠ PREVENTION

Closely monitor patients taking antidepressants for suicidal thoughts, especially during the first 4 weeks of starting therapy.

⚠ ALERT

Although they are less commonly prescribed, patients taking MAOIs must avoid foods and beverages that contain tyramine. Tyramine is found in aged cheeses, smoked meats, and wine and may trigger a hypertensive crisis.

SPECIAL CONSIDERATIONS

● Help the patient maintain integrity of the affected system. Regularly exercise paralyzed limbs to prevent muscle wasting and contractures.

● Frequently change the patient's position to prevent pressure ulcers.

● Ensure adequate nutrition, even if the patient is complaining of GI distress.

● Provide a supportive environment, and encourage the patient to explore the stressful event or conflict that preceded her disorder.

● Don't force the patient to talk, but convey a caring attitude to help her share her feelings.

● Don't insist that the patient use the affected system. This will lead to distrust and prevent the formation of a therapeutic relationship.

● Add your support to the recommendation for psychiatric care.

● Include the patient's family in all care. They're essential to help her regain normal functioning.

D

Delusional disorders

According to the *Diagnostic and Statistical Manual of Mental Disorders,* Fourth Edition, Text Revision, delusional disorders are marked by false beliefs that have a plausible basis in reality. Formerly referred to as paranoid disorders, delusional disorders involve erotomanic, grandiose, jealous, somatic, or persecutory themes. (See *Delusional themes.*)

Some patients experience several types of delusions, whereas others experience unspecified delusions with no dominant theme. Typically chronic, these disorders commonly interfere with social and marital relationships, but seldom impair intellectual or occupational functioning.

CAUSES AND INCIDENCE

Delusional disorders of later life suggest a hereditary predisposition. An individual is more likely to develop it if there is another family member who also has delusional disorder or schizophrenia. At least one study has linked the development of delusional disorder to feelings of inferiority within the family. Some researchers suggest that delusional disorders are the product of specific early childhood experiences with an authoritarian family structure. Predisposing factors include social isolation (and isolation caused by vision or hearing impairment), lack of stimulating interpersonal relationships, and physical illness. Severe stress (such as a move to a foreign country) may make an individual vulnerable to developing delusional disorder. Imbalances in neurotransmitters have been shown to cause delusional symptoms, and research continues into studying the effects of such imbalances and the potential to develop delusional disorder.

Delusional disorders commonly begin in middle or late adulthood, usually between ages 40 and 55, but they can occur at a younger age. The disorders affect less than 1% of the population; the incidence is about equal in men and women.

SIGNS AND SYMPTOMS

The psychiatric history of a delusional patient may be unremarkable, aside from behavior related to his delusions. He's likely to report problems with:
- social and marital relationships
- depression
- sexual dysfunction
- social isolation
- hostility
- accepting treatment.

Gathering accurate information from a delusional patient may prove difficult. His responses and behavior

DELUSIONAL THEMES

In a patient with a delusional disorder, the delusions usually are well systematized and follow a predominant theme. Common delusional themes are discussed below.

Erotomanic delusions

This prevalent delusional theme concerns romantic or spiritual love. The patient believes that he shares an idealized (rather than sexual) relationship with someone of higher status—a superior at work, a celebrity, or an anonymous stranger.

The patient may keep this delusion secret, but more commonly will try to contact the object of his delusion by phone calls, letters (including e-mail), gifts, or even stalking. He may attempt to rescue his beloved from imagined danger. Many patients with erotomanic delusions harass public figures and come to the attention of the police.

Grandiose delusions

The patient with grandiose delusions believes that he has great, unrecognized talent, special insights, prophetic power, or has made an important discovery. To achieve recognition, he may contact government agencies such as the Federal Bureau of Investigation. The patient with a religion-oriented delusion of grandeur may become a cult leader. Less commonly, he believes that he shares a special relationship with some well-known personality, such as a rock star or a world leader. He may believe himself to be a famous person, his identity usurped by an imposter.

Jealous delusions

Jealous delusions focus on infidelity. For example, a patient may insist that his spouse or lover has been unfaithful, and may search for evidence to justify the delusion such as spots on bed sheets. He may confront his partner, try to control her movements, follow her, or try to track down her suspected lover. He may physically assault her or, less likely, his perceived rival.

Somatic delusions

Somatic delusions center on an imagined physical defect or deformity. The patient may perceive a foul odor coming from his skin, mouth, rectum, or another body part. Other delusions involve skin-crawling insects, internal parasites, or physical illness.

Persecutory delusions

The patient suffering from persecutory delusions, the most common type of delusion, believes that he's being followed, harassed, plotted against, poisoned, mocked, or deliberately prevented from achieving his long-term goals. These delusions may evolve into a simple or complex persecution scheme, in which even the slightest injustice is interpreted as part of the scheme.

Such a patient may file numerous lawsuits or seek redress from government agencies (querulous paranoia). A patient who becomes resentful and angry may lash out violently against the alleged offender.

during the assessment interview provide clues that can help to identify his disorder. Family members may confirm your observations—for example, by reporting that the patient is chronically jealous or suspicious. He may deny feeling lonely, relentlessly criticizing or placing unreasonable demands on others.

When assessing the patient, look for:

• unusual communication patterns—he may be evasive, overly talkative with grandiose themes, or make contradictory, jumbled, or irrational statements

• expressions of denial, projection, and rationalization (Once delusions become firmly entrenched, the patient will no longer seek to justify his beliefs. However, if he's still struggling to maintain his delusional defenses, he may make statements that reveal his condition, such as "People at work won't talk to me because I'm smarter than them.")

• accusatory statements—these are characteristic of the delusional patient

• pervasive delusional themes (grandiose or persecutory)

• nonverbal cues, such as excessive vigilance or obvious apprehension when people enter the room.

COMPLICATIONS

• Violent behavior
• Suicide
• Legal problems

DIAGNOSTIC CRITERIA

For characteristic findings in patients with this condition, see *Diagnosing delusional disorders.*

Assessment also includes:

• neurologic evaluation
• psychological evaluation
• laboratory blood and urine tests, which are used to exclude organic causes of delusions, such as amphetamine-induced psychoses, electrolyte imbalances, hyperadrenalism, pernicious anemia, and thyroid disorders.

TREATMENT

Therapy options that have shown effectiveness consist of:

• individual therapy
• cognitive behavioral therapy to recognize and change inappropriate thought patterns
• family therapy
• mobilization of support system for the isolated elderly patient.

Drugs

• Antipsychotics appear to work by blocking postsynaptic dopamine receptors. These drugs reduce the incidence of psychotic symptoms, such as hallucinations and delusions, and relieve anxiety and agitation. Some of the conventional antipsychotics include chlorpromazine (Thorazine), haloperidol (Haldol), and fluphenazine (Prolixin). Haloperidol and fluphenazine are depot formulations that can be implanted I.M. to release the drug gradually over a 30-day period, thus improving compliance. Usually, however, this type of treatment isn't needed. Newer, atypical antipsy-

DIAGNOSING DELUSIONAL DISORDERS

In an individual with suspected delusional disorder, psychiatric examination confirms the diagnosis. The examiner bases the diagnosis on the following criteria set forth in the *Diagnostic and Statistical Manual of Mental Disorders*, Fourth Edition, Text Revision:

■ Nonbizarre delusions of at least 1 month's duration are present, involving real-life situations, such as being followed, poisoned, infected, loved at a distance, or deceived by one's spouse or lover.

■ The patient's symptoms have never met the criteria known as *characteristic symptoms* of schizophrenia. However, tactile and olfactory hallucinations may be present if they're related to a delusional theme.

■ Apart from being affected by the delusion or its ramifications, the patient is neither markedly impaired functionally nor is his behavior obviously odd or bizarre.

■ If mood disturbances have occurred concurrently with delusions, their total duration has been brief relative to the duration of the delusional disturbance.

■ The disturbance isn't caused by the direct physiologic effects of a substance or a general medical condition.

Delusional disorder or paranoid schizophrenia?

To distinguish between these two disorders, consider the following characteristics.

Delusional disorder

In a delusional disorder, the patient's delusions reflect reality and are arranged into a coherent system. They're based on misinterpretations of, or elaborations on, reality. The patient doesn't experience hallucinations, and his affect and behavior are normal.

Paranoid schizophrenia

In paranoid schizophrenia, the patient's delusions are scattered, illogical, and incoherently arranged with no direct relation to reality. The patient may have hallucinations, his affect is inappropriate and inconsistent, and his behavior is bizarre.

chotics may be more effective in treating symptoms by blocking dopamine and serotonin brain receptors. Some of these newer drugs include risperidone (Risperdal), clozapine (Clozaril), and olanzapine (Zyprexa).

⚠ ALERT

Agranulocytosis, a potentially fatal blood disorder characterized by a low white blood cell count and pronounced neutropenia, may also occur when taking clozapine. Routine blood monitoring is essential to detect the estimated 1% to 2% of all patients who develop agranulocytosis. This disorder is reversible if it's detected in the early stages.

● Antidepressants are commonly prescribed if the patient develops symptoms of depression. Selective serotonin reuptake inhibitors act on the brain to help balance the levels of serotonin. Tricyclic antidepressants and monoamine oxidase inhibitors (MAOIs) help to balance serotonin and norepineph-rine. Other medications may act to balance a combination of dopamine, norepinephrine, serotonin, and other chemicals.

⧕ PREVENTION

Closely monitor patients taking an-tidepressants for suicidal thoughts, especially during the first 4 weeks of starting therapy.

⚠ ALERT

Patients taking MAOIs must avoid foods and beverages that contain tyramine. Tyramine is found in aged cheeses, smoked meats, and wine and may trigger a hypertensive crisis.

• Anxiolytics may be used if the pa-tient has a very high level of anxiety or problems sleeping. The patient must be carefully monitored as the potential for addiction is high. For this reason, they shouldn't be pre-scribed if the patient has a history of substance abuse.

SPECIAL CONSIDERATIONS

• In dealing with the delusional pa-tient, be direct, straightforward, and dependable. Whenever possible, elicit his feedback. Move slowly and matter-of-factly and respond with-out anger or defensiveness to his hostile remarks.

• Respect the patient's privacy and space needs. Don't touch him un-necessarily.

• If the patient allows, take steps to reduce social isolation. Gradually increase social contacts after he has become comfortable with the staff.

• Watch for refusal of medication or food, resulting from the patient's irrational fear of poisoning.

• Monitor the patient carefully for the adverse effects of antipsychotic drugs: drug-induced parkinsonism, acute dystonia, akathisia, tardive dyskinesia, and malignant neurolep-tic syndrome.

• If the patient is taking clozapine, stress the importance of returning weekly to the hospital or an outpa-tient setting to have his blood count monitored.

• Involve the patient's family in treatment. Teach them how to recog-nize an impending relapse, and sug-gest ways to manage symptoms. These include tension, nervousness, insomnia, decreased concentration ability, and apathy.

• Remember to consider cultural and religious beliefs. Beliefs that may be considered delusional in one culture may be culturally sanctioned in another.

Dementia, Alzheimer's type

Alzheimer's dementia is a primary type of dementia caused by an or-ganic brain disease. Dementia is characterized by a loss of brain function involving memory, learn-ing, communication, and behavior and interferes with an individual's social or occupational functioning. In Alzheimer's dementia, the indi-vidual's decline is gradual and pro-gressive. In the early-onset type, symptoms appear at age 65 or younger and in the late-onset type, symptoms appear after age 65. Alzheimer's dementia can appear along with other types of dementia, such as vascular dementia.

CAUSES AND INCIDENCE

Alzheimer's is the most common dementia in individuals age 65 and older. At least 50% to 60% of all dementias currently seen are caused by Alzheimer's disease. In the United States, slightly more than 5 million individuals have Alzheimer's disease and 4.9 million of those individuals are over age 65. The incidence of Alzheimer's dementia increases as people age. It's estimated that 2% of the population ages 65 to 75 have Alzheimer's dementia, which increases to 42% of the population by age 85 and older.

Alzheimer's disease is the fifth leading cause of death among older American adults.

The cause of Alzheimer's dementia is unknown and can only be diagnosed with complete accuracy by the microscopic examination of brain tissue after death. Researchers continue to investigate the influence of biologic, environmental, and genetic factors in attempt to identify the cause of the disease. Studies show that there's a familial pattern with early-onset cases of Alzheimer's dementia. Researchers have found that after death, the brain tissue of Alzheimer's patients exhibits abnormal clusters of beta-amyloid proteins that form plaques, which are found outside and around the neurons in the hippocampus. When the brain tissue is stained, neurofibrillary tangles (twisted nerve cell fibers) are also evident. These tangles impair communication between neurons. It isn't known if these plaques and tangles are the cause of or the result of the disease, however. Other gross changes in the brain include thickening of the leptomeninges, enlarging ventricles, shrinking of the hippocampus and gyri, widening sulci, and generalized atrophy. There are also lower levels of acetylcholine in the brains of individuals with Alzheimer's dementia.

SIGNS AND SYMPTOMS

The patient with Alzheimer's dementia typically exhibits four stages of progressive decline in intellectual function, personality changes, behavioral changes, and impairment in judgment. These stages consist of the following:
• Preclinical Alzheimer's dementia—The hippocampus structure is affected and shrinks over time resulting in both short- and long-term memory loss.
• Stage 1 (mild Alzheimer's dementia)—The cerebral cortex continues to shrink and additional cognitive losses occur. The patient is usually cooperative and can follow basic instructions. The patient may show signs of:
– memory disturbance, and inability to recall events, which is noticed by others

- apathy
- poor judgment and problem-solving skills
- new carelessness in habits and personal appearance
- poor concentration and short attention span
- disorientation to time
- mild aphasia
- inability to retain new memories
- gradual withdrawal from activities
- wandering and becoming easily lost
- denial of or hiding impairment
- suspiciousness
- irritability
- uncharacteristic motor behavior.
● Stage 2 (moderate Alzheimer's dementia)—Continued impairment is characterized by:
- language disturbance with impaired word finding and circumlocution (talking around a topic)
- increased apraxia, agnosia, and aphasia
- continuous repetitive behaviors such as pacing
- disorientation to person, place, and time
- worsening irritability
- depression
- delusions and psychosis (possibly)
- inability to perform normal activities without assistance
- altered sleep-wake cycles and wandering at night (possibly)
- motor skill lack of coordination with poor balance and gait.
● Stage 3 (severe Alzheimer's dementia)—Marked by pervasive

plaques and tangles in the brain with severe cognitive impairment. This final stage is characterized by:
- inability to recognize family and friends
- frequent inability to communicate at all (incoherence)
- decreased response to stimuli
- less voluntary movement, leading to complete immobility
- frequent urinary and fecal incontinence
- frequent aspiration
- swallowing problems
- emaciation.

COMPLICATIONS
● Loss of ability to care for self
● Increased trauma from falls, wandering, and environmental hazards
● Increased risk of infection caused by aspiration and immobility
● Reduced lifespan
● Increased caregiver and family stress
● Increased societal costs

DIAGNOSTIC CRITERIA
The diagnosis of Alzheimer's dementia requires that alternative causes of dementia, some of which may be reversible, must be excluded. Other such causes include the following:
● metabolic disorders, such as vitamin B_{12}, B_1, and B_3 deficiencies
● endocrine disorders, such as hypothyroidism or hypoglycemia
● vascular disorders
● infections that affect the central nervous system, such as human

immunodeficiency virus, Creutzfeldt-Jakob disease, and syphilis
- substance abuse such as with chronic drug and alcohol abuse
- brain injury, such as tumors, hydrocephalus, and trauma
- Huntington's disease
- Parkinson's disease
- Pick's disease, a degenerative disease of the frontal and temporal lobes of the brain.

Tests to aid in diagnosis include:
- cognitive assessment evaluation
- functional dementia scale
- EEG
- computed axial tomography of the head
- magnetic resonance imaging of the head
- cerebrospinal fluid analysis, which may show beta-amyloid deposits
- laboratory tests:
– serum electrolytes
– serum glucose, calcium, blood chemistry
– serum thyroid function tests
– vitamin B_{12} level
– serum ammonia level
– toxicology screen for drugs or alcohol
– urinalysis
– blood gas analysis.

Once alternative causes of Alzheimer's dementia have been excluded, a diagnosis can be made if the patient's symptoms match the criteria in the *Diagnostic and Statistical Manual of Mental Disorders,* Fourth Edition, Text Revision. (See *Diagnosing dementia of the Alzheimer's type,* page 60.)

TREATMENT

There is no cure for Alzheimer's dementia. Treatment centers on activities to prevent or minimize the patient's behavioral problems, enhance his cognition, and provide a safe, supportive environment for the patient and caregivers.

Drugs

- Cholinesterase inhibitors, such as donepezil (Aricept) and rivastigmine tartrate (Exelon), increase acetylcholine levels in the brain, maintain neuron function, and help improve cognition.
- N-methyl-D-aspartate receptor antagonists, such as memantine (Namenda), block glutamate receptors in the brain and have been shown to improve cognitive function in some patients.
- Antipsychotics, such as haloperidol (Haldol) and risperidone (Risperdal), may be used to calm agitated behavior.
- Anxiolytics (benzodiazepines), such as alprazolam (Xanax), may be used to decrease anxiety.
- Central nervous system stimulants, such as methylphenidate (Ritalin), promote nerve impulse transmission to increase activity and spontaneity.
- Antidepressants are commonly prescribed to treat depression. Selective serotonin reuptake inhibitors act on the brain to help balance the levels of serotonin. Tricyclic antidepressants and monoamine oxidase inhibitors (MAOIs) help to balance serotonin and norepinephrine. Other medications may act to balance a

DIAGNOSING DEMENTIA OF THE ALZHEIMER'S TYPE

The following criteria described in the *Diagnostic and Statistical Manual of Mental Disorders*, Fourth Edition, Text Revision, are used to diagnose dementia of the Alzheimer's type.

The person with Alzheimer's dementia has developed multiple cognitive deficits manifested by both:
- memory impairment (impaired ability to learn new information or to recall previously learned information
- one (or more) of the following cognitive disturbances:
  – aphasia
  – apraxia (impaired ability to carry out motor activities despite intact motor function)
  – agnosia (failure to recognize or identify objects despite intact sensory function)
  – disturbance in executive functioning (i.e., planning, organizing, sequencing, abstracting).

The cognitive deficits each cause significant impairment in social or occupational functioning and represent a significant decline from a previous level of functioning.

The course is characterized by gradual onset and continuing cognitive decline.

The cognitive deficits aren't caused by any of the following:
- other central nervous system conditions that cause progressive deficits in memory and cognition
- systemic conditions that are known to cause dementia
- substance-induced conditions.

The deficits don't occur exclusively during the course of delirium.

The disturbance isn't better accounted for by another axis 1 disorder (major depressive disorder, schizophrenia).

combination of dopamine, norepinephrine, serotonin, and other chemicals.

⊠ PREVENTION

Closely monitor patients taking antidepressants for suicidal thoughts, especially during the first 4 weeks of starting therapy.

⚠ ALERT

Patients taking MAOIs must avoid foods and beverages that contain tyramine. Tyramine is found in aged cheeses, smoked meats, and wine and may trigger a hypertensive crisis.

SPECIAL CONSIDERATIONS

- The patient may require assistance at home and possibly within an institution.

- Hospitalization should be avoided whenever possible to decrease confusion caused by unfamiliar environment and lack of understanding.

- Teach caregivers how to provide a safe home environment for the individual.

- Encourage the individual with Alzheimer's dementia to participate in normal activities to enhance his functioning and self-esteem. Individualize his care as his condition declines. Cuing may be needed to perform daily activities.

- Minimize confusion by maintaining consistent, structured verbal and nonverbal communication.

- Add reorienting details to all con-versations.
- Monitor the patient for adverse drug reactions and interactions.
- Memory should be tested on ad-mission to and discharge from an inpatient setting using evidence-based standardized instruments.
- Monitor the patient's swallowing ability to prevent aspiration.
- Monitor the patient's intake to promote adequate nutrition and hy-dration.
- Provide support and education to home caregivers, referring them to respite and social services, as needed.

Dementia, vascular type

Vascular dementia is a primary type of dementia caused by a decrease in the blood supply to the brain, which results in damage to brain tissue. Dementia is characterized by a loss of brain function involving memory, learning, communication, and be-havior and interferes with an indi-vidual's social or occupational func-tioning. The cognitive changes in vascular dementia can begin abrupt-ly and progress less predictably than in Alzheimer's dementia. Unlike Alzheimer's dementia, memory loss may not occur early in the disease. Vascular dementia may also com-monly occur with Alzheimer's de-mentia.

CAUSES AND INCIDENCE

Vascular dementia is caused by re-duced blood supply to brain tissue.

Conditions that affect blood flow in-clude thrombosis, embolus, arterial occlusive disease, low blood pres-sure, and brain hemorrhages; or dis-eases such as lupus erythematosus, which damages arteries. Other con-ditions associated with development of vascular dementia include hyper-tension, leading to cerebral vascular events; diabetes, which causes dam-age to small and medium-sized ar-teries; and cardiac diseases, which can cause thromboembolic events. Not all strokes result in vascular de-mentia, but the risk increases with each infarction. Indeed, about 30% of individuals who suffer a stroke will exhibit signs of dementia with-in 6 months.

The risk of developing vascular dementia increases with age, but is rare in patients younger than age 65. Vascular dementia accounts for ap-proximately 20% of patients with dementia and is more common in men than in women.

SIGNS AND SYMPTOMS

Signs and symptoms are directly re-lated to the portion of the brain that's affected. Each episode of in-farction often leads to a step-wise progression of decline. Signs and symptoms include:

- symptoms that appear abruptly
- symptoms that wax and wane in intensity
- memory impairment (later in the disease)
- language impairment (not as pro-nounced as with Alzheimer's dementia)

- slurred speech
- agitation
- unsteady gait and falls
- mood or personality changes
- difficulty processing instructions
- dizziness
- weakness in the extremities
- incontinence
- sensory deficits.

COMPLICATIONS

- Loss of ability to perform self care
- Death from stroke, cardiovascular disease, pneumonia, or infections

DIAGNOSTIC CRITERIA

- Computed tomography scans or magnetic resonance imaging identify areas of brain infarction.

- Duplex ultrasound scanning or magnetic resonance angiography or arteriography identify occlusive disease of the carotid arteries.
- Echocardiography helps identify the origin of emboli and valvular disease.
- Electrocardiography identifies rhythm disturbances, such as atrial fibrillation.
- Neuropsychological tests may be performed.

A diagnosis can be made if the patient's symptoms match those in the *Diagnostic and Statistical Manual of Mental Disorders,* Fourth Edition, Text Revision. (See *Diagnosing vascular dementia.*)

DIAGNOSING VASCULAR DEMENTIA

The following criteria described in the *Diagnostic and Statistical Manual of Mental Disorders*, Fourth Edition, Text Revision, are used to diagnose a person with vascular dementia.

The development of multiple cognitive deficits manifested by both:
- memory impairment (impaired ability to learn new information or to recall previously learned information)
- one or more of the following cognitive disturbances:
  – aphasia
  – apraxia (impaired ability to carry out motor activities despite intact motor function)
  – agnosia (failure to recognize or identify objects despite intact sensory function)

  – disturbance in executive function (planning, organizing, sequencing, abstracting).
- The cognitive deficits each cause significant impairment in social or occupational functioning and represent a significant decline from a previous level of functioning.
- Focal neurologic signs and symptoms or laboratory evidence indicative of cerebrovascular disease (e.g., multiple infarctions involving the cortex and underlying white matter) are judged to be directly related to the disturbance.
- The deficits don't occur exclusively during the course of a delirium.

TREATMENT

Although there's no cure for vascular dementia, treatment goals include:

- strategies to minimize risk factors for cardiovascular disease such as:
  – controlling hypertension
  – maximizing cardiac function
  – controlling hypercholesteremia
  – controlling obesity
  – controlling serum glucose levels
  – stopping smoking
- carotid endarterectomy or stenting, if indicated, to reduce obstructions and potential sources of emboli.

Drugs

- Cholinesterase inhibitors (such as donepezil [Aricept]), which were approved for use in Alzheimer's dementia to improve cognition, may sometimes be prescribed for the patient with vascular dementia.
- N-methyl-D-aspartate receptor antagonists, such as memantine (Namenda), block glutamate receptors in the brain and have shown modest benefit in improving information processing, storage, and retrieval functions in some patients.
- Acetylsalicylic acid (aspirin) inhibits clotting formation by preventing platelet aggregation. It's used to treat acute ischemic stroke and to prevent recurrent transient ischemic attacks.

SPECIAL CONSIDERATIONS

- Teach caregivers how to minimize hazards in the home, thus ensuring a safe environment.

- Encourage the patient to perform self-care activities to his ability.
- Reorient and cue patient, as needed, when performing tasks.
- Teach caregivers how to monitor the patient's intake to prevent dehydration and nutritional deficiencies.
- Teach caregivers how to monitor the patient's swallowing ability and teach strategies to prevent aspiration.
- Teach caregivers about ways to reduce the patient's cardiovascular risk factors.

Depersonalization disorder

Persistent or recurrent episodes of detachment characterize depersonalization disorder. During these episodes, self-awareness is temporarily altered or lost; the patient in many cases perceives this alteration in consciousness as a barrier between himself and the outside world. The sense of depersonalization may be restricted to a single body part, such as a limb, or it may encompass the whole self. The patient with this disorder may feel that he's mechanical, in a dream, or detached from his body.

Although the patient seldom loses touch with reality completely, the episodes of depersonalization may cause him severe distress. Depersonalization disorder usually has a sudden onset in adolescence or early in adult life. It follows a chronic course, with periodic exacerbations and remissions, and resolves gradually.

CAUSES AND INCIDENCE

Chronic depersonalization disorder is rarely diagnosed and commonly untreated. It's believed that about 0.8% to 2.4% of the general population may be affected and that about 40% to 60% of the population have experienced the symptoms at some time in their lives. Depersonalization disorder is thought to be a reaction to overwhelming stress, including war experiences, accidents, and natural disasters, which becomes chronic and dysfunctional. Neurobiological research has shown that the limbic system in these patients is suppressed in response to emotional stimuli. Other research suggests a dysregulation of the opioid system in the brains of such patients.

SIGNS AND SYMPTOMS

The patient with depersonalization disorder may complain of:
• feeling detached from his entire being and body, as if he were watching himself from a distance or living in a dream
• sensory anesthesia
• loss of self control
• difficulty speaking
• feelings of losing touch with reality
• disturbed sense of time
• memory disturbance and prolonged recall time.

Common findings during the assessment interview include:

• symptoms of depression
• obsessive rumination
• somatic concerns
• physical complaints such as dizziness
• anxiety and fear of going insane.

COMPLICATIONS

• Diminished ability to cope with activities of daily living
• Poor work performance

DIAGNOSTIC CRITERIA

For characteristic findings in patients with this condition, see *Diagnosing depersonalization disorder.*

TREATMENT

Psychotherapy aims to establish a trusting, therapeutic relationship in which the patient recognizes the traumatic event that triggered the disorder and the anxiety it evoked. The therapist subsequently teaches the patient to use reality-based coping strategies rather than to detach himself from the situation.

Drugs

• Antidepressants, such as selective serotonin reuptake inhibitors, act on the brain to help balance levels of serotonin and have been shown to benefit patients who have a great deal of background anxiety.

⊠ PREVENTION

Closely monitor patients taking antidepressants for suicidal thoughts, especially during the first 4 weeks of starting therapy.

DIAGNOSING DEPERSONALIZATION DISORDER

The depersonalization disorder diagnosis is made when the patient's symptoms match the following criteria put forth in the *Diagnostic and Statistical Manual of Mental Disorders*, Fourth Edition, Text Revision:
- The person has persistent or recurrent experiences of feeling detached from mind or body (as if he were an outside observer) or feeling like an automaton (as if he were in a dream).
- During the depersonalization experience, reality testing remains intact.
- The depersonalization causes clinically significant distress or impairment in social, occupational, or other important areas of functioning.
- The depersonalization experience doesn't occur exclusively during the course of another mental disorder, such as schizophrenia, panic disorder, acute stress disorder, or another dissociative disorder, and isn't caused by the direct physiologic effects of a substance or a general medical condition.

• Opioid receptor antagonists, such as naltrexone (Vivitrol), help to regulate the opioid system in the brain.

SPECIAL CONSIDERATIONS
• Assist the patient in using reality-based coping strategies under stress rather than those strategies that distort reality.
• Help the patient recognize and deal with the experiences that produce anxiety.
• Establish a therapeutic, nonjudgmental relationship with the patient.

Dissociative amnesia

The essential feature of dissociative amnesia is a sudden inability to recall important personal information that can't be explained by ordinary forgetfulness. The patient typically is unable to recall all events that occurred during a specific period, but other types of recall disturbance are also possible.

The *Diagnostic and Statistical Manual of Mental Disorders,* Fourth Edition, Text Revision, recognizes five types of amnesia, based on the time period and amount of information lost to recall:
• localized amnesia—failure to recall all events that occurred during a circumscribed time period
• selective amnesia—failure to recall some of the events that occurred during a circumscribed time period
• generalized amnesia—failure to recall all events over the entire lifespan
• continuous amnesia—failure to recall events subsequent to a specific time up to and including the present
• systematized amnesia—failure to recall certain categories of information.

Dissociative amnesia is linked to severe stress and is thought to result when the brain's executive control system operates to repress the retrieval of information. This disorder commonly occurs during war and natural disasters. Although it's more common in adolescents and young adult women, it's also seen in young men after combat experience. The amnesic event typically ends abruptly, and recovery is complete, with rare recurrences.

CAUSES AND INCIDENCE

Dissociative amnesia follows severe psychosocial stress, commonly involving a threat of physical injury or death. Amnesia may also occur after thinking about or engaging in unacceptable behavior such as an extramarital affair. Neuroimaging studies are being used to investigate brain activity and the formation of memory. Research using magnetic resonance imaging has shown that the anterior cingulated and dorsolateral prefrontal cortex areas are activated when subjects try to suppress unwanted memories. Studies of the neurochemicals of the brain show that alterations in neuropeptides and neurotransmitters affect an individual's ability to retain information and recall memories. Research on the brain and memory will help practitioners to develop treatment strategies for this disorder.

SIGNS AND SYMPTOMS

Commonly the patient with amnesia is brought to the emergency depart-

ment after having been found wandering.

During the assessment interview, the amnesic patient may appear:
● alert but perplexed
● disoriented
● unable to recall the event that precipitated the amnesia
● unable to recognize her inability to recall information.

After the episode has ended, the patient is usually unaware that she has suffered what's known as a *recall disturbance.*

COMPLICATIONS

● Risk of social or occupational problems

DIAGNOSTIC CRITERIA

There are no specific laboratory tests to diagnose this condition. However, radiographic imaging and laboratory tests may be used to exclude:
● medication toxicity
● substance abuse
● head injury
● sleep deprivation.

For characteristic findings in patients with this condition, see *Diagnosing dissociative amnesia.*

TREATMENT

Psychotherapy aims to help the patient recognize the traumatic event that triggered the amnesia and the anxiety it produced. A trusting, therapeutic relationship is essential to achieving this goal. The therapist subsequently attempts to teach

---

DIAGNOSING DISSOCIATIVE AMNESIA

A diagnosis of dissociative amnesia is made when the patient's symptoms meet the following criteria put forth in the *Diagnostic and Statistical Manual of Mental Disorders*, Fourth Edition, Text Revision:

■ The predominant disturbance is at least one episode of inability to recall important personal information, usually of a traumatic or stressful nature, that is too extensive to be explained by ordinary forgetfulness.

■ The disturbance isn't caused by dissociative identity disorder, dissociative fugue, posttraumatic stress disorder, acute stress disorder, or somatization disorder. It also isn't caused by the direct physiologic effects of a substance or a neurologic or other general medical condition.

■ The symptoms cause clinically significant distress or impairment in social, occupational, or other important areas of functioning.

---

the patient reality-based coping strategies.

Drugs

● Anxiolytics, such as benzodiazepines, may be prescribed to treat anxiety, help the patient relax, and is sometimes used to assist in the recovery of repressed memories. The patient must be carefully monitored because the potential for addiction is high. For this reason, they shouldn't be prescribed if the patient has a history of substance abuse.

SPECIAL CONSIDERATIONS

● When providing care, teach the patient effective coping strategies to use in stressful situations rather than those strategies that distort reality.

● Help the patient recognize and deal with experiences that produce anxiety.

● Establish a therapeutic, nonjudgmental relationship with the patient.

Dissociative fugue

The word fugue is derived from the Latin word for flight. The patient suffering from dissociative fugue wanders or travels while unconsciously blocking out a traumatic event. During the fugue state, he usually assumes a different identity and later can't recall what has happened. The degree of impairment varies, depending on the duration of the fugue and the nature of the personality state it invokes. Dissociative fugue may be related to dissociative identity disorder, narcissistic personality disorder, and sleepwalking.

Although the age of onset varies, it almost always affects adults only. The fugue state is usually brief (hours to days); however, it can last for months and carry the patient far from home. The prognosis for complete recovery is good, and recurrences are rare.

CAUSES AND INCIDENCE

The prevalence of dissociative fugue in the general population is estimated at 0.2%.

Dissociative fugue typically follows an extremely stressful event, such as combat experience, a natural disaster, a violent or abusive confrontation, or personal rejection. Heavy alcohol or other substance abuse may constitute predisposing factors.

SIGNS AND SYMPTOMS

Psychiatric examination of the patient with dissociative fugue may reveal that he has assumed a new, more uninhibited identity. His psychosocial history may include episodes of violent behavior. He may also show signs of:

• unplanned travel far from home
• inability to recall important biographical information and past events
• identity confusion

• anxiety
• inability to recall events during his fugue state.

COMPLICATIONS

• Impaired social, occupational, and daily functioning caused by the fugue state
• Legal problems from assuming another identity

DIAGNOSTIC CRITERIA

There are no specific laboratory tests to diagnose this condition. However, radiographic imaging and laboratory tests may be used to exclude:

• medication toxicity
• substance abuse
• head injury
• sleep deprivation.

For characteristic findings in patients with this condition, see *Diagnosing dissociative fugue.*

DIAGNOSING DISSOCIATIVE FUGUE

The diagnosis of dissociative fugue is made when the patient's symptoms match the following criteria put forth in the *Diagnostic and Statistical Manual of Mental Disorders*, Fourth Edition, Text Revision:

■ The predominant disturbance is sudden, unexpected travel away from home or the patient's customary place of work, with an inability to recall the past.

■ The person experiences confusion about personal identity or assumption of a new partial or complete identity.

■ The disturbance isn't caused by dissociative identity disorder, physiologic effects of a substance, or a general medical condition.

■ The symptoms cause clinically significant distress or impairment in social, occupational, or other important areas of functioning.

TREATMENT

Psychotherapy aims to help the patient recognize the traumatic event that triggered the fugue state and develop reality-based strategies for coping with anxiety. A trusting, therapeutic relationship is essential for success. Other treatments may include:

- cognitive behavioral therapy
- family therapy
- hypnosis, to recall memories from the unconscious mind.

Drugs

- Antidepressants are commonly prescribed to treat anxiety and depression, which are commonly associated with dissociative fugue. Selective serotonin reuptake inhibitors act on the brain to help balance levels of serotonin. Tricyclic antidepressants and monoamine oxidase inhibitors (MAOIs) help to balance serotonin and norepinephrine. Other drugs may act to balance a combination of dopamine, norepinephrine, serotonin, and other chemicals.

⧉ PREVENTION

Closely monitor patients taking antidepressants for suicidal thoughts, especially during the first 4 weeks of starting therapy.

⚠ ALERT

Patients taking MAOIs must avoid foods and beverages that contain tyramine. Tyramine is found in aged cheeses, smoked meats, and wine and may trigger a hypertensive crisis.

- Anxiolytics (benzodiazepines), such as alprazolam (Xanax), may be prescribed to treat anxiety in the short term. The patient must be carefully monitored because the potential for addiction is high. For this reason, they should not be prescribed if the patient has a history of substance abuse.

SPECIAL CONSIDERATIONS

- When providing care, teach the patient effective coping strategies to use in stressful situations rather than strategies that distort reality.
- Help the patient recognize and deal with anxiety-producing experiences.
- Establish a therapeutic, nonjudgmental relationship with the patient.

Dissociative identity disorder

A complex disturbance of identity and memory, dissociative identity disorder (formerly referred to as *multiple personality disorder*) is characterized by the existence of two or more distinct, fully integrated personalities in the same person. The personalities alternate in dominance. Each comprises unique memories, behavior patterns, and social relationships; in many cases, rigid and flamboyant personalities are combined. Usually, one personality is unaware of the existence of the other.

CAUSES AND INCIDENCE

The exact cause isn't known. However, it's theorized that the disorder results from the unconscious mind's effort to protect the self from traumatic events or memories. The patient typically has experienced physical or sexual abuse or some form of emotional trauma in childhood. A child may develop multiple personalities to dissociate herself from traumatic situations. The dissociated contents become linked with one of many possible shaping influences for personality organization. Dissociative identity disorder usually begins in childhood, but patients seldom seek treatment until much later in life. The disorder is three to nine times more common in women than in men. Researchers theorize that there may be a genetic predisposition to dissociation as it seems to have a familial link.

SIGNS AND SYMPTOMS

The patient may seek treatment for a concurrent psychiatric disorder present in one of the personalities. She may have a history of unsuccessful psychiatric treatment, or she may report periods of amnesia and disturbances in time perception. Family members may describe incidents that the patient can't recall as well as alterations in facial presentation, voice, and behavior. The patient may find items that she doesn't remember purchasing.

Stress or idiosyncratically meaningful social or environmental cues commonly trigger the transition from one personality to another. Although usually sudden, the transition can occur over hours or days. Other signs and symptoms include:

- changes in daily functioning, ranging from being highly effective to almost disabled
- headaches or pain in other body parts
- feelings of detachment from reality or one's body
- labile moods
- depression
- anxiety and panic attacks
- alterations in patterns of eating and sleeping
- self-injurious behavior
- evidence of suicide attempt
- substance abuse
- problems with sexual function.

COMPLICATIONS

- Impaired social, occupational, and daily functioning caused by the fugue state
- Legal problems from assuming another identity
- Suicide attempt or self injury
- Victimization by others
- Substance abuse

DIAGNOSTIC CRITERIA

There are no specific laboratory tests to diagnose this condition. However, radiographic imaging and laboratory tests may be used to exclude:

- medication toxicity
- substance abuse
- head injury
- sleep deprivation.

For characteristic findings in patients with this condition, see *Diagnosing dissociative identity disorder.*

DIAGNOSING DISSOCIATIVE IDENTITY DISORDER

The diagnosis of dissociative identity disorder is based on fulfillment of the following criteria established in the *Diagnostic and Statistical Manual of Mental Disorders*, Fourth Edition, Text Revision:

■ Two or more distinct personalities or personality states (each with its own relatively enduring pattern of perceiving, relating to, and thinking about the environment and self) are present.

■ At least two of these personalities or personality states recurrently take full control of the person's behavior.

■ The person can't recall important personal information that's too extensive to be explained by ordinary forgetfulness.

■ The disturbance isn't caused by the direct physiologic effects of a substance or a general medical condition.

TREATMENT

Psychotherapy is essential to uniting the personalities and preventing the personality from splitting again. Treatment is usually intensive and prolonged, with success linked to the strength of the patient-therapist relationship with each of the personalities, all of which require equal respect and concern. Other treatments may include:

• cognitive behavioral therapy
• family therapy
• hypnosis, to recall memories from the unconscious mind and to facilitate personality transitions.

Drugs

• Antidepressants are commonly prescribed to treat anxiety and depression, which are commonly associated with this disorder. Selective serotonin reuptake inhibitors act on the brain to help balance levels of serotonin. Tricyclic antidepressants and monoamine oxidase inhibitors (MAOIs) help to balance serotonin and norepinephrine. Other drugs may act to balance a combination of dopamine, norepinephrine, serotonin, and other chemicals.

⊠ PREVENTION

Closely monitor patients taking antidepressants for suicidal thoughts, especially during the first 4 weeks of starting therapy.

⚠ ALERT

Patients taking MAOIs must avoid foods and beverages that contain tyramine. Tyramine is found in aged cheeses, smoked meats, and wine and may trigger a hypertensive crisis.

• Anxiolytics (benzodiazepines), such as alprazolam (Xanax), may be prescribed to treat anxiety in the short term. The patient must be carefully monitored because the potential for addiction is high. For this reason, they shouldn't be prescribed if the patient has a history of substance abuse.

SPECIAL CONSIDERATIONS

● Establish an empathetic relationship with each emerging personality.

⚠ ALERT

Monitor the patient's actions for evidence of self-directed violence or violence directed at others.

● Recognize even small gains.

● Stress the importance of continuing psychotherapy. Point out that the therapy can be prolonged, with alternating successes and failures, and that one or more of the personalities may resist treatment.

Dyspareunia

Dyspareunia is one of several sexual pain disorders and is defined as genital pain associated with intercourse. The disorder can occur in both men and women. It may be mild, or it may be severe enough to affect enjoyment of intercourse. Dyspareunia is commonly associated with physical problems; less commonly, with a psychological disorder. The prognosis is good if the underlying disorder can be treated successfully.

CAUSES AND INCIDENCE

Physical causes of dyspareunia in women include an intact hymen; deformities or lesions of the introitus or vagina; marked retroversion of the uterus; genital, rectal, or pelvic scar tissue; acute or chronic infections of the genitourinary tract; disorders of the surrounding viscera (including residual effects of pelvic inflammatory disease or disease of the adnexal and broad ligaments);

and postmenopausal vaginal atrophy.

Among the many other possible physical causes are:

● endometriosis

● benign and malignant growths and tumors

● insufficient lubrication

● radiation to the area

● allergic reactions to diaphragms, condoms, or other contraceptives.

Physical causes of dyspareunia in men include urinary tract infections, sexually transmitted diseases, genital deformities, and pelvic pathology and scarring from previous surgery or irradiation.

Psychological causes include fear of pain or of injury during intercourse, recollection of a previous painful experience, and guilty feelings about sex; fear of pregnancy or of injury to the fetus during pregnancy; anxiety caused by a new sexual partner or technique; and mental or physical fatigue.

SIGNS AND SYMPTOMS

● Persistent genital or pelvic pain before, during, or after intercourse

● Vaginal itching or burning

COMPLICATIONS

● Impaired interpersonal relationships

● Anxiety

● Depression

DIAGNOSTIC CRITERIA

Physical examination, laboratory tests, and radiologic tests, such as ultrasound, help to exclude any underlying physical disorder or other cause. For example, painful orgasm has been reported as a side effect of drug therapy with fluphenazine (Prolixin). Diagnosis also depends on obtaining a detailed sexual history with such questions as:

- When does the pain occur?
- Does it occur with certain positions or techniques or at certain times during the sexual response cycle?
- Where does the pain occur?
- What's the quality, frequency, and duration of the pain?
- What factors relieve or aggravate the pain?

When the disorder causes marked distress or interpersonal difficulty, and is not caused by a general medical condition, psychiatric disorder, or substance, it may fulfill the diagnostic criteria from the *Diagnostic and Statistical Manual of Mental Disorders,* Fourth Edition, Text Revision.

TREATMENT

- Treatment of physical causes may include creams and water-soluble gels for inadequate lubrication, appropriate medications for infections, excision of hymenal scars, and gentle stretching of painful scars at the vaginal opening. The patient may be advised to change her coital position to reduce pain on deep penetration.
- Methods of treating psychological causes vary with the particular patient. Sensate focus exercises deem-

phasize intercourse itself and teach appropriate foreplay techniques.
- Education about contraception methods can reduce fear of pregnancy.
- Education about sexual activity during pregnancy can relieve fear of harming the fetus.

Drugs

- Antidepressants are commonly prescribed to treat anxiety and depression, which are commonly associated with this disorder. Selective serotonin reuptake inhibitors act on the brain to help balance levels of serotonin. Tricyclic antidepressants and monoamine oxidase inhibitors (MAOIs) help to balance serotonin and norepinephrine. Other medications may act to balance a combination of dopamine, norepinephrine, serotonin, and other chemicals.

▧ PREVENTION

Closely monitor patients taking antidepressants for suicidal thoughts, especially during the first 4 weeks of starting therapy.

⚠ ALERT

Patients taking MAOIs must avoid foods and beverages that contain tyramine. Tyramine is found in aged cheeses, smoked meats, and wine and may trigger a hypertensive crisis.

- Anxiolytics (benzodiazepines), such as alprazolam (Xanax), may be prescribed to treat anxiety in the short term. The patient must be carefully monitored because the potential for addiction is high. For this reason, they shouldn't be prescribed if the patient has a history of substance abuse.

SPECIAL CONSIDERATIONS

• Provide the patient with instruction concerning anatomy and physiology of the reproductive system, contraception, and the human sexual response cycle.

• When appropriate, provide advice and information on drugs that may affect the patient sexually.

• Listen to the patient's complaints of sex-related pain, and maintain a sympathetic, nonjudgmental attitude toward her, which will encourage her to express her feelings without embarrassment.

E

Erectile disorder

Erectile disorder, or impotence, refers to a male's inability to attain or maintain penile erection sufficient to complete intercourse. There are two forms of erectile disorder: the patient with the *primary* form has never achieved a sufficient erection; the patient with the *acquired* form, which is more common and less serious than the primary form, implies that, despite present inability, the patient has succeeded in completing intercourse in the past. Transient periods of erectile dysfunction aren't considered pathological and probably occur in half of adult males. Erectile disorder affects all age-groups but increases in frequency with age. The prognosis depends on the severity and duration of impotence and the underlying cause.

CAUSES AND INCIDENCE

In about 50% to 80% of men who have erectile disorder, statistics point to an organic basis; psychological causes account for the remainder. In many patients, organic and psychogenic factors may coexist, making isolation of the primary cause difficult. It's estimated that 30 million men are affected by erectile disorder.

Organic causes may include cardiovascular occlusive disease, diabetes, anemia, multiple sclerosis, renal failure, neurologic disease, complications from surgery, alcohol or substance abuse, genital anomalies, incompetent penile venous valves, nicotine abuse, or hormonal disorders. Many drugs prescribed to treat other conditions also have side effects that may affect sexual functioning.

✄ PREVENTION

Some drugs known to cause erectile disorder include antihypertensives, antihistamines, tranquilizers, appetite suppressants, some antidepressants, and cimetidine (Tagamet), an H_2 receptor antagonist.

Psychogenic causes may be intrapersonal, reflecting personal sexual anxieties, or interpersonal, reflecting a disturbed sexual relationship. Intrapersonal factors generally involve guilt, fear, depression, or feelings of inadequacy resulting from previous traumatic sexual experience, rejection by parents or peers, exaggerated religious orthodoxy, or abnormal mother-son intimacy. Interpersonal factors may stem from differences in sexual preferences between partners, lack of communication, insufficient knowledge of sexual function, or nonsexual personal conflicts.

Situational impotence, a temporary condition, may develop in response to stress, as in performance anxiety. Erectile disorder is commonly reported by patients who also have eating and personality disorders.

SIGNS AND SYMPTOMS

Secondary erectile disorder is classified as follows:

• *Partial*—The patient is unable to achieve a full erection.

• *Intermittent*—The patient is sometimes able to complete intercourse with the same partner.

• *Selective*—The patient is only able to achieve intercourse in certain situations or only with certain types of partners.

The pattern of erectile dysfunction varies greatly. Some men report sudden loss of erectile function, whereas others lose it more gradually. If the cause isn't organic, erection may still be achieved through masturbation.

Patients with psychogenic impotence may:

• appear anxious, with sweating and palpitations

• lose interest in sexual activity

• suffer from depression

• report severe fatigue

• report severe stress.

COMPLICATIONS

• Interpersonal relationship problems

• Fertility problems

• Depression

• Anxiety

DIAGNOSTIC CRITERIA

A detailed sexual history helps differentiate between organic and psychogenic factors and between primary and secondary impotence. Questions should include the following:

• Does the patient have intermittent, selective, nocturnal, or early-morning erections?

• Can he achieve erections through other sexual activity?

• When did his problem begin, and what was his life situation at that time?

• Did erectile problems occur suddenly or gradually?

• What medications, alcohol, or substances is he taking?

Test that may be ordered to help identify or exclude organic causes for erectile disorder include:

• duplex ultrasound to identify penile blood flow patterns

• nocturnal penile tumescence studies to document the presence of nighttime erections

• nerve conduction studies

• dynamic infusion cavernosometry and cavernosography to check penile blood pressures and blood flow

• arteriography to check patency of the arteries.

Laboratory studies that may be ordered to help identify or exclude medical conditions affecting erectile function include:

• glucose tolerance tests to check for diabetes

• serum hormone assays to check testosterone, prolactin, and follicle-stimulating hormone levels

- liver, renal, and thyroid function tests
- complete blood count.

When erectile disorder causes marked distress or interpersonal difficulty and is not caused by another mental disorder, medical condition, or ingestion of a substance, it may fulfill diagnostic criteria from the *Diagnostic and Statistical Manual of Mental Disorders,* Fourth Edition, Text Revision.

TREATMENT

Treatment of organic impotence focuses on reversing the cause, if possible. Surgery may be necessary to reduce blockages in arteries. Patients suffering from erectile disorder may benefit from surgically inserted implants or vacuum devices.

Sex therapy, which should include both partners, may effectively treat psychogenic impotence. The course and content of such therapy depend on the specific cause of the dysfunction and the nature of the couple's relationship. Usually, therapy includes sensate focus exercises, which restrict the couple's sexual activity and encourage them to become more attuned to the physical sensations of touching. Sex therapy also includes improving verbal communication skills, eliminating unreasonable guilt, and reevaluating attitudes toward sex and sexual roles.

Drugs

- Phosphodiesterase inhibitors, such as sildenafil (Viagra) and tadalafil (Cialis), help to relax smooth muscle and increase blood flow to the penis.
- Prostaglandins, such as alprostadil (Caverject, Edex), are either injected into the corpus cavernosum of the penis or administered as a urethral suppository. Prostaglandins relax smooth muscle and dilate cavernosal arteries and increase blood flow into the penis.
- Antidepressants, such as nefazodone and bupropion (Wellbutrin), are less likely to cause erectile dysfunction than selective serotonin reuptake inhibitors such as citalopram (Celexa). Patients who have anxiety or depression may benefit from switching medications or from decreasing dosages.

☒ PREVENTION

Closely monitor the patient taking antidepressants for suicidal thoughts, especially during the first 4 weeks of starting therapy.

SPECIAL CONSIDERATIONS

- When you identify a patient with impotence or with a condition that may cause impotence, help him feel comfortable about discussing his sexuality. Assess his sexual health during your initial nursing history. When appropriate, refer him for further evaluation or treatment.
- Help the patient identify stressors and develop stress management skills.
- Monitor the patient for the development of erectile dysfunction when initiating drug therapy for anxiety and depression.

• After penile implant surgery, tell the patient to avoid intercourse until the incision heals—usually in 6 weeks.

To help prevent impotence:

• Promote establishment of responsible health and sex education programs at primary, secondary, and college levels.

• Promote healthy lifestyles, discouraging nicotine use and substance abuse.

• Provide information about resuming sexual activity as part of discharge instructions for patients with conditions that require modification of daily activities. Such patients include those with cardiac disease, renal disease, neurologic disease, diabetes, hypertension, and chronic obstructive pulmonary disease and all postoperative patients.

F

Female arousal and orgasmic disorders

Female arousal and orgasmic disorders are characterized by an inability or persistent delay to achieve orgasm following a phase of normal sexual excitement. They may be classified as (1) primary anorgasmia, when a female has never experienced sexual arousal or orgasm; (2) secondary anorgasmia, when some physical, mental, or situational condition has inhibited or obliterated a female's previously normal sexual function; and (3) situational anorgasmia, when a female is only able to achieve orgasm in certain situations. For temporary or mild disorders that result from misinformation or situational stress, the prognosis is good; however, for disorders that result from intense anxiety, chronically discordant relationships, psychological disturbances, or drug or alcohol abuse in either partner, the prognosis is guarded.

CAUSES AND INCIDENCE

In the United States, it's estimated that 15% of women have difficulty achieving orgasm and approximately 10% have never had an orgasm. Problems with arousal and orgasm may result from medical conditions, psychological factors, or a combination of the two; therefore, it may be difficult to isolate the cause of the disorder. In addition, female sexual function and response may decline because of decreasing estrogen levels in the perimenopausal period. This decrease in estrogen affects nerve transmission and response in the peripheral vascular system. As a result, the timing and degree of vasoconstriction during the sexual response is affected, vasocongestion decreases, muscle tension decreases, and contractions are fewer and less intense during orgasm.

Medical conditions that may affect arousal and orgasm include side effects of drugs prescribed to treat other conditions, alcohol and substance abuse, cardiovascular occlusive disease, endocrine disorders, neurologic disorders, genitourinary tract infections and surgery, severe fatigue, and inadequate sexual stimulation.

Psychological factors that may cause arousal and orgasmic disorders include relationship problems, communication problems, unresolved conflict, anxiety, depression, severe stress, fear of pregnancy, fear of sexually transmitted disease, guilt about sexual enjoyment, religious and cultural beliefs, and fear of losing control.

SIGNS AND SYMPTOMS

The female with arousal and orgasmic disorder may experience:

- limited or absent sexual desire
- little or no pleasure from sexual stimulation
- lack of vaginal lubrication
- absence of signs of genital vaso-congestion
- inability to achieve orgasm, either totally or under certain circumstances
- ability to achieve orgasm through masturbation or other means but not through intercourse
- ability to achieve orgasm with some partners but not with others.

COMPLICATIONS

- Interpersonal relationship problems
- Anxiety
- Depression

DIAGNOSTIC CRITERIA

A thorough physical examination is necessary to identify or exclude medical conditions and medications that may affect arousal. Laboratory and imaging tests may include:

- complete blood count
- liver, renal, and thyroid function studies
- serum hormonal assays
- imaging studies of the pelvis to identify anatomy and pathology
- duplex ultrasound to identify vascular problems.

A detailed psychosexual history is essential to differentiate between organic and psychogenic factors influencing arousal and orgasm. A psychosexual history should include:

- detailed information concerning the patient's knowledge of sexual response and reproductive health
- previous sexual response patterns
- level of family stress or fatigue
- patient's feelings (during childhood and adolescence) about sex in general and, specifically, about masturbation, incest, rape, sexual fantasies, and homosexual or heterosexual practices
- contraceptive practices and reproductive goals
- patient's present relationship, including her partner's attitude toward sex
- assessment of patient's self-esteem and body image
- treatment for other psychological disorders.

When the disorder causes marked distress or interpersonal difficulty and is not attributed to another psychological disorder, it may fulfill criteria from the *Diagnostic and Statistical Manual of Mental Disorders,* Fourth Edition, Text Revision.

TREATMENT

Arousal disorder is difficult to treat, especially if the female has never experienced sexual pleasure. Therapy is designed to help the patient relax and become aware of her feelings about sex and to eliminate guilt and fear of rejection. The goal in treating orgasmic disorder is to decrease or eliminate involuntary inhibition of the orgasmic reflex. Treatment may include experiential therapy, psychoanalysis, or behavior modification.

Specific measures may include the following:

• Sensate focus exercises similar to those developed by Masters and Johnson are commonly used. In these exercises, the therapist should communicate an accepting attitude and help the patient and partner understand that satisfactory sexual experiences don't always require coital orgasm. Sensate focus exercises emphasize touching and an awareness of sensual feelings all over the body—not just genital sensations—and minimize the importance of intercourse and orgasm.

• Psychoanalytic treatment consists of free association, dream analysis, and discussion of life patterns to achieve greater sexual awareness. One behavioral approach attempts to correct maladaptive patterns through systematic desensitization to situations that provoke anxiety, partially by encouraging the patient to fantasize about these situations.

• Treatment of primary orgasmic disorder may involve teaching the patient self-stimulation. Also, the therapist may teach distraction techniques, such as focusing attention on fantasies, breathing patterns, or muscle contractions to relieve anxiety. The patient learns new behavior through exercises she does privately between sessions. Gradually, the therapist involves the patient's sexual

partner in the treatment sessions; some therapists treat the couple as a unit from the outset.

• Treatment of secondary orgasmic disorder is designed to decrease anxiety and depression and promote the factors needed for the patient to experience orgasm.

Drugs

Treatment may consist of treating underlying anxiety or depression.

• Antidepressants, such as nefazodone and bupropion (Wellbutrin), are less likely to cause orgasmic dysfunction than selective serotonin reuptake inhibitors, such as citalopram (Celexa). Patients who have anxiety or depression may benefit from switching medications or from decreasing dosages.

⊠ PREVENTION

When the patient is taking antidepressants, closely monitor her for suicidal thoughts, especially during the first 4 weeks of starting therapy.

SPECIAL CONSIDERATIONS

• Be alert for clues to arousal or orgasmic disorder when taking a health history.

• Maintain an open, nonjudgmental attitude toward the patient.

• Instruct the patient in anatomy and physiology of the reproductive system and in sexual response patterns.

• Refer the patient to a physician, nurse, psychologist, social worker, or counselor trained in sex therapy. Inform the patient that the therapist's certification by the American Association of Sex Educators, Counselors, and Therapists or by the Society for Sex Therapy and Research usually ensures quality treatment.

If the therapist isn't certified by these organizations, advise the patient to ask about the therapist's credentials.

Gender identity disorder

Gender identity is defined as the psychological state reflecting a sense of being male or female. It's culturally based on determined sets of attitude and behavioral patterns as well as other attributes usually associated with masculinity or femininity. Gender identity disorder involves persistent cross-gender identification (longer than 2 years) and feelings of discomfort and dissatisfaction (gender dysphoria). The disorder shouldn't be confused with the more common feelings of inadequacy in fulfilling the expectations normally associated with a particular sex. Among some practitioners and transgender people, the diagnosis of gender identity disorder is controversial because it creates a pathologic label. Indeed, some believe the label should be eliminated.

CAUSES AND INCIDENCE

The incidence of gender identity disorder is relatively rare—it affects only 1 in 10,000 males and 1 in 30,000 females in the United States. Current theories about gender identity disorder and its causes suggest a combination of predisposing factors, such as heredity, prenatal hormone influences (occurring particularly during brain formation *in utero*), and environmental and social influences. Research shows that the number of neurons in the limbic nucleus of female-to-male transgender individuals is in the male range. This suggests that there may be changes in hormone levels in the brain that drive some individuals to be males.

SIGNS AND SYMPTOMS

Gender identity disorder may emerge at an early age. A child may express the desire to be—or insist that he or she is—the opposite sex. For example, a male child may express disgust with his genitalia.

Men with gender identity disorder may describe a lifelong history of feeling feminine and pursuing feminine activities. Women report similar propensities for opposite-sex activities and discomfort with the female role. For both sexes, the conflict intensifies during puberty and can cause intense anxiety and depression.

COMPLICATIONS

● Anxiety
● Depression
● Social isolation
● Legal problems (many states do not recognize gender reassignment)
● Discrimination (Individuals are not legally protected from discrimination

DIAGNOSING GENDER IDENTITY DISORDERS

The diagnosis of gender identity disorder is confirmed when the patient's symptoms meet the following criteria established in the *Diagnostic and Statistical Manual of Mental Disorders,* Fourth Edition, Text Revision:

■ A strong and persistent cross-gender identification (not merely a desire for any perceived cultural advantages of being the other sex).

In children, the disturbance is manifested by at least four of the following:
– repeatedly stated desire to be, or insistence that he or she is, the other sex
– in boys, preference for cross-dressing or simulating female attire; in girls, insistence on wearing only stereotypical masculine clothing
– strong and persistent preferences for cross-sex roles in make-believe play or persistent fantasies of being the other sex
– intense desire to participate in the stereotypical games and pastimes of the other sex
– strong preference for playmates of the other sex.

In adolescents and adults, the disturbance is manifested by such symptoms as a stated desire to be the other sex, frequent passing as the other sex, desire to live or be treated as the other sex, or the conviction that he or she has the typical feelings and reactions of the other sex.

■ Persistent discomfort with his or her sex or sense of inappropriateness in the gender role of that sex.

In children, the disturbance is manifested by any of the following:
– in boys, assertion that his penis or testes are disgusting or will disappear or he'd be better off not to have a penis, rejection of rough-and-tumble play, and rejection of male stereotypical toys, games, and activities
– in girls, rejection of urinating in a sitting position, assertion that she has or will grow a penis, or assertion that she doesn't want to grow breasts or menstruate, or marked aversion toward feminine clothing.

In adolescents and adults, the disturbance is manifested by such symptoms as preoccupation with getting rid of primary and secondary sex characteristics or the belief that he or she was born the wrong sex.

■ The disturbance isn't concurrent with a physical intersex condition.

■ The disturbance causes clinically significant distress or impairment in social, occupational, or other important areas of functioning.

in employment or housing based on gender identity or gender expression.)

DIAGNOSTIC CRITERIA

For specific diagnostic criteria from the *Diagnostic and Statistical Manual of Mental Disorders,* Fourth Edition,

Text Revision, see *Diagnosing gender identity disorders.*

TREATMENT

Treatment may include:
• psychotherapy to consider the range of options, set realistic life goals, and define conflicts

• individual and family therapy, which is especially indicated for childhood gender identity disorder
• individual and couples therapy for adult patients
• gender reassignment, which consists of various combinations of real-life experiences, such as living the gender for at least 12 months, hormonal therapy (for at least 12 months), and gender reassignment surgery
– Not every individual desires or is a candidate for gender reassignment surgery. Patients are carefully evaluated in order to individually tailor treatments. In some patients, severe psychological problems may persist after sex reassignment surgery. Further, for some patients, the gender identity disorder may be part of a larger depression and personality disorder pattern.
• appropriate psychiatric management, including hospitalization, if the patient displays the potential for violent behavior, such as suicide or self-mutilation.

Drugs

• Estrogens are used for male-to-female patients to increase breast growth, soften the skin, decrease body hair, and redistribute body fat. Estrogens cause the testicles to become smaller and penile erections to be less firm and less frequent. Upper-body strength also decreases. Drugs that interfere with testosterone production, such as spironolactone (Aldactone), and testosterone metabolization, such as finasteride

(Proscar), may also be added to the regimen.
• Androgens, such as testosterone, are given to masculinize female-to-male patients. Females experience voice deepening, some breast atrophy, increased hair growth and distribution, clitoral enlargement, and increased sexual interest. Upper-body strength also increases and body fat decreases.

SPECIAL CONSIDERATIONS

• Adopt a nonjudgmental approach in facial expression, tone of voice, and choice of words to convey your acceptance of the patient's choices.
• Respect the patient's privacy and sense of modesty, particularly during procedures or examinations.
• Monitor the patient for related or compounded problems, such as suicidal thoughts or intent, depression, and anxiety.
• Refer the patient to a physician, nurse, psychologist, social worker, or counselor trained in transgender health.
• Refer the patient and his family to the World Professional Association for Transgender Health for education and support.

Generalized anxiety disorder

Anxiety is a feeling of apprehension that some describe as an exaggerated feeling of impending doom, dread, or uneasiness. Unlike fear—a reaction to danger from a specific external source—anxiety is a reaction to an internal threat, such as an unacceptable impulse or a repressed thought that's straining to reach a conscious level.

A rational response to a real threat, occasional anxiety is a normal part of life. Overwhelming anxiety, however, can result in generalized anxiety disorder—uncontrollable, unreasonable worry that persists for at least 6 months and narrows perceptions or interferes with normal functioning. Recent evidence indicates that the prevalence of generalized anxiety disorder is greater than previously thought and may be even greater than that of depression.

CAUSES AND INCIDENCE

Generalized anxiety disorder has a 1-year prevalence range from 3% to 8%. It's more common in women than in men, and half of all cases begin in childhood or adolescence.

Research into generalized anxiety disorder suggests that it may be caused by dysregulation in the neurotransmitters serotonin and norepinephrine and by a combination of other factors such as genetics and an individual's biologic processes, environment, and life situation. Higher rates of generalized anxiety disorder are seen in patients who have suffered childhood hardships, severe illnesses, and who have unmet psychological needs. It's more common in patients who also have borderline personality disorder.

SIGNS AND SYMPTOMS

Generalized anxiety disorder can begin at any age, but typically has an onset in the 20s and 30s. Psychological or physiologic symptoms of anxiety states vary with the degree of anxiety. Mild anxiety mainly causes psychological symptoms, with unusual self-awareness and alertness to the environment. Moderate anxiety leads to selective inattention but with the ability to concentrate on a single task. Severe anxiety causes an inability to concentrate on more than scattered details of a task. A panic state with acute anxiety causes a complete loss of concentration, typically with unintelligible speech.

Physical examination of the patient with generalized anxiety disorder may reveal:
- motor tension, including trembling and muscle aches and spasms
- headaches
- shortness of breath and tachypnea
- tachycardia and sweating
- abdominal pain
- diarrhea.

The individual may also report:
- startling easily
- feelings of restlessness
- feelings of apprehension and fear
- difficulty concentrating
- sleeping disturbances
- eating disturbances.

Medical conditions that should be excluded before making a diagnosis include hyperthyroidism, pheochromocytoma, coronary artery disease, cardiac arrhythmias, cardiac valvular disease, Ménière's disease, hypocalcemia, substance abuse, and GI disease.

COMPLICATIONS

- Depression
- Insomnia
- Alcohol and substance abuse
- Digestive problems
- Teeth grinding

DIAGNOSTIC CRITERIA

For characteristic findings in patients with this condition, see *Diagnosing generalized anxiety disorder*.

The diagnostic and laboratory tests commonly ordered to exclude organic causes of the patient's signs and symptoms include:

- electrocardiography
- echocardiography
- cardiac enzymes
- complete blood count with white blood cell count and differential
- serum lactate and calcium levels
- serum toxicology screen.

Because anxiety is the central feature of other mental disorders, psychiatric evaluation must rule out phobias, obsessive-compulsive disorder, depression, and acute schizophrenia.

TREATMENT

The treatment plan for individuals with generalized anxiety disorder often includes a combination of psychotherapy, relaxation techniques, cognitive behavioral therapy, and drug therapy. Treatment may include:

DIAGNOSING GENERALIZED ANXIETY DISORDER

When the patient's symptoms match criteria documented in the *Diagnostic and Statistical Manual of Mental Disorders,* Fourth Edition, Text Revision, the diagnosis of generalized anxiety disorder is confirmed. The criteria include:

- Excessive anxiety and worry about numerous events or activities occur more days than not for at least 6 months.
- The person finds it difficult to control the worry.
- The anxiety and worry are associated with at least three of the following six symptoms:
  – restlessness or feeling keyed up or on edge
  – being easily fatigued
  – difficulty concentrating or mind going blank
  – irritability
  – muscle tension
  – sleep disturbances (difficulty falling or staying asleep, or restless, unsatisfying sleep).
- The focus of the anxiety and worry isn't confined to features of an axis I disorder.
- The anxiety, worry, or physical symptoms cause clinically significant distress or impairment in social, occupational, or other important areas of functioning.
- The disturbance isn't due to the direct physiologic effects of a substance or a general medical condition and doesn't occur exclusively during a mood disorder, a psychotic disorder, or a pervasive developmental disorder.

• psychotherapy, which helps the patient identify and deal with the cause of the anxiety and eliminates environmental factors that precipitate an anxious reaction

• relaxation techniques such as deep breathing, progressive muscle relaxation, focused relaxation, and visualization

• cognitive behavioral therapy, which can help the patient identify negative thought patterns and behaviors and replace them with more healthy ones.

Drugs

• Anxiolytics (benzodiazepines), such as alprazolam (Xanax) and lorazepam (Ativan), may be prescribed to treat anxiety in the short term. However, the patient must be carefully monitored because the potential for addiction to sedatives is high. For this reason, benzodiazepines should not be prescribed if the patient has a history of substance abuse.

– Buspirone (BuSpar), a different type of anxiolytic, causes the patient less sedation and poses less risk of physical and psychological dependence than the benzodiazepines. It may also help to regulate serotonin in the brain.

⚠ ALERT

Buspirone shouldn't be given in combination with a monoamine oxidase inhibitor because severe hypertension may result.

• Antidepressants, such as tricyclic antidepressants, may relieve severe anxiety and panic attacks. Venlafaxine (Effexor), a selective serotonin and norepinephrine reuptake inhibitor, is approved by the Food and Drug Administration for the treatment of generalized anxiety disorder.

▣ PREVENTION

When the patient is taking antidepressants, closely monitor him for suicidal thoughts, especially during the first 4 weeks of starting therapy.

SPECIAL CONSIDERATIONS

• Stay with the patient when he's anxious, and encourage him to discuss his feelings.

• Reduce environmental stimuli and remain calm.

• Give anxiolytic or antidepressant, as prescribed, and evaluate the patient's response. Teach the patient about prescribed medications, including the need for adherence with the medication regimen. Review adverse reactions.

• Teach the patient effective coping strategies and relaxation techniques. Help him identify stressful situations that trigger his anxiety, and provide positive reinforcement when he uses alternative coping strategies.

• Encourage the patient to participate in anxiety support groups.

Hypochondriasis

The dominant feature of hypochondriasis is an unrealistic misinterpretation of the severity and significance of physical signs or sensations
as abnormal. This leads to preoccupation with fear of having a serious
disease, which persists despite medical reassurance to the contrary. It
isn't due to other mental disorders,
such as schizophrenia, mood disorder, or somatization disorder.

The course of hypochondriasis is
usually chronic, although the severity
of symptoms may vary.

CAUSES AND INCIDENCE

Estimates place the incidence of
hypochondriasis in the general population at about 5%. Hypochondriasis occurs in men and women with
equal frequency. It can begin at any
age, even in children, but onset usually occurs between ages 20 and 30.

Although the cause of hypochondriasis is unknown, some research
suggests an inherited susceptibility.
It's more commonly seen in individuals who suffered a serious illness as
a child, who have a loved one who is
seriously ill, who recently suffered a
stressful event such as a death, who
find it difficult to express emotions,
and who have anxiety disorder. Few
individuals fully recover.

SIGNS AND SYMPTOMS

The dominant feature of hypochondriasis is the misinterpretation of
symptoms—usually multiple complaints that involve a single organ
system—as signs of serious illness.
As the medical evaluation proceeds,
complaints may shift and change.
Symptoms, which can range from
specific to general, typically are associated with a preoccupation with
normal body functions.

The hypochondriacal patient will
relate a chronic history of:
- waxing and waning symptoms
- excessive concern about a body
part or system
- anxiety or depression
- frequent changing of health care
providers
- belief that the diagnosis of the
health care provider is wrong
- excessive concern about illness
that interferes with his social, family, and occupational functioning
- unfounded belief that he's especially vulnerable to disease
- multiple evaluations and diagnostic testing for similar symptoms.

DIAGNOSTIC CRITERIA

For characteristic findings in
patients with this condition, see
Diagnosing hypochondriasis,
page 90.

DIAGNOSING HYPOCHONDRIASIS

A diagnosis of hypochondriasis is made when the patient's symptoms meet the following criteria put forth in the *Diagnostic and Statistical Manual of Mental Disorders,* Fourth Edition, Text Revision:

- Preoccupation with the fear of having or the belief that one has a serious disease is based on the person's misinterpretation of bodily symptoms.
- The preoccupation persists despite appropriate medical evaluation and reassurance.
- The fear of having or the belief that one has a serious disease isn't of delusional intensity (as in delusional disorder, somatic type) and isn't restricted to a circumscribed concern about appearance (as in body dysmorphic disorder).
- The preoccupation causes clinically significant distress or impairment in social, occupational, or other important areas of functioning.
- The disturbance has persisted for at least 6 months.
- The preoccupation isn't better accounted for by generalized anxiety disorder, obsessive-compulsive disorder, panic disorder, a major depressive episode, separation anxiety, or another somatoform disorder.

TREATMENT

The goal of treatment is to help the patient continue to lead a productive life, despite what the patient sees as distressing symptoms and fears. After a thorough medical evaluation is complete, the patient should be told clearly that he doesn't have a serious disease. Although providing a diagnosis of hypochondriasis won't make it disappear, it may ease the patient's anxiety.

One of the treatment goals should also be for the patient to develop a trusting relationship with his health care provider in order to accurately help monitor his symptoms. Regular outpatient follow-up can help the patient deal with his symptoms and is needed to detect organic illness; up to 30% of these patients develop an organic disease. However, because the patient can be demanding and distrustful, follow-up may be difficult. Further, most patients don't acknowledge any psychological basis for their symptoms and may resist psychiatric treatment.

Drugs

- Antidepressants can help relieve anxiety associated with hypochondriasis. Selective serotonin reuptake inhibitors act on the brain to help balance levels of serotonin. Tricyclic antidepressants help to balance both serotonin and norepinephrine.

⚠ ALERT

The patient with hypochondriasis may consider common side effects of antidepressant therapy as evidence of disease. Side effects may increase his anxiety about his health.

⊠ PREVENTION

When the patient is taking antidepressants, closely monitor him for suicidal thoughts, especially during the first 4 weeks of initiating therapy.

SPECIAL CONSIDERATIONS

• Provide a supportive relationship that enables the patient to feel cared for and understood. The patient with hypochondriasis feels real pain and distress; so, don't deny his symptoms or challenge his behavior.

• Firmly state that medical test results are normal. Instead of reinforcing his symptoms, encourage him to discuss his other problems and express his feelings and urge his family to do the same.

• Recognize that the patient may never be symptom-free, and don't become upset when he won't give up his disease. Such anger can drive him to yet another unnecessary medical evaluation.

• Help the patient and his family find new ways to deal with stress other than the development of physical symptoms.

Kleptomania

Kleptomania was first described in 1838 and is classified as one of the impulse control disorders. The patient with kleptomania has an irresistible urge to steal objects, but isn't motivated by monetary gain, anger, or revenge. Many times he doesn't need the items and also has the ability to pay for them. Sometimes the patient keeps and hides the objects or may simply give them away. These behaviors are highly ritualistic. Indeed, the patient with kleptomania shares similar characteristics with the patient who has obsessive-compulsive disorder.

Stealing initially brings the patient gratification but is quickly followed by feelings of guilt, shame, and remorse. The theft is solitary and is usually unplanned, and the patient won't usually steal when it's obvious that he would be arrested.

CAUSES AND INCIDENCE

It's estimated that the prevalence of kleptomania is about 0.6% in the general population. However, the true incidence of kleptomania is probably underreported because patients are often ashamed to seek help and often only receive help after they have been referred by the criminal justice system following their arrest. Of those arrested for shoplifting, the incidence is about 5%.

Kleptomania affects three times as many females as males. It may begin in childhood but is more typical in adolescence and adulthood. The exact cause of kleptomania isn't known. Sometimes patients develop it after suffering brain trauma. Research into the neurobiology of the brain has shown that there may be dysfunction in the regulation of dopamine and of circuits that modulate human motivation. Research also continues into identifying dysfunction in the regulation of levels of serotonin. In some patients, episodes of kleptomania are linked to substance abuse, which may increase impulsivity and diminish inhibition. Some studies have demonstrated that patients with kleptomania have a higher-than-normal incidence of having a close relative with obsessive-compulsive disorder. Kleptomania is also associated with having mood, eating, and personality disorders.

SIGNS AND SYMPTOMS

The patient with kleptomania may report:

- powerful urges to steal
- feelings of tension before stealing
- pleasure while stealing

- remorse after stealing
- stealing items that have no value to the individual
- stealing only one type of item (fetishism)
- stealing from public places and stores
- stealing from family and friends.

There are several typical patterns of kleptomania. The patient may exhibit:

- sporadic episodes of stealing followed by a long period of remission
- lengthy periods of stealing followed by a period of remission
- chronic patterns of stealing that may continue for several years despite multiple criminal convictions.

COMPLICATIONS

- Legal problems, arrest, and imprisonment
- Occupational problems
- Social isolation
- Family problems
- Anxiety
- Depression
- Suicidal thoughts
- Substance and alcohol abuse

DIAGNOSTIC CRITERIA

For characteristic findings in patients with this condition, see *Diagnosing kleptomania*.

TREATMENT

Treatment plans may include:
- cognitive behavioral therapy to change unhealthy thoughts and behavior

---

DIAGNOSING KLEPTOMANIA

The diagnosis of kleptomania is based on criteria from the *Diagnostic and Statistical Manual of Mental Disorders,* Fourth Edition, Text Revision. The criteria are:
- recurrent failure to resist impulses to steal objects that aren't needed for personal use or for their monetary value
- increasing sense of tension immediately before committing the theft
- pleasure, gratification, or relief at the time of committing the theft
- notion that stealing isn't committed to express anger or vengeance and isn't in response to a delusion or a hallucination
- fact that stealing isn't better accounted for by Conduct Disorder, a Manic Episode, or Antisocial Personality Disorder.

- appropriate self-help groups
- 12-step groups such as Alcoholics Anonymous (AA)
- family therapy.

Drugs

- Anxiolytics such alprazolam (Xanax), a benzodiazepine, may be prescribed to treat anxiety in the short term. However, the patient must be carefully monitored because the potential for addiction is high. Benzodiazepines shouldn't be prescribed if the patient has a history of substance abuse.

• Antidepressants, such as fluoxetine (Prozac), sertraline (Zoloft), and paroxetine (Paxil), are approved to treat depression and obsessive-compulsive disorder and have been shown to benefit patients with kleptomania.

⊁ PREVENTION

Carefully monitor the patient for patterns of kleptomania. In some patients, selective serotonin reuptake inhibitors (SSRIs) may actually trigger episodes.

⊁ PREVENTION

Closely monitor the patient for signs of increasing depression or suicidal thoughts, especially during the first 4 weeks of starting therapy with SSRIs.

• Mood stabilizers, such as lithium (Eskalith), may help prevent mood changes that can trigger stealing episodes.

• Anticonvulsants, such as topiramate (Topamax) and valproate (Depakene), have shown benefit in decreasing the urge to steal.

• Opioid blockers, such as naltrexone (ReVia), have been shown to reduce urges and pleasurable feelings associated with stealing.

SPECIAL CONSIDERATIONS

• Monitor the patient and help him identify triggers for stealing behavior.

• Help the patient identify techniques to decrease his anxiety and channel his urges to steal.

• Because relapses are common even with treatment, encourage the patient to stay focused on his goals.

• Help the patient obtain treatment for substance abuse problems when appropriate.

Major depressive disorder

Also known as *unipolar disorder,* major depressive disorder is characterized by persistently sad, dysphoric mood, accompanied by disturbances in sleep and appetite, lethargy, and an inability to experience pleasure (anhedonia) that lasts longer than 2 weeks.

About half of all depressed patients experience a single episode and recover completely; the rest have at least one recurrence. Major depression can profoundly alter social, family, and occupational functioning. However, suicide is the most serious consequence of major depression—feelings of worthlessness, guilt, and hopelessness are so overwhelming that patients no longer consider life worth living. Nearly twice as many women as men attempt suicide, but men are far more likely to succeed.

CAUSES AND INCIDENCE

Depression occurs in up to 18 million Americans, affecting all racial, ethnic, and socioeconomic groups (more common in lower socioeconomic groups). It affects both sexes, but is more commonly diagnosed in women.

Children and the elderly can also be affected and are often not diagnosed. According to the United States Department of Health and Human Services, 1 in every 12 adolescents experiences major depression each year, and more than twice as many females than males are affected.

The causes of depression aren't completely understood and are probably due to a combination of genetic, familial, biochemical, psychological, and social factors as well as medical conditions. The incidence of depression is higher among people who also have a family member with depression or who have attempted suicide, which suggests an inherited predisposition. Research using brain imaging suggests that depressed people have physical brain changes. Other research suggests that dysregulation in neurotransmitters and hormones influences the development of depression. Psychological causes (the focus of many nursing interventions) may include the feelings of helplessness, vulnerability, anger, hopelessness and pessimism, and low self-esteem. Developing depression may be related to dysfunctional character and behavior patterns and troubled personal relationships. In many cases, the individual identifies a specific personal loss or severe stressor that probably combines

DYSTHYMIC DISORDER

Dysthymic disorder is characterized by a chronic dysphoric mood (irritable mood in children), persisting at least 2 years in adults and 1 year in children and adolescents.

Signs and symptoms
During periods of depression, the patient may also experience poor appetite or overeating, insomnia or hypersomnia, low energy or fatigue, low self-esteem, poor concentration or difficulty making decisions, and feelings of hopelessness.

Diagnosis
Dysthymic disorder is confirmed when the patient exhibits at least two of the signs or symptoms listed above nearly every day, with intervening normal moods lasting no more than 2 months during a 2-year period.

The disorder typically begins in childhood, adolescence, or early adulthood and causes only mild social or occupational impairment. In adults, it's more common in women; in children and adolescents, it's equally common in both sexes.

with the person's predisposition to provoke major depression.

Depression may be secondary to a specific medical condition—for example, metabolic disturbances, such as hypoxia and hypercalcemia; endocrine disorders, such as diabetes and Cushing's syndrome; neurologic diseases, such as Parkinson's and Alzheimer's diseases; cancer (especially of the pancreas); viral and bacterial infections, such as influenza and pneumonia; cardiovascular disorders, such as heart failure; pulmonary disorders, such as chronic obstructive lung disease; musculoskeletal disorders, such as degenerative arthritis; GI disorders, such as irritable bowel syndrome; genitourinary problems, such as incontinence; collagen vascular diseases, such as lupus; and anemia.

Drugs prescribed for medical and psychiatric conditions as well as many commonly abused substances can also cause depression. Examples include some antihypertensives, psychotropics, opioid and nonopioid analgesics, antiparkinsonian drugs, numerous cardiovascular medications, oral antidiabetics, antimicrobials, steroids, chemotherapeutic agents, cimetidine, and alcohol.

SIGNS AND SYMPTOMS

The primary features of major depression are a predominantly sad mood and a loss of interest or pleasure in daily activities. The patient may complain of feeling "down in the dumps," express doubts about his self-worth or ability to cope, or simply appear unhappy and apathetic. Symptoms tend to be more severe than those caused by dysthymic disorder, which is a milder, chronic form of depression. (See *Dysthymic disorder*.)

Other common signs and symptoms include:

● difficulty concentrating or thinking clearly

- distractibility and indecisiveness
- reduced psychomotor activity (for example, slowed speech)
- agitation and restlessness
- anxiety
- crying for no reason
- hostility and irritability (in men)
- lack of energy
- anhedonia (inability to experience pleasure)
- severe stress or loss
- sleep disturbances (for example, insomnia or early wakening)
- weight loss or gain for no reason
- constipation or diarrhea
- loss of interest in sex and sexual dysfunction
- suicidal thoughts or preoccupation with death.

The patient's medical history may implicate a physical disorder or the use of prescription, nonprescription, or illegal drugs that can cause depression. Note that many of the characteristics of depression, such as changes in eating and sleeping patterns, fatigue, and problems with concentration, may also occur in chronic medical conditions.

COMPLICATIONS

- Suicide
- Anxiety
- Heart disease—patients are twice as likely to develop cardiac disease within 10 years of being diagnosed with depression (Depressed patients are more likely to die after having a myocardial infarction.)
- Depressed immune response
- Substance and alcohol abuse

- Occupational and school problems
- Interpersonal relationship problems
- Social isolation

DIAGNOSTIC CRITERIA

For characteristic findings in patients with this condition, see *Diagnosing major depression,* page 98.

- Psychological tests, such as the Beck Depression Inventory, may help determine the onset, severity, duration, and progression of depressive symptoms.
- Laboratory tests to exclude medical conditions may include:
  – complete blood count
  – thyroid function studies
  – toxicology tests to detect alcohol and other substances
  – cytochrome P450 test: pharmacogenetic test that indicates an individual's ability to metabolize certain medications. (It's used to help tailor and predict the patient's response to antidepressants and other drugs.)

TREATMENT

About 70% to 80% of people with depression demonstrate improvement in symptoms within a few months of starting treatment. Treatment may include:

- psychotherapy to help identify stressors, conflicts, and losses and to problem solve
- cognitive behavioral therapy to help the patient identify and change negative thoughts, beliefs, and behavior
- group and family therapy

DIAGNOSING MAJOR DEPRESSION

A patient is diagnosed with major depression when he fulfills the following criteria for a single major depressive episode put forth in the *Diagnostic and Statistical Manual of Mental Disorders,* Fourth Edition, Text Revision:

■ At least five of the following symptoms must have been present during the same 2-week period and must represent a change from previous functioning; one of these must be either depressed mood or loss of interest in previously pleasurable activities:
– depressed mood (irritable mood in children and adolescents) most of the day, nearly every day, as indicated by either subjective account or observation by others
– markedly diminished interest or pleasure in all, or almost all, activities most of the day, nearly every day
– significant weight loss or weight gain when not dieting or decrease or increase in appetite nearly every day (in children, consider failure to make expected weight gains)
– insomnia or hypersomnia nearly every day
– psychomotor agitation or retardation nearly every day
– fatigue or loss of energy nearly every day

– feelings of worthlessness or excessive or inappropriate guilt nearly every day
– diminished ability to think or concentrate, or indecisiveness, nearly every day
– recurrent thoughts of death, recurrent suicidal ideation without a specific plan, a suicide attempt, or a specific plan for committing suicide.
■ The symptoms don't meet criteria for a mixed episode.
■ The symptoms cause clinically significant distress or impairment in social, occupational, or other important areas of functioning.
■ The symptoms aren't due to the direct physiologic effects of a substance or a general medical condition.
■ The symptoms aren't better accounted for by bereavement, the symptoms persist for longer than 2 months, or the symptoms are characterized by marked functional impairment, morbid preoccupation with worthlessness, suicidal ideation, psychotic symptoms, or psychomotor retardation.

● electroconvulsive therapy (ECT), which may be considered in particularly severe or drug-resistant depression (Researchers hypothesize that ECT affects the same receptor sites as antidepressants. ECT has been associated with later short-term memory loss, heart arrhythmias, and seizure activity.)

● transcranial magnetic stimulation, which uses magnets to change the electrical currents in the areas of the brain that control mood (It's used for patients who don't respond well to drug therapy, but it's not a replacement for ECT. Research continues to determine long-term safety and side effects.)

● vagal nerve stimulation, which involves a mild electrical impulse applied to the left vagus nerve. (It's believed that these electrical impulses affect neurotransmission and may be helpful in treating those patients who haven't responded to other treatment. Research continues to evaluate the safety and effectiveness of this treatment.)

Drugs

• Antidepressants may include tricyclic antidepressants (TCAs) such as amitriptyline; and monoamine oxidase inhibitors (MAOIs), such as isocarboxazid (Marplan), maprotiline, and trazodone. A newer class of drugs, the selective serotonin reuptake inhibitors (SSRIs), such as fluoxetine (Prozac), paroxetine (Paxil), sertraline (Zoloft), bupropion (Zyban), venlafaxine (Effexor), and mirtazapine (Remeron), are equally effective and have more tolerable adverse effect profiles. Drugs that target serotonin and norepinephrine as well as dopamine include bupropion (Wellbutrin), venlafaxine (Effexor), and duloxetine (Cymbalta). These varied psychopharmacologic drugs allow for increased specificity of action. So, for example, a patient who shows neurovegetative signs of depression may benefit from bupropion, whereas the patient who's experiencing both anxiety and depression may benefit more from venlafaxine.
– TCAs, the oldest class of antidepressants, prevent the reuptake of norepinephrine or serotonin (or both) into the presynaptic nerve endings, resulting in increased synaptic concentrations of these neurotransmitters. Although often

effective, these drugs have significant side effects. Because of their effect on cardiac conduction, TCAs may be lethal in overdoses. They also cause a gradual loss in the number of beta-adrenergic receptors.
– MAOIs block the enzymatic degradation of norepinephrine and serotonin. These drugs commonly are prescribed for patients with atypical depression (for example, depression marked by an increased appetite and need for sleep, rather than anorexia and insomnia) and for some patients who fail to respond to other classes of antidepressants. MAOIs are associated with a high risk of toxicity; patients treated with one of these drugs must be able to comply with the necessary dietary restrictions.

≫ PREVENTION

When the patient is taking antidepressants, monitor him closely for suicidal thoughts, especially during the first 4 weeks of starting therapy.

⚠ ALERT

The patient taking MAOIs must avoid foods and beverages that contain tyramine, which is found in aged cheeses, smoked meats, and wine, because they may trigger a hypertensive crisis.

SPECIAL CONSIDERATIONS

• Share your observations of the patient's behavior with him. For instance, you might say, "You're sitting all by yourself, looking very sad. Is that how you feel?" Because the patient may think and react sluggishly, speak slowly and allow ample time for him to respond. Avoid feigned cheerfulness. However, don't hesitate to laugh with the patient and point out the value of humor.

• Show the patient he's important by listening attentively and respectfully, preventing interruptions, and avoiding judgmental responses.

• Provide a structured routine, including noncompetitive activities, to build the patient's self-confidence and encourage interaction with others. Urge him to join group activities and to socialize.

• Inform the patient that he can help ease depression by expressing his feelings, participating in pleasurable activities, and improving grooming and hygiene.

• Ask the patient if he thinks of death or suicide. Such thoughts signal an immediate need for consultation and assessment. The risk of suicide increases as the depression lifts, typically in the early stages of treatment with antidepressants. The Food and Drug Administration has issued "black box" warnings on antidepressants because of this increased risk. (See *Suicide prevention guidelines*.)

• To prevent possible drug interactions, encourage the patient to inform his practitioner if he's taking antidepressants.

• While tending to the patient's psychological needs, don't forget his physical needs. If he's too depressed to take care of himself, help him with personal hygiene. Encourage

him to eat, or feed him if necessary. If he's constipated, add high-fiber foods to his diet; offer small, frequent meals; and encourage physical activity and fluid intake. Offer warm milk or back rubs at bedtime to improve sleep.

• Inform the patient that antidepressants may take several weeks (8 to 12) to produce full effect.

• Teach the patient about depression. Emphasize that effective methods are available to relieve his symptoms. Help him to recognize distorted perceptions that may contribute to his depression. After the patient learns to recognize depressive thought patterns, he can consciously begin to substitute self-affirming thoughts.

• Instruct the patient about prescribed medications. Stress the need for compliance, and review adverse effects. For drugs that produce strong anticholinergic effects, such as amitriptyline and amoxapine, suggest sugarless gum or hard candy to relieve dry mouth. Many antidepressants are sedating (for example, amitriptyline and trazodone); warn the patient to avoid activities that require alertness, including driving and operating mechanical equipment until the central nervous system (CNS) effects of the drug are known.

• Caution the patient taking a TCA to avoid drinking alcoholic beverages or taking other CNS depressants during therapy.

• Because alcohol acts as a CNS depressant, recommend avoiding

SUICIDE PREVENTION GUIDELINES

When the patient is diagnosed with major depression, keep in mind these guidelines.

Assess for clues to suicide
Watch for the patient's suicidal thoughts, threats, and messages; describing a suicide plan; hoarding medication; talking about death and feelings of futility; giving away prized possessions; and changing behavior, especially as depression begins to lift.

Provide a safe environment
Check patient areas and correct dangerous conditions, such as exposed pipes, windows without safety glass, and access to the roof or balconies.

Remove dangerous objects
Take away potentially dangerous objects, such as belts, razors, suspenders, light cords, glass, knives, nail files and clippers, metal and hard plastic objects, and cleaning fluids and other toxic chemicals.

Consult with staff
Recognize and document verbal and nonverbal suicidal behaviors, keep the physician informed, share data with all staff members, clarify the patient's specific restrictions, assess risk and plan for observation, and clarify day and night staff responsibilities and the frequency of consultations.

Observe the suicidal patient
Be alert when the patient is using a sharp object (such as a razor), taking medication, or using the bathroom (to prevent hanging or other injury). Assign the patient to a room near the nurses' station and with another patient. Continuously observe the acutely suicidal patient.

Maintain personal contact
Help the suicidal patient feel that he isn't alone or without resources or hope. Encourage continuity of care and consistency of primary nurses. Building emotional ties to others is the ultimate technique for preventing suicide.

---

alcohol to a patient who's experiencing depression.

• When assessing a patient, ask about herbal remedies that he may be using for depression. A common herbal remedy, St. John's Wort, can interact with many other antidepressants.

Mental retardation

The American Association on Intellectual and Developmental Disabilities (AAIDD) defines mental retardation and intellectual disability as "significantly sub average general intellectual function existing concurrently with deficits in adaptive behavior manifesting itself during the developmental period (before age 18)." Intellectual disability is commonly accompanied by other physical and emotional disorders that may constitute disabilities in themselves.

CAUSES OF MENTAL RETARDATION

- Chromosomal abnormalities (Down syndrome, Klinefelter's syndrome)
- Disorders resulting from unknown prenatal influences (hydrocephalus, hydraencephaly, microcephaly)
- Disorders of metabolism or nutrition (phenylketonuria, hypothyroidism, Hurler's syndrome, galactosemia, Tay-Sachs disease)
- Environmental influences (cultural-familial retardation, poor nutrition, lack of medical care)
- Gestational disorders (prematurity)
- Gross brain disorders that develop after birth (neurofibromatosis, intracranial neoplasm)
- Infection and intoxication (congenital rubella, syphilis, lead poisoning, meningitis, encephalitis, insecticides, drugs, maternal viral infection, toxins)
- Psychiatric disorders (autism)
- Trauma or physical conditions (mechanical injury, asphyxia, hyperpyrexia)

CAUSES AND INCIDENCE

An estimated 1% to 3% of the population has intellectual disability, demonstrating an IQ below 70 and associated difficulty in carrying out tasks required for personal independence. A specific cause is identifiable in only about 25% of people and, of these, only 10% have the potential for cure. (See *Causes of mental retardation.*)

In the remaining 75% of individuals, the causes remain unknown, but predisposing factors, such as deficient prenatal or perinatal care, inadequate nutrition, poor social environment, and poor child-rearing practices, may contribute significantly to the development of intellectual disability.

⊠ PREVENTION

Prenatal screening for genetic defects (such as Tay-Sachs disease) and counseling for families at risk for specific defects have reduced the incidence of genetically transmitted intellectual disability. Other preventive measures include programs to promote nutrition and decrease substance and alcohol abuse during pregnancy, efforts to reduce environmental exposure to lead and mercury, and measures to prevent congenital rubella. Decreasing exposure to known infectious material such as cat litter help prevent acquiring toxoplasmosis during pregnancy.

SIGNS AND SYMPTOMS

The observable effects of mental retardation include:
- deviations from normal adaptive behaviors, ranging from learning disabilities and uncontrollable behavior to severe cognitive and motor skill impairment
- failure to achieve developmental milestones
- diminished ability to learn
- lack of curiosity.

Occasionally children are not diagnosed until they enter school.

The earlier a child's adaptive deficit is recognized and he's placed in a special learning program, the more likely he is to achieve age-appropriate adaptive behaviors. If the patient is older, review his adaptation to his environment.

The family of an individual with mental retardation may report many problems stemming from the individual's needs, frustration, and fear. Family problems, such as financial difficulties, abuse, and divorce, can compromise the child's care. Physical examination may reveal signs of abuse or neglect.

Patients who have mental retardation may exhibit signs and symptoms of other disorders, such as:

- cleft lip
- congenital heart defects
- cerebral palsy
- diminished resistance to infection.

COMPLICATIONS

- Impaired self-care ability
- Impaired social interaction and isolation
- Impaired family relationships
- Occupational and educational difficulties

DIAGNOSTIC CRITERIA

There are several different tools used to diagnose mental retardation. Common tests include:

- Standardized IQ test—a score of less than 70 confirms the diagnosis of mental retardation. The IQ test primarily predicts school performance and must be supplemented by other diagnostic evaluations.

- Adaptive Behavior Scale—evaluates behaviors important to activities of daily living. This test evaluates self-help skills (toileting and eating), physical and social development, language, socialization, and time and number concepts. It also examines inappropriate behaviors, such as violent or destructive acts, withdrawal, and self-abusive or sexually aberrant behavior.

- Denver Developmental Screening Test—assesses age-appropriate adaptive behaviors. This test compares the patient's functional level with the normal level for the same chronologic age. The greater the discrepancy between chronologic and developmental age determines the severity of disability.

- Vineland Social Maturity Scale—determines social competence. In children, the functional level is based on sensorimotor skills, self-help skills, and socialization. In adolescents and adults, it's based on academic skills, reasoning and judgment skills, and social skills.

TREATMENT

Effective management requires an interdisciplinary team approach to assist the patient and his family on primary, secondary, and tertiary levels. A major goal is to develop the patient's strengths. Another important goal is the development of social adaptive skills. The amount of care and help necessary for the individual to perform activities of daily living should be determined and emphasized rather than the degree of intellectual impairment.

Children who have mental retardation require special education and training, ideally beginning in infancy. An individualized, effective education program can optimize the quality of life for even those with profound intellectual disability. The prognosis for people who have mental retardation may be determined by:

• child's age when intervention is started

• aggressiveness of treatment

• individual and family motivation and support

• training opportunities

• social integration and behavior management.

Many people with mental retardation are productive members of society. Successful treatment can lead to independent functioning and occupational skills for some and a sheltered environment for others.

Drugs

Drug therapy is not used to cure mental retardation but to help manage behavior problems.

• Antipsychotics, such as risperidone (Risperdal), have been increasingly prescribed to successfully decrease aggressive, destructive, and disruptive behavior in both adults and children. Research continues in order to determine the long-term safety and efficacy of these drugs in children.

⚠ ALERT

More than 50% of patients taking atypical antipsychotics will have significant weight gain and should be monitored for the development of metabolic syndrome and type 2 diabetes.

⚠ ALERT

Monitor the patient taking atypical antipsychotics for the development of neuroleptic malignant syndrome (hyperthermia, autonomic disturbances, and extrapyramidal symptoms), which can be fatal.

SPECIAL CONSIDERATIONS

• Support the parents of a child diagnosed with mental retardation. They may be overwhelmed by caretaking and financial concerns and may have difficulty accepting and bonding with their child.

• Remember that a child has all the ordinary needs of an intellectually average child plus those created by his intellectual disability. All children need affection, acceptance, stimulation, and prudent, consistent discipline. The child is less able to cope if rejected, overprotected, or forced beyond his abilities.

• When caring for a hospitalized patient with mental retardation, promote continuity of care by acting as a liaison for parents and other practitioners.

• During hospitalization, continue behavioral treatment programs already in place, but remember that illness may bring on some regression.

• For the parents of a child with severe intellectual disability, promote healthy family relationships and support. The parents may need an extensive teaching and discharge planning program, including physical care procedures, stress reduction techniques, support services, and referral to developmental programs. Refer them to the social services department to identify community resources.

• Teach parents how to care for the special needs of their child. Suggest they contact AAIDD.

• Teach adolescents and family how to deal with physical changes and sexual maturation. Encourage them to participate in appropriate sex education classes. People may have difficulty expressing sexual concerns because of limited verbal skills.

Obsessive-compulsive disorder

Obsessive thoughts and compulsive behaviors represent recurring efforts to control overwhelming anxiety, guilt, or unacceptable impulses that persistently enter the consciousness. The word obsession refers to a recurrent idea, thought, impulse, or image that's intrusive and inappropriate, causing marked anxiety or distress. A compulsion is a ritualistic, repetitive, and involuntary defensive behavior. Performing a compulsive behavior reduces the patient's anxiety and increases the probability that the behavior will recur.

Patients with obsessive-compulsive disorder (OCD) may abuse psychoactive substances, such as alcohol and anxiolytics, in an attempt to relieve anxiety. In addition, other anxiety disorders and major depression commonly coexist with OCD.

OCD is typically a chronic condition with remissions and flare-ups. Mild forms of the disorder are relatively common in the general population.

CAUSES AND INCIDENCE

According to the National Institutes of Health, about 2.2 million people in the United States have OCD, although it tends to be under-reported, under-recognized, and under-treated. Patients may not be correctly diagnosed for many years. About one-third of adults suffering from OCD report that their symptoms began in childhood.

The cause of OCD is unknown. Some genetic research, however, suggests that there may be an inherited tendency to develop OCD because the development of childhood OCD seems to run in families. Neurobiologic studies suggest that OCD may be caused by abnormally low levels of serotonin. Other research suggests that some maladaptive behaviors are learned from the patient's environment, and some controversial research suggests OCD may be linked to group A beta-hemolytic streptococcus infection. Some studies suggest the possibility of brain lesions. In addition, major depression, organic brain syndrome, and schizophrenia may occur with OCD. Some researchers find that depression may occur when the individual is no longer able to cope with his symptoms of OCD. Some authorities think that OCD is closely related to some eating disorders. Symptoms usually are noticed between ages 20 and 30, with 75% of patients displaying symptoms before age 30.

SIGNS AND SYMPTOMS

The psychiatric history of a patient with OCD may reveal the presence of obsessive thoughts, words, or mental images that persistently and involuntarily invade the consciousness. The patient recognizes that the obsessions are a product of his own mind and they interfere with normal daily activities.

Some common obsessions include:
• thoughts of violence (such as stabbing, shooting, maiming, or hitting)
• thoughts and fears of contamination (images of dirt, germs, or feces)
• repetitive doubts and worries about a tragic event
• repeating or counting images, words, or objects in the environment
• recurrent rituals
• thoughts about maintaining symmetry in his environment.

The patient's history may also reveal the presence of compulsions— irrational and recurring impulses to repeat a certain behavior. Common compulsions include:
• repetitive touching and arranging of objects, sometimes combined with counting
• doing and undoing (for instance, opening and closing doors or rearranging things)
• excessive washing (especially of hands)
• repetitive checking of the environment (to be sure no tragedy has occurred since the last time he checked)
• constant demanding of reassurance.

In many cases, the patient's anxiety is so strong that he'll avoid the situation or the object that evokes the impulse. When the obsessive-compulsive phenomena are mental, observation may reveal no behavioral abnormalities. However, compulsive acts may be observed. Feelings of shame, nervousness, or embarrassment may prompt the patient to hide his behavior and limit these acts to his own private time.

COMPLICATIONS

• Impaired functioning in work and school
• Impaired family relationships
• Impaired social functioning
• Depression
• Suicide attempt
• Substance and alcohol abuse in attempt to self-medicate his anxiety and distress
• Physical complications from compulsive behaviors (for example, dermatitis from excessive handwashing)

DIAGNOSTIC CRITERIA

There are no laboratory tests to diagnose OCD. For characteristic findings in patients with this condition, see *Diagnosing obsessive-compulsive disorder,* page 108.

Be sure to evaluate the impact of obsessive-compulsive phenomena on the patient's normal routine. He'll typically report moderate to

DIAGNOSING OBSESSIVE-COMPULSIVE DISORDER

The diagnosis of obsessive-compulsive disorder is made when the patient's signs and symptoms meet the established criteria put forth in the *Diagnostic and Statistical Manual of Mental Disorders,* Fourth Edition, Text Revision.

Either obsessions or compulsions

Obsessions are defined as all of the following:

- Recurrent and persistent thoughts, impulses, or images perceived to be intrusive and inappropriate by the patient, causing anxiety or distress at some point in time during the disturbance.
- The thoughts, impulses, or images are not simply excessive worries about real-life problems.
- The person attempts to ignore or suppress such thoughts or impulses, or to neutralize them with some other thought or action.
- The person recognizes that the obsessions are the products of his mind and not externally imposed.

Compulsions are defined as all of the following:

- Repetitive behaviors or mental acts performed by the person, who feels driven to perform them in response to an obsession or according to rules that must be applied rigidly.
- The behavior or mental acts are aimed at preventing or reducing distress or preventing some dreaded event or situation. However, either the activity isn't connected in a realistic way with what it's designed to neutralize or prevent or it's clearly excessive.
- The patient recognizes that his behavior is excessive or unreasonable (this may not be true for young children or for patients whose obsessions have evolved into overvalued ideas).

Additional criteria

- At some point, the person recognizes that the obsessions or compulsions are excessive or unreasonable.
- The obsessions or compulsions cause marked distress, are time-consuming (take more than 1 hour per day), or significantly interfere with the person's normal routine, occupational functioning, or usual social activities or relationships.
- If another axis I disorder is present, the content of the obsession is unrelated to it; for example, the ideas, thoughts, or images aren't about food in the presence of an eating disorder, about drugs in the presence of a psychoactive substance abuse disorder, or about guilt in a major depressive disorder.
- The disturbance isn't due to the direct physiologic effects of a substance or a general medical condition.

severe impairment of social and occupational functioning.

TREATMENT

OCD is tenacious, but improvement occurs in 75% to 85% of patients who obtain treatment. Current treatment usually involves a combination of drug and cognitive behavioral therapy. Cognitive behavioral therapy helps the patient identify and change negative thought patterns

BEHAVIORAL THERAPIES

The following behavioral therapies are used to treat the patient with obsessive-compulsive disorder.

Aversion therapy
Application of a painful stimulus creates an aversion to the obsession that leads to undesirable behavior (compulsion).

Flooding
Flooding is frequent, full-intensity exposure (through the use of imagery) to an object that triggers a symptom. It must be used with caution because it produces extreme discomfort.

Implosion therapy
A form of desensitization, implosion therapy calls for repeated exposure to a highly feared object.

Response prevention
Preventing compulsive behavior by distraction, persuasion, or redirection of activity, response prevention may require hospitalization or involvement of the patient's family to be effective.

Thought stopping
Thought stopping breaks the habit of fear-inducing anticipatory thoughts. The patient learns to stop unwanted thoughts by saying the word "stop" and then focusing his attention on achieving calmness and muscle relaxation.

Thought switching
To replace fear-inducing self-instructions with competent self-instructions, the patient learns to replace negative thoughts with positive ones until the positive thoughts become strong enough to overcome the anxiety-provoking ones.

and behaviors. Behavioral therpies—aversion therapy, thought stopping, thought switching, flooding, implosion therapy, and response prevention—have also been effective. (See *Behavioral therapies*.)

Drugs
- Antidepressants that affect serotonin levels in the brain (selective serotonin reuptake inhibitors [SSRIs]), such as fluvoxamine (Luvox), sertraline (Zoloft), and paroxetine (Paxil), are approved by the Food and Drug Administration to treat OCD. Antidepressant therapy may take 8 to 12 weeks to show effectiveness in decreasing symptoms. Tricyclic antidepressants such as clomipramine (Anafranil) have also demonstrated benefits.

≥ PREVENTION
Closely monitor patients, especially children and adolescents, for signs of increasing depression or suicidal thoughts, particularly during the first 4 weeks of starting therapy with SSRIs.

- Antipsychotics, such as clozapine (Clozaril) and olanzapine (Zyprexa), are sometimes prescribed to help control behavioral tics in patients with OCD, but only show benefit when they are added to SSRI therapy.

⚠ **ALERT**

Fluoxetine, fluvoxamine, paroxetine, and sertraline may increase clozapine levels and toxicity.

⚠ **ALERT**

Monitor the patient taking olanzapine for the development of neuroleptic malignant syndrome (hyperthermia, autonomic disturbances, and extrapyramidal symptoms), which can be fatal.

SPECIAL CONSIDERATIONS

• Approach the patient unhurriedly.
• Provide an accepting atmosphere; don't appear shocked, amused, or critical of the ritualistic behavior.
• Keep the patient's physical health in mind. For example, compulsive handwashing may cause skin breakdown; rituals or preoccupations may cause inadequate food and fluid intake and exhaustion. If the patient becomes involved in ritualistic thoughts and behaviors to the point of self-neglect, provide for basic needs, such as rest, nutrition, and grooming.
• Let the patient know that you're aware of his behavior. For example, you might say, "I noticed you've made your bed three times today; that must be very tiring for you." Help the patient explore feelings associated with the behavior. For example, ask him, "What do you

think about while you're performing your chores?"
• Make reasonable demands and set reasonable limits, explaining their purpose clearly. Avoid creating situations that increase frustration and provoke anger, which may interfere with treatment.
• Help the patient identify and explore triggers for obsessive thoughts or compulsive behaviors.
• Work with the patient and other treatment team members to develop behavioral goals and to help the patient tolerate anxiety while pursuing these goals.
• Encourage his compliance with drug, behavioral, group, and family therapy.
• Listen attentively, offering feedback.
• Promote social activities to relieve loneliness and prevent isolation.
• Engage the patient in activities to create positive accomplishments and raise self-esteem and confidence.
• Encourage active diversionary activities, such as whistling or humming, to divert attention from the unwanted thoughts and to promote a pleasurable experience.
• Help the patient develop new ways to solve problems and cultivate more effective coping skills by setting limits on unacceptable behavior (for example, by limiting the number of times per day he may

indulge in compulsive behavior). Gradually shorten the time allowed for compulsive behavior. Help him focus on other feelings or problems for the remainder of the time.

• Identify insight and improved behavior (reduced compulsive behavior and fewer obsessive thoughts). Evaluate behavioral changes by your own observations and the patient's reports.

• Evaluate interventions and, if unsuccessful, develop new goals and pursue alternative strategies.

• Help the patient identify progress and set realistic expectations.

• Explain how to channel emotional energy to relieve stress (for example, through sports and creative endeavors). In addition, teach the patient relaxation and breathing techniques to help reduce anxiety.

• Teach the patient to avoid intoxicating substances and alcohol as a means to decrease his anxiety.

• Encourage the individual and family to contact the Obsessive Compulsive Foundation for additional educational resources and support.

P

Pain disorder

The striking feature of pain disorder is a persistent complaint of pain in the absence of appropriate physical findings. The symptoms are either inconsistent with the normal anatomic distribution of the nervous system or they mimic a disease (such as angina) in the absence of diagnostic validation. Although the pain has no identifiable physical cause, it's real to the patient. The pain is usually chronic and disabling and may, in many cases, interfere with interpersonal relationships or employment.

CAUSES AND INCIDENCE

The true incidence of pain disorder is unknown, but some research suggests that it's quite common. Pain disorder has no specific cause, but it may be related to severe psychological stress or internal conflict. The patient is not aware that psychological factors are central to the onset, severity, and exacerbation of the pain. The patient does not consciously create or fabricate the symptoms, and he's not malingering.

Pain disorder is thought to be more common in women than in men and usually has an onset between ages 30 and 40.

Researchers are using positron emission tomography (PET) scanning and functional magnetic resonance imaging (fMRI) to explore the anatomy and metabolic activity of the brain during the experience of pain in order to understand it and develop better treatments.

SIGNS AND SYMPTOMS

The cardinal feature of pain disorder is a history of chronic, consistent complaints of pain without confirming physical disease. The patient's history and physical may reveal:

- long history of evaluations and procedures at multiple settings
- multiple treatment without much pain relief
- familiarity with pain medications and tranquilizers and knowledge of correct dosages and administration routes
- impaired motor movements
- normal laboratory and diagnostic results
- pain that does not follow anatomic pathways
- absence of typical nonverbal signs of pain, such as grimacing or guarding (Sometimes such reactions are absent in the patient with chronic organic pain. Palpation, percussion, and auscultation may not reveal expected associated signs.)

• anger with practitioners because they have failed to relieve the pain

• anger with the suggestion that psychological factors may be impacting the patient's experience of pain.

COMPLICATIONS

• Impaired work and school functioning
• Impaired family relationships
• Impaired social functioning
• Potential addiction to prescription pain medication
• Potential injury from undergoing multiple diagnostic tests and procedures

DIAGNOSTIC CRITERIA

For characteristic findings in patients with this condition, see *Diagnosing pain disorder*.

TREATMENT

In pain disorder, the goal of treatment is to decrease the pain and help the patient resume activities of daily living. Thus, long, invasive evaluations and surgical interventions are generally avoided. Treatment at a comprehensive pain center may be indicated. Cognitive behavioral therapy helps the individual to identify negative thoughts and behaviors and helps him develop strategies to manage his pain.

A continuing, supportive relationship with an understanding practitioner is essential for effective management; regularly scheduled follow-up appointments are helpful.

DIAGNOSING PAIN DISORDER

The diagnosis of pain disorder is difficult because the perception of pain is subjective. Diagnosis is based on fulfillment of the following criteria put forth in the *Diagnostic and Statistical Manual of Mental Disorders,* Fourth Edition, Text Revision:

■ Pain in one or more body sites is the predominant focus of the patient and is sufficiently severe to warrant clinical attention.
■ The pain causes clinically significant distress or impairment in social, occupational, or other important areas of functioning.
■ Psychological factors are judged to have an important role in the onset, severity, exacerbation, and maintenance of the pain.
■ The symptom or deficit isn't intentionally produced or feigned.
■ The pain isn't better accounted for by a mood, anxiety, or psychotic disorder and doesn't meet criteria for dyspareunia.

Additional supportive measures for pain relief may include:
• hot or cold packs
• exercise and physical therapy
• distraction techniques
• cutaneous stimulation with massage
• transcutaneous electrical nerve stimulation
• acupuncture
• meditation techniques
• relaxation techniques
• yoga.

Drugs

- Regularly scheduled analgesic doses can be more effective than scheduling medication as needed. Regular doses combat pain by reducing anxiety about asking for medication and eliminate unnecessary confrontations.
- Antidepressants—selective serotonin reuptake inhibitors—act on the brain to help balance levels of serotonin. Tricyclic antidepressants help to balance serotonin and norepinephrine. They help to improve sleep, decrease pain, and also relieve depression. The dosages given to treat pain disorder are often lower than dosages required to treat depression.

⊠ PREVENTION

When the patient is taking antidepressants, closely monitor him for suicidal thoughts, especially during the first 4 weeks of starting therapy.

SPECIAL CONSIDERATIONS

- Observe and record characteristics of the pain: severity, duration, and any precipitating factors.
- Provide a caring atmosphere in which the patient's complaints are taken seriously and every effort is made to provide relief. This means communicating to the patient that you'll collaborate on a plan of treatment, clearly stating the limitations.
- Don't tell the patient that she's imagining the pain or can wait longer for medication that's due. Assess her complaints and help her understand what's contributing to the pain.
- Develop a collaborative treatment plan to provide other comfort measures, such as repositioning or massage, relaxation techniques, and distraction when appropriate.
- Encourage the patient to maintain independence and normal daily activities despite pain.
- Refer the patient to a comprehensive pain control clinic.
- Consider psychiatric referrals; however, realize that the patient may resist psychiatric intervention, and don't expect it to replace analgesic measures.

Panic disorder

Characterized by recurrent episodes of intense apprehension, terror, and impending doom, panic attacks represent anxiety in its most severe form. Initially unpredictable, panic attacks may become associated with specific situations or tasks and, if they become debilitating, are considered panic disorder. The disorder commonly exists concurrently with other phobias such as agoraphobia. Equal numbers of men and women are affected by panic disorder alone, whereas panic disorder with agoraphobia occurs in about twice as many women.

Without treatment, panic disorder can persist for years, with alternating exacerbations and remissions. The patient with panic disorder is at high risk for a psychoactive substance abuse disorder: He may resort to alcohol or anxiolytics in an attempt to relieve his extreme anxiety.

CAUSES AND INCIDENCE

Between 2 and 6 million people in the United States are affected by panic disorder. The typical age of onset is late adolescence through the late 30s. Like other anxiety disorders, panic disorder may stem from a combination of genetic, environmental, or biological factors. Recent evidence indicates that alterations in brain biochemistry, especially in norepinephrine, serotonin, and gamma-aminobutyric acid activity, may contribute to panic disorder. Panic disorder is more common in individuals who have a childhood history of sexual or physical abuse, have suffered a severely traumatic event or accident, or have a severely ill loved one. It may also be triggered by severe childhood separation anxiety.

SIGNS AND SYMPTOMS

The patient with panic disorder typically complains of repeated episodes of unexpected apprehension, fear or, rarely, intense discomfort. These panic attacks may last for minutes or hours and leave the patient shaken, fearful, and exhausted. They may occur several times a week, sometimes even daily. Because the attacks occur spontaneously, without exposure to a known anxiety-producing situation, the patient generally worries between attacks about when the next episode will occur. This is referred to as anticipatory anxiety.

Physical examination of the patient during a panic attack may reveal signs of intense anxiety, such as:

- hyperventilation
- tachycardia
- trembling
- profuse sweating
- difficulty breathing
- digestive disturbances
- chest pain or pressure.

COMPLICATIONS

- Additional phobias
- Depression
- Suicidal thoughts
- Work and school problems
- Impaired social and family relationships
- Substance or alcohol abuse

DIAGNOSTIC CRITERIA

For characteristic findings in patients with this condition, see *Diagnosing panic disorder,* page 116.

Because many medical conditions can mimic panic disorder, a thorough physical examination is necessary to rule out an organic basis for the symptoms. Diagnostic tests may include:

- serum glucose levels to rule out hypoglycemia
- urine levels of catecholamine and vanillylmandelic acid to rule out pheochromocytoma
- thyroid function tests to rule out hyperthyroidism
- electrocardiography, cardiac enzymes, and echocardiography to exclude myocardial infarction and other cardiac diseases
- urine and serum toxicology tests to check for psychoactive substances, such as alcohol, barbiturates, and amphetamines.

DIAGNOSING PANIC DISORDER

The diagnosis of panic disorder is confirmed when the patient meets the criteria put forth in the *Diagnostic and Statistical Manual of Mental Disorders,* Fourth Edition, Text Revision.

Panic attack

A discrete period of intense fear or discomfort in which at least four of the following symptoms develop abruptly and reach a peak within 10 minutes:

- palpitations, pounding heart, or tachycardia
- sweating
- trembling or shaking
- shortness of breath or smothering sensations
- feeling of choking
- chest pain or discomfort
- nausea or abdominal distress
- dizziness or faintness
- depersonalization or derealization
- fear of losing control or going crazy
- fear of dying
- numbness or tingling sensations (paresthesia)
- hot flashes or chills.

Panic disorder without agoraphobia

- The person experiences recurrent unexpected panic attacks and at least one of the attacks has been followed by 1 month (or more) of one (or more) of the following:
  – persistent concern about having additional attacks
  – worry about the implications of the attack or its consequences
  – a significant change in behavior related to the attacks.

- The panic attacks aren't caused by the direct physiologic effects of a substance or a general medical condition.
- The panic attacks aren't better accounted for by another mental disorder, such as social phobia, specific phobia, obsessive-compulsive disorder, posttraumatic stress disorder, or separation anxiety disorder.

Panic disorder with agoraphobia

- The person experiences recurrent unexpected panic attacks and at least one of the attacks has been followed by 1 month (or more) of one (or more) of the following:
  – persistent concern about having additional attacks
  – worry about the implications of the attack or its consequences
  – a significant change in behavior related to the attacks.
- The person exhibits agoraphobia.
- The panic attacks aren't caused by the direct physiologic effects of a substance or a general medical condition.
- The panic attacks aren't better accounted for by another mental disorder, such as social phobia, specific phobia, obsessive-compulsive disorder, posttraumatic stress disorder, or separation anxiety disorder.

TREATMENT

The goal of treatment is to eliminate all of the symptoms of panic disorder. Treatment is individual and may include:

- cognitive behavioral therapy to identify and change negative thoughts and behaviors
- supportive psychotherapy

• behavioral therapy, which works best when agoraphobia accompanies panic disorder because the identification of anxiety-inducing situations is easier.

Drugs

• Antidepressants—SSRIs such as paroxetine (Paxil)—act on the brain to help regulate levels of serotonin. Selective serotonin and norepinephrine reuptake inhibitors (SSNRIs) such as duloxetine (Cymbalta), and tricyclic antidepressants such as clomipramine (Anafranil) help regulate norepinephrine and serotonin.

⊠ PREVENTION

When the patient is taking antidepressants, closely monitor him for suicidal thoughts, especially during the first 4 weeks of starting therapy.

• Anxiolytics, such lorazepam (Ativan), a benzodiazepine, may be prescribed to treat anxiety in the short term. However, the patient must be carefully monitored because the potential for addiction is high. For this reason, they should not be prescribed if the patient has a history of substance abuse.

SPECIAL CONSIDERATIONS

• Stay with the patient until the attack subsides. If left alone, he may become even more anxious.
• Maintain a calm, serene approach. Statements such as "I won't let anything here hurt you," and "I'll stay with you," can assure the patient that you're in control of the immediate situation. Avoid giving him insincere expressions of reassurance.

• The patient's perceptual field may be narrowed, and excessive stimuli may cause him to feel overwhelmed. Dim bright lights or raise dim lights as needed.
• If the patient loses control, move him to a smaller, quieter space.
• The patient may be so overwhelmed that he can't follow lengthy or complicated instructions. Speak in short, simple sentences, and slowly give one direction at a time. Avoid giving lengthy explanations and asking too many questions.
• Allow the patient to pace around the room (provided he isn't belligerent) to help expend energy. Show him how to take slow, deep breaths if he's hyperventilating.
• Avoid touching the patient until you've established a rapport. Unless he trusts you, he may be too stimulated or frightened to find touch reassuring.
• Administer drugs as prescribed.
• During and after a panic attack, encourage the patient to express his feelings. Discuss his fears, and help him identify situations or events that trigger the attacks.
• Teach the patient relaxation techniques, and explain how he can use them to relieve stress or avoid a panic attack.
• Review with the patient any adverse effects of the drugs he'll be taking. Caution him to notify the practitioner before discontinuing any drug because abrupt withdrawal could cause severe symptoms.

- Encourage the patient and his family to use community resources such as the Anxiety Disorders Association of America.

Paraphilias

Characterized by a dependence on unusual behaviors or fantasies to achieve sexual excitement, paraphilias are complex psychosexual disorders. Some paraphilias are considered sex offenses or crimes because they violate social mores, norms, and laws. However, sexual fantasies are common, and sexual behavior between consenting adults that isn't physically or psychologically harmful isn't considered a paraphilia.

CAUSES AND INCIDENCE

The cause of paraphilia is unknown, but multiple contributing factors have been identified. These include changes in the neurobiology and anatomy of the brain, abnormal hormonal levels, neurologic disorders, chromosomal abnormalities, poor socialization, and environment. For example, many people with these disorders come from dysfunctional families and have childhoods characterized by isolation and sexual, emotional, or physical abuse. Many individuals have poor social skills, and others suffer from personality or psychoactive substance use disorders.

SIGNS AND SYMPTOMS

The patient's history will reveal the particular pattern of abnormal sexual behaviors associated with one of the eight recognized paraphilias.

COMPLICATIONS

- Impaired work and school function
- Impaired family and social function
- Legal problems and incarceration
- Substance and alcohol abuse
- Death from dangerous behavior such as autoasphyxiation

DIAGNOSTIC CRITERIA

A paraphiliac has ongoing, intense, sexually arousing fantasies, urges, or behaviors involving various aberrant sexual expressions that cause clinically significant distress or impairment in social, occupational, or other important areas of functioning. The *Diagnostic and Statistical Manual of Mental Disorders,* Fourth Edition, Text Revision (*DSM-IV-TR*), recognizes eight paraphilias. The standard diagnostic criteria for paraphilias include not only specific criteria for each paraphilia but also general features. (See *Diagnosing paraphilias.*)

Sex offenders who have committed crimes may be required to undergo various diagnostic tests such as:

- sex hormone profiles
- sexual history and questionnaires
- physiological sexual preference testing.

TREATMENT

Paraphilias require mandatory treatment when the patient's sexual

DIAGNOSING PARAPHILIAS

The most commonly diagnosed paraphilias are exhibitionism, fetishism, frotteurism, pedophilia, sexual masochism, sexual sadism, transvestic fetishism, and voyeurism. Criteria for diagnosis are in the *Diagnostic and Statistical Manual of Mental Disorders,* Fourth Edition, Text Revision.

Exhibitionism
The person with this paraphilia obtains sexual gratification from publicly exposing his genitalia to others—principally female passersby. The problem occurs mostly in men (who may achieve erection while exposing themselves and may masturbate to orgasm at the time).

A diagnosed exhibitionist has had at least 6 months of recurrent, intense, sexually arousing fantasies, urges, or behaviors that involve exposing his genitalia to an unsuspecting stranger.

Fetishism
The term *fetish* describes a recurrent and intense sexual arousal from an inanimate object (usually clothing, such as panties or boots) or from nonsexual body parts. The person typically masturbates while holding, rubbing, or smelling the fetish object—or asks a sexual partner to wear the object during a sexual encounter. Fetishism is usually chronic and occurs primarily in men.

A diagnosed fetishist has had at least 6 months of recurrent, intense, sexually arousing fantasies, urges, or behaviors evoked by inanimate objects. The fetish objects aren't restricted to clothing used in cross-dressing or devices designed for tactile genital stimulation.

Frotteurism
The frotteur achieves sexual arousal by touching or rubbing a nonconsenting person. A male frotteur may rub his genitals against a woman's thigh or fondle her breasts. The behavior may occur in crowded places (for example, buses), where it's easier to avoid detection. It's most common between ages 15 and 25.

A diagnosed frotteur has had at least 6 months of recurrent, intense, sexually arousing fantasies, urges, or behaviors involving touching and rubbing against a nonconsenting person.

Pedophilia
The pedophile (almost always a man) is aroused by, and seeks sexual gratification from, children. This urge forms his preferred or exclusive sexual activity. Prepubescent children are common targets, and attraction to girls is more common than attraction to boys. The pedophile may sexually abuse his own children or those of a friend or relative. Rarely, he may abduct a child. Some pedophiles are also attracted to adults.

A diagnosed pedophile has had at least 6 months of recurrent, intense, sexually arousing fantasies, urges, or behaviors involving a prepubescent child or children (usually age 13 or younger). The pedophile is at least age 16 and at least 5 years older than the desired child. (This excludes a person in late adolescence engaged in an ongoing sexual relationship with a child of age 12 or 13.)

(*continued*)

DIAGNOSING PARAPHILIAS *(continued)*

Sexual masochism

A sexual masochist achieves sexual gratification by submitting to physical or psychological pain, such as being beaten, tortured, or humiliated.

Infantilism, a form of sexual masochism, is a desire to be treated as a helpless infant, including wearing diapers.

A dangerous form of this paraphilia, *sexual hypoxyphilia,* relies on oxygen deprivation to induce sexual arousal. The person uses a noose, mask, plastic bag, or chemical to temporarily reduce cerebral oxygenation. Equipment malfunction or other mistakes can cause accidental death.

A diagnosed sexual masochist has had at least 6 months of recurrent, intense, sexually arousing fantasies, urges, or behaviors involving the act (real, not simulated) of being beaten, humiliated, or otherwise made to suffer.

Sexual sadism

The converse of a sexual masochist, a sadist has recurrent, intense, sexual urges and fantasies that involve inflicting physical or psychological suffering. The sadist derives sexual gratification from this behavior.

A diagnosed sexual sadist has had at least 6 months of recurrent, intense, sexually arousing fantasies, urges, or behaviors involving acts (real, not simulated) that cause another person pain and suffering and that evoke sexual excitement in the sadist.

Transvestic fetishism

The transvestite is a heterosexual man who obtains sexual pleasure from cross-dressing (dressing in women's clothing). He may select a single article of apparel, such as a garter or bra, or he may dress entirely as a woman. This behavior is usually accompanied by masturbation and mental images of other men being attracted to him as a woman.

A diagnosed transvestic fetishist is a heterosexual male who has had at least 6 months of recurrent, intense, sexually arousing fantasies, urges, or behaviors involving cross-dressing.

Voyeurism

The voyeur derives sexual pleasure from looking at sexual objects or situations such as an unsuspecting couple engaged in sexual intercourse. Onset of this disorder, which tends to be chronic, occurs before age 15.

A diagnosed voyeur is a heterosexual male who has had at least 6 months of recurrent, intense, sexually arousing fantasies, urges, or behaviors involving the act of observing an unsuspecting person who's naked, disrobing, or engaging in sexual activity.

---

preferences result in socially unacceptable, harmful, or criminal behavior. Depending on the paraphilia, treatment may include:

- individual psychotherapy
- group therapy

- cognitive behavioral therapy and restructuring (to change deviant sexual interests and behavior and break down the individual's justification for sexual victimization)

• pharmacologic therapy to suppress deviant sexual urges and behavior and prevent further victimization.

Drugs

• Luteinizing hormone-releasing hormone (LHRH) agonists, such as goserelin (Zoladex) and leuprolide (Lupron), reduce plasma testosterone.
• Medroxyprogesterone acetate (Cycrin) is a progestin that also may be given to reduce plasma testosterone.
• SSRIs, such as fluoxetine (Prozac) and sertraline (Zoloft), increase serotonin levels in the brain and are given to decrease sexual interest and to cause erectile dysfunction. This chemical castration may be required as a condition of a criminal sentence.

SPECIAL CONSIDERATIONS

• Use a nonjudgmental approach when dealing with the patient.
• Realize that treating such a patient with empathy doesn't threaten your own sexuality.
• Encourage the patient to express his emotions in an appropriate manner.
• As needed, refer the patient to a practitioner, nurse, psychologist, social worker, or counselor trained in sex therapy.
• As a helpful guideline, inform the patient that a therapist's certification by the American Association of Sex Educators, Counselors, and Therapists or by the Society for Sex Therapy and Research usually ensures quality treatment.

Personality disorders

Defined as individual traits that reflect chronic, inflexible, and maladaptive patterns of behavior, personality disorders cause social discomfort and impair social and occupational functioning. The *DSM-IV-TR* groups personality disorders into three clusters:
• Cluster A—paranoid, schizoid, and schizotypal personality disorders. These disorders share odd or eccentric behavior.
• Cluster B—antisocial, borderline, histrionic, and narcissistic personality disorders. Dramatic, emotional, or erratic behavior highlights these disorders.
• Cluster C—avoidant, dependent, and obsessive-compulsive personality disorders. These disorders are marked by anxious or fearful behavior.

Personality disorders are lifelong conditions with an onset in adolescence or early adulthood. Cluster A and B disorders tend to grow less intense in middle age and late life, whereas cluster C disorders tend to become exaggerated. Patients with cluster B disorders are susceptible to substance abuse, poor impulse control, and suicidal behavior, which may shorten lives.

Personality disorders overlap with other psychiatric disorders, such as substance abuse disorders, mood disorders, and anxiety disorders.

CAUSES AND INCIDENCE

Various theories attempt to explain the origin of personality disorders. Genetic factors influence the biological basis of brain function as well as basic personality structure. In turn, personality structure affects how a person responds to life experiences and interacts with the social environment. Over time, each person develops distinctive ways of perceiving the world and of feeling, thinking, and behaving.

Some researchers suspect that poor regulation of the areas controlling emotion within the brain increases the risk of a personality disorder, especially when combined with such factors as abuse, neglect, separation, and childhood trauma. For a biologically predisposed person, the major developmental challenges of adolescence and early adulthood may trigger a personality disorder.

Social theories hold that disorders reflect learned responses, having much to do with reinforcement, modeling, and aversive stimuli as contributing factors. According to psychodynamic theories, personality disorders reflect deficiencies in ego and superego development and are related to poor mother-child relationships characterized by unresponsiveness, overprotectiveness, or early separation.

Personality disorders are common and affect 10% to 15% of the population in the United States. Individuals who have a family member with schizophrenia or personality disorder have an increased risk of developing personality disorders.

Gender also factors into the type of personality disorder present. For example, antisocial and obsessive-compulsive personality disorders are more common in men, whereas borderline, dependent, and histrionic personality disorders are more prevalent in women.

SIGNS AND SYMPTOMS

Each specific personality disorder produces characteristic signs and symptoms, which may vary among patients and within the same patient at different times. In general, the history of the patient with a personality disorder will reveal:
- long-standing difficulties in interpersonal relationships, ranging from dependency to withdrawal
- problems in occupational functioning, ranging from compulsive perfectionism to intentional sabotage
- symptoms that generally become apparent in early adulthood
- lack of insight about his personality.

The patient with a personality disorder may show any degree of self-confidence, ranging from no self-esteem to arrogance. Convinced that his behavior is normal, he avoids responsibility for its consequences, commonly resorting to projections and blame.

COMPLICATIONS
- Occupational or school problems
- Schizophrenia

- Anxiety, phobic, or panic disorders
- Major depression
- Additional personality disorders
- Suicide

DIAGNOSTIC CRITERIA

Diagnosis is made by clinical interview. Individuals must not meet the criteria for schizophrenia. For characteristic findings in patients with this condition, see *Diagnosing personality disorders,* page 124.

TREATMENT

Personality disorders are difficult to treat. Successful therapy requires a trusting relationship in which the therapist can use a direct approach. The type of therapy chosen depends on the patient's symptoms and may include:

- psychotherapy
- behavioral therapy to learn interpersonal skills and behavior
- cognitive behavioral therapy to identify and change maladaptive thoughts and behaviors
- family therapy
- group therapy
- dialectical behavioral therapy to help the individual develop strategies to deal with life's problems.

Hospital inpatient milieu therapy can be effective in crisis situations and, possibly, for long-term treatment of some disorders. Inpatient treatment is controversial, however, because most patients with personality disorders don't comply with extended therapeutic regimens; for such patients, outpatient therapy may be more helpful.

Drugs

- Antipsychotics, such as olanzapine (Zyprexa) and risperidone (Risperdal), are given to help diminish distorted or delusional thinking and to treat agitation.

⚠ ALERT

Monitor the patient taking atypical antipsychotics for the development of neuroleptic malignant syndrome (hyperthermia, autonomic disturbances, and extrapyramidal symptoms), which may be fatal.

⚠ ALERT

More than 50% of patients taking atypical antipsychotics will have significant weight gain and should be monitored for the development of metabolic syndrome and type 2 diabetes.

- SSRIs, such as fluoxetine, may be used to treat irritability, anger, and obsessional thinking.

⊠ PREVENTION

When the patient is taking antidepressants, closely monitor him for suicidal thoughts, especially during the first 4 weeks of starting therapy.

- Anxiolytics may be used to treat severe anxiety that interferes with normal thinking.

SPECIAL CONSIDERATIONS

- Provide consistent care. Take a direct, consistent approach to ensure trust. Keep in mind that many of these patients don't respond well to interviews, whereas others are charming and convincing.
- Teach the patient social skills, and reinforce appropriate behavior.

(*Text continues on page 128*)

DIAGNOSING PERSONALITY DISORDERS

The diagnosis of a recognized personality disorder is made when a patient's symptoms match the diagnostic criteria put forth in the *Diagnostic and Statistical Manual of Mental Disorders,* Fourth Edition, Text Revision.

Antisocial personality disorder

■ This disorder manifests as a pervasive disregard for and violation of the rights of others occurring since age 15, as indicated by at least three of the following:

– The person fails to conform to social norms with respect to lawful behavior, as demonstrated by repeatedly performing acts that are grounds for arrest.

– The person exhibits deceitfulness, as indicated by repeated lying, using aliases, or conning others for personal profit or pleasure.

– The person demonstrates impulsivity or failure to plan ahead.

– The person is irritable and aggressive, as indicated by repeated physical fights or assaults.

– The person has reckless disregard for the safety of self or others.

– The person shows consistent irresponsibility, as indicated by repeated failure to sustain consistent work behavior or honor financial obligations.

– The person lacks remorse, as indicated by being indifferent to or rationalizing having hurt, mistreated, or stolen from others.

■ The person is at least age 18.

■ The person's history includes evidence of a conduct disorder with an onset before age 15.

■ The antisocial behavior doesn't occur exclusively during the course of schizophrenia or a manic episode.

Avoidant personality disorder

This pervasive pattern of social inhibition, feelings of inadequacy, and hypersensitivity to negative evaluation, beginning by early adulthood and present in a variety of contexts, is indicated by at least four of the following:

■ The person avoids social or occupational activities that involve significant interpersonal contact because of fears of criticism, disapproval, or rejection.

■ The person is unwilling to get involved with people unless he's certain that they will like him.

■ The person shows restraint within intimate relationships because of the fear of being shamed or ridiculed.

■ The person is preoccupied with being criticized or rejected in social situations.

■ The person's feelings of inadequacy inhibit him in new interpersonal situations.

■ The person views himself as socially inept, personally unappealing, or inferior to others.

■ The person is unusually reluctant to take personal risks or to engage in any new activities because they may prove embarrassing.

Borderline personality disorder

This pervasive pattern of instability of interpersonal relationships, self-image and affect, and marked impulsivity, beginning by early adulthood and present in various contexts, is indicated by at least five of the following features:

■ The person makes frantic efforts to avoid real or imagined abandon-

DIAGNOSING PERSONALITY DISORDERS (*continued*)

ment (excluding suicidal or self-mutilating behavior).

■ The person has a pattern of unstable and intense interpersonal relationships characterized by alternating extremes of overidealization and devaluation.

■ The person has an identity disturbance characterized by a markedly and persistently unstable self-image or sense of self.

■ The person shows impulsiveness in at least two areas that are potentially self-damaging, such as spending, sexual activity, substance abuse, shoplifting, reckless driving, and binge eating (excluding suicidal or self-mutilating behavior).

■ The person engages in recurrent suicidal threats, gestures, or behavior or in self-mutilating behavior.

■ The person has affective instability resulting from marked mood reactivity (for example, depression, irritability, or anxiety, lasting usually a few hours and seldom more than a few days).

■ The person has chronic feelings of emptiness or boredom.

■ The person has inappropriate intense anger or difficulty controlling anger.

■ The person has transient, stress-related paranoid ideation or severe dissociative symptoms.

Dependent personality disorder

This pervasive and excessive need to be taken care of that leads to submissive and clinging behavior and fears of separation, beginning by early adulthood and present in several contexts, is indicated by at least five of the following:

■ The person has difficulty making everyday decisions without an excessive amount of advice or reassurance from others.

■ The person needs others to assume responsibility for most major areas of his life.

■ The person has difficulty expressing disagreement with others because of fear of loss of support or approval (excluding realistic fears of retribution).

■ The person has difficulty initiating projects or doing things on his own (because of a lack of self-confidence in his judgment or abilities rather than a lack of motivation or energy).

■ The person goes to excessive lengths to obtain nurture and support from others, to the point of volunteering to do things that are unpleasant.

■ The person feels uncomfortable or helpless when alone because of exaggerated fears of inability to care for himself.

■ The person urgently seeks another relationship as a source of care and support when a close relationship ends.

■ The person is unrealistically preoccupied with fears of being left to take care of himself.

Histrionic personality disorder

This pervasive pattern of excessive emotionality and attention-seeking behavior, beginning by early adulthood and present in various contexts, is indicated by at least five of the following:

■ The person is uncomfortable in situations in which he isn't the center of attention.

(*continued*)

DIAGNOSING PERSONALITY DISORDERS (*continued*)

- The person's interaction with others is commonly characterized by inappropriately sexually seductive or provocative behavior.
- The person displays rapidly shifting and shallow expression of emotions.
- The person consistently uses physical appearance to draw attention to self.
- The person has a style of speech that is excessively impressionistic and lacking in detail.
- The person shows theatricality, self-dramatization, and exaggerated emotional expression.
- The person is suggestible (easily influenced by others or circumstances).
- The person considers relationships to be more intimate than they actually are.

Narcissistic personality disorder

This pervasive pattern of grandiosity, need for admiration, and lack of empathy, beginning by early adulthood and present in various contexts, is indicated by at least five of the following:

- The person has a grandiose sense of self-importance.
- The person is preoccupied with fantasies of unlimited success, power, brilliance, beauty, or ideal love.
- The person believes that he's special and unique and can only be understood by, or should associate with, other special or high-status people (or institutions).
- The person requires excessive admiration.
- The person has a sense of entitlement (an unreasonable expectation of especially favorable treatment or automatic compliance with his expectations).
- The person is interpersonally exploitive, taking advantage of others to achieve his own ends.
- The person lacks empathy.
- The person is typically envious of others or believes that others are envious of him.
- The person shows arrogant, haughty behaviors or attitudes.

Obsessive-compulsive personality disorder

This pervasive pattern of preoccupation with orderliness, perfectionism, and mental and interpersonal control at the expense of flexibility, openness, and efficiency, beginning by early adulthood and present in various contexts, is indicated by at least four of the following:

- The person is preoccupied with details, rules, lists, order, organization, or schedules to the extent that the core point of the activity is lost.
- The person shows perfectionism that interferes with task completion.
- The person is excessively devoted to work and productivity to the exclusion of leisure activities and friendships (not accounted for by obvious economic need).
- The person exhibits overconscientiousness, scrupulousness, and inflexibility about matters of morality, ethics, or values (not accounted for by cultural or religious identification).
- The person can't discard worn-out or worthless objects even when they have no sentimental value.
- The person is reluctant to delegate tasks or to work with others unless they submit exactly to his way of doing things.

DIAGNOSING PERSONALITY DISORDERS (*continued*)

■ The person adopts a miserly spending style toward self and others; money is viewed as something to be hoarded in preparation for future catastrophes.
■ The person shows rigidity and stubbornness.

Paranoid personality disorder
■ The person must exhibit a pervasive and unwarranted tendency, beginning by early adulthood and present in various contexts, to interpret the actions of people as deliberately demeaning or threatening, as indicated by at least four of the following:
– The person suspects, without sufficient basis, that he's being exploited, deceived, or harmed by others.
– The person questions without justification the loyalty or trustworthiness of friends or associates.
– The person is reluctant to confide in others because of unwarranted fear that the information will be used against him.
– The person finds hostile or evil meanings in benign remarks.
– The person bears grudges or is unforgiving of insults or slights.
– The person is easily slighted and quick to react with anger or to counterattack.
– The person questions without justification the fidelity of a spouse or sexual partner.
■ The symptoms don't occur exclusively during the course of schizophrenia or other psychotic disorders and aren't the direct physiologic effect of a general medical condition.

Schizoid personality disorder
■ The patient must exhibit a pervasive pattern of indifference to social

relationships and a restricted range of emotional experience and expression, beginning by early adulthood and present in various contexts, as indicated by at least four of the following:
– The person neither desires nor enjoys close relationships, including being part of a family.
– The person almost always chooses solitary activities.
– The person seldom, if ever, claims or appears to experience strong emotions, such as anger and joy.
– The person indicates little, if any, desire to have sexual experiences with another person.
– The person is indifferent to the praise and criticism of others.
– The person has no close friends or confidants other than immediate relatives.
– The person displays flat affect.
■ The symptoms don't occur exclusively during the course of schizophrenia, another psychotic disorder, or a pervasive developmental disorder and aren't the direct physiologic effect of a general medical condition.

Schizotypal personality disorder
■ This pervasive pattern of social and interpersonal deficits is marked by acute discomfort with, and reduced capacity for, close relationships as well as by cognitive or perceptual distortions and eccentricities of behavior, beginning by early adulthood and present in various contexts. The person with schizotypal personality disorder has at least five of the following:
– ideas of reference (excluding delusions of reference)

(*continued*)

DIAGNOSING PERSONALITY DISORDERS (*continued*)

– odd beliefs or magical thinking, influencing behavior and inconsistent with subcultural norms
– unusual perceptual experiences, including bodily illusions
– odd thinking and speech
– suspiciousness or paranoid thinking
– inappropriate or flat affect
– odd behavior or appearance
– no close friends or confidants other than first-degree relatives

– excessive social anxiety that doesn't diminish with familiarity and tends to be associated with paranoid fears rather than negative self-judgment.
■ The symptoms don't occur exclusively during the course of schizophrenia, a mood disorder with psychotic features, another psychotic disorder, or a pervasive developmental disorder.

● Encourage expression of feelings, self-analysis of behavior, and accountability for actions.
● Set appropriate boundaries with the patient who may push limits and blame others for his feelings and behaviors.

Specific care measures vary with the particular personality disorder.

For antisocial personality disorder:
● Be clear about your expectations and the consequences of failing to meet them.
● Use a straightforward, matter-of-fact approach to set limits on unacceptable behavior. Encourage and reinforce positive behavior.
● Expect the patient to refuse to cooperate so that he can gain control.
● Avoid power struggles and confrontations to maintain the opportunity for therapeutic communication.
● Avoid defensiveness and arguing.
● Observe for physical and verbal signs of agitation.
● Help the patient manage anger.

● Teach the patient social skills, and reinforce appropriate behavior.

For avoidant personality disorder:
● Assess for signs of depression. Impaired social interaction increases the risk of affective disorders.
● Establish a trusting relationship with the patient. Be aware that he may become dependent on the few staff members whom he believes he can trust.
● Make sure that the patient has plenty of time to prepare for all upcoming procedures because he has difficulty with changes in routine.
● Inform the patient when you will and won't be available if he needs assistance.

For borderline personality disorder:
● Deliberate self-harm is different from a suicide attempt. Self-harm involves such activities as cutting oneself, burning oneself, hitting one's head or other body part, or inserting objects into the body with

the intent of causing pain. Self-harm is often used as a way to modulate affect or to control uncomfortable feelings. Although some patients die from serious self-harm, the patient's intent isn't to die, but rather to decrease emotional pain. Self-harm behavior is often seen in patients with borderline personality disorder.

• Encourage the patient to take responsibility for himself. Don't attempt to rescue him from the consequences of his actions (except for suicidal and self-mutilating behaviors).

• Help the patient develop problem-solving strategies.

• Maintain a consistent approach in all interactions with the patient, and ensure that other staff members do so as well.

• Recognize behaviors that the patient uses to manipulate people so that you can avoid unconsciously reinforcing them.

• Set appropriate expectations for social interactions, and praise the patient when expectations are met.

• To promote trust, respect the patient's personal space.

• Recognize that the patient may idolize some staff members and devalue others.

• Don't take sides in the patient's disputes with other staff members.

For dependent personality disorder:

• Encourage the patient to make decisions. Continue to provide support and reassurance as his decision-making ability improves.

• Give the patient as much opportunity to control treatment as possible. Offer options and allow choices, even if all are chosen.

• Encourage activities that require decision-making to promote autonomy.

For histrionic personality disorder:

• Give the patient choices in care strategies, and incorporate his wishes into the plan of treatment as much as possible. By increasing his sense of self-control, his anxiety will decrease.

• Be aware that the patient will want to "win over" caregivers and, at least initially, will be responsive and cooperative.

For narcissistic personality disorder:

• Convey respect and acknowledge the patient's sense of self-importance so that a coherent sense of self can be reestablished. Don't reinforce either pathologic grandiosity or weakness.

• If the patient makes unreasonable demands or has unreasonable expectations, tell him in a matter-of-fact way that he's being unreasonable. Remain nonjudgmental because a critical attitude may make the patient more demanding and difficult. Don't avoid him because this could increase maladaptive attention-seeking behavior.

• Focus on positive traits, or on feelings of pain, loss, or rejection.

For obsessive-compulsive personality disorder:

- Allow the patient to participate in his own treatment plan by offering choices whenever possible.

- Adopt a professional approach in your interactions with the patient. Avoid informality because this type of patient expects strict attention to detail.

For paranoid personality disorder:

- Avoid situations that threaten the patient's autonomy or challenge his beliefs.

- Approach the patient in a straightforward and candid manner, adopting a professional, rather than a casual or friendly, attitude. Remember that the paranoid patient easily misinterprets remarks intended to be humorous.

- Encourage the patient to take part in social interactions to expose him to others' perceptions and realities and to promote social skills development.

- Help the patient identify negative behaviors that interfere with his relationships so that he can see how his behavior affects others.

- Provide a supportive and nonjudgmental environment in which the patient can safely explore and verbalize his feelings.

For schizoid personality disorder:

- Remember that the patient with schizoid personality disorder needs close human contact but is easily overwhelmed. Respect the patient's need for privacy, and slowly build a trusting, therapeutic relationship, so that he finds more pleasure than fear in relating to you.

- Give the patient plenty of time to express his feelings. Keep in mind that if you push him to do so before he's ready, he may retreat.

- Recognize the patient's need for physical and emotional distance.

For schizotypal personality disorder:

- Recognize that the patient with this disorder is easily overwhelmed by stress. Allow him plenty of time to make difficult decisions.

- Avoid defensiveness and arguing.

- Recognize the patient's need for physical and emotional distance.

- Be aware that the patient may relate unusually well to certain staff members and not at all to others.

Phobias

Phobias are persistent and irrational fears of a specific object, activity, or situation that results in a compelling desire to avoid the perceived hazard. The patient recognizes that his fear is out of proportion to any actual danger, but he can't control it or explain it away. Three types of phobias exist: agoraphobia, the fear of being alone or of open space; social, the fear of embarrassing oneself in public; and specific, the fear of a single, specific object, such as animals or heights.

Agoraphobia and social phobia tend to be chronic, but new treatments are improving the prognosis. A social phobia typically begins in late childhood or early adolescence; a specific phobia may begin in childhood, but may resolve as the child matures.

CAUSES AND INCIDENCE

A phobia develops when anxiety about an object or a situation compels the patient to avoid it. The precise cause of most phobias is unknown, but research into the neurobiology of the brain and genetic and environmental factors have been implicated. Psychoanalytic theory holds that the phobia is actually repression and displacement of an internal conflict. Behavior theorists view phobia as a stimulus-response reflex, avoiding a situation or object that causes anxiety. Twin studies indicate that there may be a genetic component to developing phobias. Children can also learn phobias from their parents.

Brain imaging research shows that when a fear response is stimulated, there is increased activity in the amygdala and hippocampus areas of the brain. The amygdala processes sensory signals and alerts the rest of the brain to threats. It also stores emotional memories and may be involved in the development of distinct phobias. The hippocampus is involved in coding traumatic events into memories. Research shows that the hippocampus becomes smaller in size in people who have suffered child abuse and in individuals who have served in the military. Research continues into identifying why and how the hippocampus changes.

About 19 million adults in the United States suffer from a phobic disorder. In fact, phobias are the most common psychiatric disorders in women and the second most common in men. Twice as many women as men are affected by phobias. More men than women experience social phobias, whereas agoraphobia and specific phobias are more common in women.

SIGNS AND SYMPTOMS

The phobic patient typically reports signs of severe anxiety when confronted with the feared object or situation. A patient with a phobia may complain of:
- dizziness
- feeling of unreality (depersonalization)
- shortness of breath
- heart pounding
- tachycardia
- profuse sweating
- dizziness
- GI distress.

Generally, the patient realizes that his fear and anxiety are out of proportion to the situation. His self-esteem may suffer, and he may have feelings of weakness, cowardice, or ineffectiveness.

COMPLICATIONS
- Impaired social, school, or work functioning
- Development of other anxiety disorders
- Depression
- Eating disorders
- Alcohol or substance abuse

DIAGNOSING PHOBIAS

Phobias are classified as agoraphobia, social phobias, and specific phobias. The diagnosis of all three is based on criteria put forth in the *Diagnostic and Statistical Manual of Mental Disorders,* Fourth Edition, Text Revision.

Agoraphobia

Fear of being in places or situations from which escape might be difficult or embarrassing or in which help might be unavailable if an unexpected or situationally predisposed panic attack or paniclike symptom occurs. Agoraphobic fears typically involve characteristic clusters of situations that include being outside the home alone, being in a crowd or standing in a line, being on a bridge, and traveling in a bus, train, or automobile.

■ The situations are avoided or endured with marked distress or with anxiety about having a panic attack or paniclike symptoms, or the person requires the presence of a companion.

■ The anxiety or phobic avoidance isn't better accounted for by mental disorder, such as social phobia, specific phobia, obsessive-compulsive disorder, posttraumatic stress disorder, or separation anxiety disorder.

Social phobia

A persistent fear of one or more social or performance situations in which the person is exposed to unfamiliar people or possible scrutiny by others. The person fears that he may act in a way that will be humiliating or embarrassing.

■ Exposure to the feared social situation almost invariably provokes anxiety, which may take the form of a situationally bound or situationally predisposed panic attack.

■ The person recognizes that the fear is excessive or unreasonable.

■ The feared social or performance situations are avoided or endured with intense anxiety or distress.

■ The avoidance, anxious anticipation, or distress in the feared social or performance situation interferes with the person's normal routine, occupational functioning, or social activities or relationships. There may be marked distress about having the phobia.

■ In individuals younger than age 18, the duration is at least 6 months.

■ The fear or avoidance isn't due to the direct physiologic effects of a substance or a general medical condition and isn't better accounted for by another mental disorder.

■ If the person has a general medical condition or another mental disorder, the person's social fear is unrelated to the medical or mental condition.

Specific phobia

Marked and persistent fear that's excessive or unreasonable and cued

DIAGNOSTIC CRITERIA

For characteristic findings in this condition, see *Diagnosing phobias.*

TREATMENT

The effectiveness of treatment depends on the severity of the patient's phobia. Because phobic behavior may never be completely cured, the

by the presence or anticipation of a specific object or situation.
- Exposure to the phobic stimulus almost invariably provokes an immediate anxiety response, which may take the form of a situationally bound or situationally predisposed panic attack.
- The person recognizes that the fear is excessive or unreasonable.
- The person avoids the situation or endures it with intense anxiety or distress.
- The avoidance, anxious anticipation, or distress in the feared situation significantly interferes with the person's normal routine, occupational functioning, or social activities or relationships. There may be marked distress about having the phobia.
- In individuals younger than age 18, the duration is at least 6 months.
- The anxiety, panic attacks, or phobic avoidance associated with the specific object or situation isn't better accounted for by another mental disorder, such as posttraumatic stress disorder, obsessive-compulsive disorder, separation anxiety disorder, social phobia, panic disorder with agoraphobia, or agoraphobia without a history of panic disorder.

goal of treatment is to help the patient function effectively. Several types of therapy have been shown to be effective.

- Behavioral therapy exposes and desensitizes the patient to the phobic trigger, lessening his anxious response.
- Cognitive behavioral therapy helps the patient identify and change his maladaptive thoughts and behavior.

Drugs
- Anxiolytics such as alprazolam (Xanax), a benzodiazepine, may be prescribed to treat anxiety in the short term. However, the patient must be carefully monitored because the potential for addiction is high. For this reason, the drug shouldn't be prescribed if the patient has a history of substance abuse.
- Antidepressants such as SSRIs act on the brain to help balance levels of serotonin. Tricyclic antidepressants and MAOIs help to balance serotonin and norepinephrine. Other medications may act to balance a combination of dopamine, norephinephrine, serotonin, and other chemicals.

▷ PREVENTION
When the patient is taking antidepressants, closely monitor him for suicidal thoughts, especially during the first 4 weeks of starting therapy.

⚠ ALERT
The patient taking MAOIs must avoid foods and beverages that contain tyramine, which is found in aged cheeses, smoked meats, and wine, because they may trigger a hypertensive crisis.

- Beta-adrenergic blockers such propranolol (Inderal) effectively diminish the stimulating effects of epinephrine and help alleviate such symptoms as tachycardia, sweating, and increased blood pressure for patients with performance anxiety and phobias.

SPECIAL CONSIDERATIONS

• Provide for the patient's safety and comfort, and monitor fluid and food intake, as needed. Certain phobias may inhibit food or fluid intake, disturb hygiene, and disrupt the patient's ability to rest.

• No matter how illogical the patient's phobia seems, avoid the urge to trivialize his fears. Remember that this behavior represents an essential coping mechanism.

• Ask the patient how he normally copes with the fear. When he's able to face the fear, encourage him to verbalize and explore his personal strengths and resources with you.

• Don't let the patient withdraw completely. If an agoraphobic patient is being treated as an outpatient, suggest small steps to overcome his fears such as planning a brief shopping trip with a supportive family member or friend.

• In social phobias, the patient fears criticism. Encourage him to interact with others, and provide continuous support and positive reinforcement.

• Support participation in psychotherapy, including desensitization therapy. However, don't force insight. Challenging the patient may aggravate his anxiety or lead to panic attacks.

• Teach the patient specific relaxation techniques, such as listening to music and meditating.

• Suggest ways to channel the patient's energy and relieve stress (such as running and creative activities).

• Teach the patient deep breathing and other relaxation techniques.

• In some cities, phobia clinics and group therapy are available. People who have recovered from phobias can usually help other phobic patients.

Posttraumatic stress disorder

Characteristic psychological consequences that persist for at least 1 month after a traumatic event outside the range of usual human experience are classified as posttraumatic stress disorder (PTSD). This disorder can follow almost any distressing event, including a natural or manmade disaster, physical or sexual abuse, an assault, a rape, or combat. It may even occur in rescuers. Psychological trauma, which accompanies the physical trauma, is characterized by intense fear, feelings of helplessness and guilt, and loss of control. PTSD can be acute, chronic, or delayed. When the precipitating event is of human design, the disorder is more severe and more persistent. Onset can occur at any age, even during childhood.

CAUSES AND INCIDENCE

It's estimated that up to 8% of Americans will suffer from PTSD at some time in their lives and about 5 million people are affected in any given year. PTSD occurs in response to an extremely distressing event, including a serious threat of harm to the patient or his family, such as war, abuse, or violent crime. It may be triggered by sudden destruction of his home or community by a bombing, fire, flood, tornado, earthquake, or similar disaster. It may also follow witnessing the death or serious injury of another person by torture, in a death camp, by natural disaster, or by a motor vehicle or airplane crash. Research continues into neurobiological and anatomic changes that occur in patients with PTSD in order to identify individuals and develop new treatment strategies.

Preexisting psychopathology can predispose some patients to this disorder, but anyone can develop it, especially if the stressor is extreme and long lasting. PTSD is more common among individuals who have a family member with PTSD or who have a history of depression. Higher incidences of PTSD can also be found among inner city citizens who live in violent environments. PTSD can occur at any age, even among children. More women than men appear to be affected. It's estimated that between 15% and 30% of the individuals who served in the military during the Vietnam War have suffered from PTSD. Many cases resolve within 3 months after the traumatic event, but some cases can last for years. Any person who has experienced traumatic relocation due to such events as rioting or other civil strife, extreme natural disasters, or war should be assessed for signs of PTSD.

SIGNS AND SYMPTOMS

The psychosocial history of a patient with PTSD may reveal early life experiences, interpersonal factors, military experiences, or other incidents that suggest the precipitating event. Typically, the patient may report that his symptoms began immediately or soon after the trauma, although they may not develop until months or years later. In such a case, avoidance symptoms usually have been present during the latency period.

Typical signs and symptoms reported include:
- intrusive memories
- memory and concentration problems
- dissociative episodes (flashbacks)
- traumatic re-experiencing of the event
- sleep difficulties, disturbing dreams
- emotional numbing (diminished or constricted response)
- chronic anxiety or panic attacks (with physical signs and symptoms)
- hypervigilance and increased startling
- substance or alcohol abuse.

The patient may report feelings of emotional distress such as:
- painful emotions and unwelcome thoughts
- shame and guilt

- suicidal thoughts
- depression
- phobic avoidance of situations that arouse memories of the traumatic event (such as hot weather and tall grass for the Vietnam veteran).

COMPLICATIONS

- Family and relationship problems
- Occupational or school problems
- Cardiac disease
- Eating disorders
- Depression
- Substance or alcohol abuse

DIAGNOSTIC CRITERIA

For characteristic findings in patients with this condition, see *Diagnosing posttraumatic stress disorder*.

TREATMENT

Treatment of PTSD aims to reduce the target symptoms, prevent chronic disability, and promote occupational and social integration. Specific treatments that may be effective include:

- behavioral techniques, such as relaxation therapy to decrease anxiety and promote sleep or progressive desensitization
- cognitive behavioral therapy to help the patient gain control of his fear and identify and change his negative thoughts and behavior
- group therapy to provide a forum for individuals with similar conflicts to gain support and work through their feelings (Support groups are highly effective and are provided through many Veterans Administra-

tion centers and crisis clinics. Group settings are appropriate for most degrees of symptoms presented. Some group programs include spouses and families in their treatment process.)

- rehabilitation programs in physical, social, and occupational settings.

Many patients need treatment for depression, alcohol or drug abuse, or medical conditions before psychological healing can take place. Treatment of this disorder may be complex, and the prognosis varies.

Drugs

- Antidepressants—SSRIs such as paroxetine (Paxil)—act on the brain to help regulate levels of serotonin. Selective serotonin and norepinephrine reuptake inhibitors (SSNRIs), such as duloxetine (Cymbalta), and tricyclic antidepressants such as clomipramine (Anafranil) help regulate norepinephrine and serotonin. Antidepressants help to relieve anxiety, improve concentration, and improve sleep.

⊠ PREVENTION

When the patient is taking antidepressants, closely monitor him for suicidal thoughts, especially during the first 4 weeks of starting therapy.

- Anxiolytics such alprazolam (Xanax), a benzodiazepine, may be prescribed to treat anxiety in the short term. However, the patient must be carefully monitored because the potential for addiction is high. For this reason, the drug shouldn't be prescribed if the patient has a history of substance abuse.

DIAGNOSING POSTTRAUMATIC STRESS DISORDER

The diagnosis of posttraumatic stress disorder is made when the patient's signs and symptoms meet the following criteria documented in the *Diagnostic and Statistical Manual of Mental Disorders,* Fourth Edition, Text Revision.

■ The person was exposed to a traumatic event in which both of the following occurred:
– The person experienced, witnessed, or was confronted with an event or events that involved actual or threatened death or serious injury or a threat to the physical integrity of self or others.
– The person's response involved intense fear, helplessness, or horror (in children, the response may be expressed by disorganized or agitated behavior).
■ The person persistently reexperiences the traumatic event in at least one of the following ways:
– recurrent and intrusive distressing recollections of the event, including images, thoughts, or perceptions
– recurrent distressing dreams of the event
– acting or feeling as if the traumatic event were recurring (includes a sense of reliving the experience, illusions, hallucinations, and dissociative episodes that occur even when awakening or intoxicated)
– intense psychological distress at exposure to internal or external cues that symbolize or resemble an aspect of the traumatic event.
■ The person persistently avoids stimuli associated with the traumatic event and experiences numbing of general responsiveness (not present before the traumatic event), as indicated by at least three of the following:
– efforts to avoid thoughts or feelings associated with the trauma
– efforts to avoid activities, places, or people that arouse recollections of the trauma
– inability to recall an important aspect of the traumatic event
– markedly diminished interest in significant activities
– feeling of detachment or estrangement from other individuals
– restricted range of affect such as inability to love others
– sense of foreshortened future.
■ The person has persistent symptoms of increased arousal (not present before the trauma), as indicated by at least two of the following:
– difficulty falling or staying asleep
– irritability or outbursts of anger
– difficulty concentrating
– hypervigilance
– exaggerated startle response.
■ The disturbance must be of at least 1 month's duration.
■ The disturbance causes clinically significant distress or impairment in the patient's social, occupational, or other important areas of functioning.

SPECIAL CONSIDERATIONS

● Encourage the patient with PTSD to express his grief, complete the mourning process, and develop coping skills to relieve anxiety and de-
sensitize him to the memories of the traumatic event.

● Keep in mind that such a patient tends to sharply test your commitment and interest. Therefore, first examine your feelings about the event (war or other trauma) so you won't react with disdain and shock. Such reactions hamper the working relationship with the patient and reinforce his typically poor self-image and sense of guilt.

• Know and practice crisis intervention techniques as appropriate in PTSD.

• Establish trust by accepting the patient's current level of functioning and assuming a positive, consistent, honest, and nonjudgmental attitude toward the patient.

• Provide encouragement as the patient shows a commitment to work on his problem.

• Deal constructively with the patient's displays of anger.

• Encourage joint assessment of angry outbursts (identify how anger escalates, and explore preventive measures that family members can take to regain control).

• Provide a safe, staff-monitored room in which the patient can safely deal with urges to commit physical violence or self-abuse through displacement (such as pounding clay or destroying selected items).

• Help the patient to develop strategies to move from physical to verbal expressions of anger.

• Help the patient relieve shame and guilt precipitated by real actions (such as killing or mutilation) that violated a consciously held moral code. Help him put his behavior into perspective, to recognize his isolation and self-destructive behavior as forms of atonement, to learn to forgive himself, and to accept forgiveness from others.

• Refer the patient to a member of the clergy, as desired.

• Provide for group therapy with other victims for peer support and forgiveness, or refer the patient to such a support group.

• Refer the patient to appropriate community resources.

• Refer the patient and family to the Post Traumatic Disorder Alliance and the National Alliance on Mental Illness for additional educational resources and support.

Premature ejaculation

Premature ejaculation refers to a male's inability to control the ejaculatory reflex during intravaginal containment, resulting in persistently early ejaculation. This common sexual disorder affects all age-groups; however, it's more common in younger males and in college-educated males. Studies suggest that 20% of men ages 18 to 59 have premature ejaculation disorder.

CAUSES AND INCIDENCE

Premature ejaculation may result from a combination of psychological and biological factors. Some of the psychological factors include anxiety or guilt regarding sexual intercourse, unrealistic expectations about sexual performance, unresolved conflicts, depression, communication difficulties, unconscious fears about the vagina, and negative cultural conditioning.

However, psychological factors aren't always the cause of premature ejaculation because this disorder can occur in emotionally healthy males with stable, positive relationships. Studies have shown that men with lower levels of serotonin in the brain have a higher incidence of premature ejaculation. Rarely, premature ejaculation may be linked to an underlying degenerative neurologic disorder such as multiple sclerosis, or an inflammatory process, such as posterior urethritis or prostatitis.

SIGNS AND SYMPTOMS

Premature ejaculation may have a devastating psychological impact on some males who may exhibit signs of severe inadequacy and a lack of confidence or self-doubt in addition to general anxiety and guilt. The patient may report that he is:

• unable to prolong foreplay
• able to prolong foreplay but ejaculates as soon as intromission occurs.

In other cases, however, premature ejaculation may have little or no psychological impact. In such cases, the complaint lies solely with the sexual partner, who may believe that the male is indifferent to her sexual needs.

COMPLICATIONS

• Reduced sexual enjoyment
• Relationship problems
• Depression

DIAGNOSTIC CRITERIA

Physical examination and laboratory test results are usually normal

---

DIAGNOSING PREMATURE EJACULATION DISORDER

The diagnosis of premature ejaculation disorder is made when the patient's signs and symptoms meet the following criteria documented in the *Diagnostic and Statistical Manual of Mental Disorders,* Fourth Edition, Text Revision.

■ Ejaculation occurs with minimal sexual stimulation or shortly after penetration. This occurs persistently or recurrently and before the patient desires.

■ Premature ejaculation causes distress or interpersonal problems.

■ Premature ejaculation isn't exclusively caused by the effects of a substance (such as an effect from opioid withdrawal).

---

because most males with this complaint are quite healthy. A detailed sexual history is necessary in order to make a diagnosis. A history of adequate ejaculatory control in the absence of precipitating psychological trauma may suggest an organic cause. See *Diagnosing premature ejaculation disorder.*

TREATMENT

• Individual psychological therapy to explore feelings and expectations about sexuality and relationships
• Behavioral therapy to learn exercises to help increase tolerance to sexual stimulation
• Couples counseling to improve communication and reduce conflict

Drugs

• SSRIs are sometimes prescribed "off label" (not approved by Food and Drug Administration) to increase serotonin levels in the brain, which prolongs the time to ejaculation and may prevent premature ejaculation. Prescribed dosages are lower than those used to treat depression.

SPECIAL CONSIDERATIONS

• Encourage a positive self-image by explaining that premature ejaculation is a common disorder that doesn't reflect on the patient's masculinity.

• Assure the patient that the condition is treatable.

• In an attempt to self-treat premature ejaculation, some men may use distraction techniques that can eventually result in secondary erectile disorder.

• Refer the patient and his partner to the Society for Sex Therapy and Research, the American Association for Marriage and Family Therapy, and the American Association of Sex Educators and Counselors for additional educational and supportive resources.

Schizophrenia

Schizophrenia is characterized by disturbances (for at least 6 months) in thought content and form, perception, affect, sense of self, volition, interpersonal relationships, and psychomotor behavior. (See *Phases of schizophrenia,* page 142.)

The *Diagnostic and Statistical Manual of Mental Disorders,* Fourth Edition, Text Revision (*DSM-IV-TR*), recognizes paranoid, disorganized, catatonic, undifferentiated, and residual schizophrenia. Onset of symptoms usually occurs during adolescence or early adulthood. The disorder produces varying degrees of impairment. Up to one-third of patients with schizophrenia have just one psychotic episode and no more. Some patients have no disability between periods of exacerbation; others need continuous institutional care. The prognosis worsens with each episode.

CAUSES AND INCIDENCE

Schizophrenia affects 1% to 2% of people in the United States and is equally prevalent in both sexes. It's thought to result from a combination of genetic, biological, cultural, and psychological factors. Some evidence supports a genetic predisposition. Close relatives of people with schizophrenia have a greater likelihood of developing schizophrenia; the closer the degree of biological relatedness, the higher the risk.

The most widely accepted biochemical theory holds that schizophrenia results from excessive activity at dopaminergic synapses. Other neurotransmitter alterations such as serotonin increases may also contribute to schizophrenic symptoms. In addition, patients with schizophrenia have structural abnormalities of the frontal and temporolimbic systems. Computed tomography scans and magnetic resonance imaging studies show various structural brain abnormalities, including frontal lobe atrophy and increased lateral and third ventricles. Positron emission tomography scans substantiate frontal lobe hypometabolism.

Numerous psychological and sociocultural causes, such as disturbed family and interpersonal patterns, also have been proposed. Schizophrenia is more common in urban areas and among lower socioeconomic groups, possibly due to downward social drift, lack of upward socioeconomic mobility, and high stress levels that may stem from poverty, social failure, illness, and inadequate social resources. Higher incidence is also linked to low birth weight and congenital deafness.

PHASES OF SCHIZOPHRENIA

Schizophrenia usually occurs in three phases: prodromal, active, and residual.

Prodromal phase
The *Diagnostic and Statistical Manual of Mental Disorders,* Fourth Edition, Text Revision (*DSM-IV-TR*), characterizes the prodromal phase as clear deterioration in functioning before the active phase of the disturbance that isn't due to a disturbance in mood or to a psychoactive substance use disorder and that involves at least two of the following signs and symptoms:
- marked social isolation or withdrawal
- marked impairment in role functioning as wage-earner, student, or homemaker
- markedly peculiar behavior
- marked impairment in personal hygiene and grooming
- blunted or inappropriate affect
- digressive, vague, overelaborate, or circumstantial speech; poverty of speech; or poverty of content of speech
- odd beliefs or magical thinking influencing behavior and inconsistent with cultural norms
- unusual perceptual experiences
- marked lack of initiative, interests, or energy.

Family members or friends may report personality changes. Typically insidious, this phase may extend over several months or years.

Active phase
During the active phase, the patient exhibits frankly psychotic symptoms. Psychiatric evaluation may reveal delusions, hallucinations, loosening of associations, incoherence, and catatonic behavior. The patient's psychosocial history may also disclose a particular stressor before the onset of this phase.

Residual phase
According to the *DSM-IV-TR*, the residual phase follows the active phase and occurs when at least two of the symptoms noted in the prodromal phase persist. These symptoms don't result from a disturbance in mood or from a psychoactive substance use disorder.

The residual phase resembles the prodromal phase, except that disturbances in affect and role functioning usually are more severe. Delusions and hallucinations may persist.

SIGNS AND SYMPTOMS

Schizophrenia is associated with many abnormal behaviors; therefore, signs and symptoms vary widely, depending on the type and phase (prodromal, active, or residual) of the illness.

Watch for these signs and symptoms:

- ambivalence—coexisting strong positive and negative feelings, leading to emotional conflict
- apathy and other affective abnormalities
- clang associations—words that rhyme or sound alike used in an illogical, nonsensical manner—for instance, "It's the rain, train, pain"

- concrete associations—inability to form or understand abstract thoughts
- delusions—false ideas or beliefs accepted as real by the patient; delusions of grandeur, persecution, and reference (distorted belief regarding the relation between events and one's self—for example, a belief that television programs address the patient on a personal level); feelings of being controlled, somatic illness, and depersonalization
- echolalia—automatic and meaningless repetition of another's words or phrases
- echopraxia—involuntary repetition of movements observed in others
- flight of ideas—rapid succession of incomplete and loosely connected ideas
- hallucinations—false sensory perceptions with no basis in reality; usually visual or auditory, but may also be olfactory (smell), gustatory (taste), or tactile (touch)
- loose associations—rapid shifts among unrelated ideas
- magical thinking—belief that thoughts or wishes can control others or events
- neologisms—bizarre words that have meaning only for the patient
- poor interpersonal relationships
- regression—return to an earlier developmental stage
- thought blocking—sudden interruption in the patient's train of thought
- withdrawal—disinterest in objects, people, or surroundings

- word salad—illogical word groupings, such as "She had a star, barn, plant."

COMPLICATIONS

- Inability to maintain employment or attend school
- Financial difficulties and poverty
- Homelessness
- Suicide or self-destructive behavior
- Victim of crime
- Legal problems from committing violent crime
- Health problems secondary to adverse reactions from drug treatment

DIAGNOSTIC CRITERIA

After a complete physical and psychiatric examination rules out an organic cause of symptoms such as an amphetamine-induced psychosis, a diagnosis of schizophrenia may be considered. A diagnosis is made if the patient's symptoms match those in the *DSM-IV-TR*. (See *Diagnosing schizophrenia,* page 144.)

TREATMENT

Treatment focuses on meeting the physical and psychosocial needs of the patient, based on his previous level of adjustment and his response to medical and nursing interventions. Treatment may combine:

- drug therapy
- long-term psychotherapy for the patient and his family
- psychosocial rehabilitation
- vocational counseling.

Clinicians disagree about the effectiveness of psychotherapy in

DIAGNOSING SCHIZOPHRENIA

The following criteria described in the *Diagnostic and Statistical Manual of Mental Disorders,* Fourth Edition, Text Revision, are used to diagnose a person with schizophrenia.

Characteristic symptoms

A person with schizophrenia has two or more of the following symptoms (each present for a significant time during a 1-month period—or less if successfully treated):

- delusions
- hallucinations
- disorganized speech
- grossly disorganized or catatonic behavior
- negative symptoms (affective flattening, alagia, anhedonia, attention impairment, apathy, and avolition).

The diagnosis requires only one of these characteristic symptoms if the person's delusions are bizarre, or if hallucinations consist of a voice issuing a running commentary on the person's behavior or thoughts or two or more voices conversing.

Social and occupational dysfunction

For a significant period since the onset of the disturbance, one or more major areas of functioning (such as work, interpersonal relations, or self-care) are markedly below the level achieved before the onset.

When the disturbance begins in childhood or adolescence, the dysfunction takes the form of failure to achieve the expected level of interpersonal, academic, or occupational development.

Duration

Continuous signs of the disturbance persist for at least 6 months. The 6-month period must include at least 1 month of symptoms (or less if

signs and symptoms have been successfully treated) that match the characteristic symptoms and may include periods of prodromal or residual symptoms.

During the prodromal or residual period, signs of the disturbance may be manifested by only negative symptoms or by two or more characteristic symptoms in a less severe form.

Schizoaffective and mood disorder exclusion

Schizoaffective disorder and mood disorder with psychotic features have been ruled out for these reasons: Either no major depressive, manic, or mixed episodes have occurred concurrently with the active-phase symptoms, or, if mood disorder episodes have occurred during active-phase symptoms, their total duration has been brief relative to the duration of the active and residual periods.

Substance and general medical condition exclusion

The disturbance isn't due to the direct physiologic effects of a substance or a general medical condition.

Relationship to a pervasive developmental disorder

If the person has a history of autistic disorder or another pervasive developmental disorder, the additional diagnosis of schizophrenia is appropriate only if prominent delusions or hallucinations are also present for at least 1 month (or less if successfully treated).

treating the patient with schizophrenia. Some consider it a useful adjunct to drug therapy. Others suggest that psychosocial rehabilitation, education, and social skills training are more effective for chronic schizophrenia. In addition to improving understanding of the disorder, these methods teach the patient and his family coping strategies, effective communication techniques, and social skills.

Because schizophrenia typically disrupts the family, family therapy may be helpful to reduce guilt and disappointment as well as improve acceptance of the patient and his bizarre behavior.

Drugs

- Antipsychotic drugs—as the primary treatment for more than 30 years, antipsychotic drugs (also called *neuroleptic drugs*) appear to work by blocking postsynaptic dopamine receptors. These drugs reduce the incidence of positive psychotic symptoms, such as hallucinations and delusions, and relieve anxiety and agitation. Newer antipsychotics are effective in relieving positive and negative symptoms of schizophrenia. Certain antipsychotic drugs are associated with numerous adverse reactions, some of which are irreversible. (See *Reviewing adverse effects of antipsychotic drugs,* page 146.)
- The newer antipsychotic drugs appear to be effective in treating the negative symptoms of schizophrenia (withdrawal, apathy, or blunted affect). However, these drugs have problematic adverse effects. Antipsychotic drugs are broken down into two major classes: dopamine-receptor antagonists (haloperidol and thorazine) and dopamine-serotonin antagonists, also called *atypical antipsychotics* (risperidone [Risperdal] and clozapine [Clozaril]). The long-acting drugs haloperidol (Haldol) and fluphenazine (Prolixin) may be given I.M. every 3 to 4 weeks to improve compliance.

– Clozapine may be prescribed for severely ill patients who fail to respond to standard treatment. This drug effectively controls more psychotic signs and symptoms without the usual adverse effects. However, clozapine can cause drowsiness, sedation, excessive salivation, tachycardia, dizziness, and seizures. Risperidone and olanzapine (Zyprexa), like clozapine, have reduced the incidence of adverse effects, including extrapyramidal symptoms and anticholinergic adverse effects.

⚠ ALERT

Monitor the patient taking antipsychotic drugs for the development of neuroleptic malignant syndrome (hyperthermia, autonomic disturbances and extrapyramidal symptoms), which can be fatal.

⚠ ALERT

The patient taking clozapine must be monitored with frequent blood counts for agranulocytosis—a potentially fatal blood disorder characterized by

REVIEWING ADVERSE EFFECTS OF ANTIPSYCHOTIC DRUGS

The newer atypical drugs, such as risperidone, olanzapine, quetiapine, sertindole, and ziprasidone, produce fewer extrapyramidal symptoms than the first, older class of antipsychotics. Risperidone is associated with increases in serum prolactin. Olanzapine, in moderate doses, induces little extrapyramidal symptoms, but has been associated with weight gain and blood glucose abnormalities. Quetiapine can cause weight gain, hypotension, and sedation.

Older classes of antipsychotic drugs (sometimes known as *neuroleptic drugs*) can cause sedative, anticholinergic, or extrapyramidal effects; orthostatic hypotension; and, rarely, neuroleptic malignant syndrome.

Sedative, anticholinergic, and extrapyramidal effects

High-potency drugs (such as haloperidol) are minimally sedative and anticholinergic but cause a high incidence of extrapyramidal adverse effects. Intermediate-potency drugs (such as molindone) are associated with a moderate incidence of adverse effects, whereas low-potency drugs (such as chlorpromazine) are highly sedative and anticholinergic but produce few extrapyramidal adverse effects.

The most common extrapyramidal effects are dystonia, parkinsonism, and akathisia. Dystonia usually occurs in young male patients within the first few days of treatment. Characterized by severe tonic contractions of the muscles in the neck, mouth, and tongue, dystonia may be misdiagnosed as a psychotic symptom. Diphenhydramine or benztropine administered I.M. or I.V. provides rapid relief from this symptom.

Drug-induced parkinsonism results in bradykinesia, muscle rigidity, shuffling or propulsive gait, stooped posture, flat facial affect, tremors, and drooling. Parkinsonism may occur from 1 week to several months after the initiation of drug treatment. Drugs prescribed to reverse or prevent this syndrome include benztropine, trihexyphenidyl, and amantadine.

Tardive dyskinesia can occur after only 6 months of continuous therapy and is usually irreversible. No effective treatment is available for this disorder, which is characterized by various involuntary movements of the mouth and jaw; flapping or writhing; purposeless, rapid, and jerky movements of the arms and legs; and dystonic posture of the neck and trunk.

Signs and symptoms of akathisia include restlessness, pacing, and an inability to rest or sit still. Akathisia may be misinterpreted as agitation or a worsening of psychotic behavior. Propranolol relieves this adverse effect.

---

a low white blood cell count and pronounced neutropenia. This disorder affects 1% to 2% of all patients and is reversible if detected early.

⚠ ALERT

More than 50% of patients taking atypical antipsychotics will have significant weight gain and should be monitored for the development of

Orthostatic hypotension

Low-potency neuroleptics can cause orthostatic hypotension because they block alpha-adrenergic receptors. If hypotension is severe, the patient is placed in the supine position and given I.V. fluids for hypovolemia. If further treatment is needed, an alpha-adrenergic agonist, such as norepinephrine or metaraminol, may be ordered to relieve hypotension. Mixed alpha- and beta-adrenergic drugs (such as epinephrine) or beta-adrenergic drugs (such as isoproterenol) shouldn't be given because they can further reduce blood pressure.

Neuroleptic malignant syndrome

Neuroleptic malignant syndrome is a life-threatening syndrome that occurs in up to 1% of patients taking antipsychotic drugs. Signs and symptoms include fever, muscle rigidity, and altered level of consciousness occurring hours to months after initiating drug therapy or increasing the dose. Treatment is symptomatic, largely consisting of dantrolene and other measures to counter muscle rigidity associated with hyperthermia. You'll need to monitor vital signs and mental status continuously.

metabolic syndrome and type 2 diabetes.
- Antidepressants, such as SSRIs, act on the brain to help balance levels of serotonin. Tricyclic anti-

depressants and MAOIs help to balance serotonin and norepinephrine. Other medications may act to balance a combination of dopamine, norephinephrine, serotonin, and other chemicals.

⚡ PREVENTION

When the patient is taking antidepressants, closely monitor him for suicidal thoughts, especially during the first 4 weeks of starting therapy.

⚠ ALERT

The patient taking an MAOI must avoid foods and beverages that contain tyramine, which is found in aged cheeses, smoked meats, and wine, because it may trigger a hypertensive crisis.

- Anxiolytics, such as alprazolam (Xanax), a benzodiazepine, may be prescribed to treat symptoms of anxiety that accompany schizophrenia and are used for short periods of time. However, the patient must be carefully monitored because the potential for addiction is high. For this reason, they should not be prescribed if the patient has a history of substance abuse.

SPECIAL CONSIDERATIONS

- Assess the patient's ability to carry out activities of daily living, paying special attention to his nutritional status. Monitor his weight if he isn't eating. If he thinks that his food is poisoned, let him fix his own food when possible or offer foods in closed containers that he can open. If you give liquid medication in a unit-dose container, allow the patient to open the container.

- Maintain a safe environment, minimizing stimuli. Administer prescribed drugs to decrease symptoms and anxiety. Adopt an accepting and consistent approach with the patient. Short, repeated contacts are best until trust has been established.

- Avoid promoting dependence. Reward positive behavior to help the patient improve his level of functioning.

- Engage the patient in reality-oriented activities that involve human contact, such as inpatient social skills training groups, outpatient day care, and sheltered workshops. Provide reality-based explanations for distorted body images or hypochondriacal complaints. Explain to the patient that his private language, autistic inventions, or neologisms aren't understood. Set limits on inappropriate behavior.

- If the patient is hallucinating, explore the content of the hallucinations. If he hears voices, find out if he believes that he must do what they command. Explore the emotions connected with the hallucinations, but don't argue about them. If possible, change the subject.

- Assist the patient to recognize the unreality of his hallucinatory experience.

- Teach the patient techniques that interrupt the hallucinations (listening to an audiocassette player, singing out loud, or reading out loud).

- Don't tease or joke with a patient with schizophrenia. Choose words and phrases that are unambiguous

and clearly understood. For instance, a patient who's told, "That procedure will be done on the floor," may become frightened, thinking he'll need to lie down on the floor.

⚠ ALERT

If the patient expresses suicidal thoughts, institute suicide precautions. Document his behavior and your actions.

⚠ ALERT

If the patient expresses homicidal thoughts (for example, "I have to kill my mother"), institute homicidal precautions according to your institution's policies.

- Don't touch the patient without telling him first exactly what you're going to do—for example, "I'm going to put this cuff on your arm so I can take your blood pressure."

- If necessary, postpone procedures that require physical contact with hospital personnel until the patient is less suspicious or agitated.

- Remember, institutionalization may produce symptoms and disabilities that aren't part of the patient's illness, so evaluate symptoms carefully.

- Mobilize community resources to provide a support system for the patient. Ongoing support is essential to his mastery of social skills.

- Encourage adherence with the medication regimen to prevent a relapse.

- Help the patient explore possible connections between anxiety and stress and the exacerbation of symptoms.

For catatonic schizophrenia:

- Assess for physical illness. Remember that the mute patient won't complain of pain or physical symptoms; if he's in a bizarre posture, he's at risk for pressure ulcers or decreased circulation to a body area.
- Meet the patient's physical needs for adequate food, fluid, exercise, and elimination; follow orders with respect to nutrition, urinary catheterization, and enema.
- Provide range-of-motion exercises for the patient, or help him ambulate every 2 hours.
- Prevent physical exhaustion and injury during periods of hyperactivity.
- Tell the patient directly, specifically, and concisely which procedures need to be done. For example, you might say to the patient, "It's time to go for a walk. Let's go." Don't offer the negativistic patient a choice.
- Spend some time with the patient even if he's mute and unresponsive. He may be acutely aware of his environment even though he seems not to be. Your presence can be reassuring and supportive.
- Verbalize for the patient the message that his nonverbal behavior seems to convey; encourage him to do so as well.
- Reorient the patient to reality. You might say, "The leaves on the trees are turning colors, and the air is cooler. It's fall!" Emphasize reality in all contacts to reduce distorted perceptions.

- Stay alert for violent outbursts; if they occur, get help promptly to ensure the patient's safety and your own.

For paranoid schizophrenia:

- When the patient is newly admitted, minimize his contact with the hospital staff.
- Don't crowd the patient physically or psychologically; he may strike out to protect himself.
- Be flexible; allow the patient some control. Approach him in a calm and unhurried manner. Let him talk about anything he wishes initially, but keep the conversation light and social. Avoid entering into power struggles.
- Respond to the patient's condescending attitudes (arrogance, put-downs, sarcasm, or open hostility) with neutral remarks.
- Don't let the patient put you on the defensive, and don't take his remarks personally. If he tells you to leave him alone, do leave but return soon. Brief contacts with the patient may be most useful at first.
- Don't make attempts to combat the patient's delusions with logic. Instead, respond to feelings, themes, or underlying needs—for example, "It seems you feel you've been treated unfairly."
- Be honest and dependable. Don't threaten the patient or make promises that you can't fulfill.
- If the patient is taking clozapine, stress the importance of returning weekly or biweekly to the hospital or an outpatient setting to have his blood count monitored.

- Teach the patient the importance of adhering to the medication regimen. Tell him to report any adverse reactions instead of discontinuing the drug. If he takes a slow-release formulation, make sure that he understands when to return to the practitioner for his next dose.
- Involve the patient's family in his treatment. Teach them how to recognize an impending relapse, and suggest ways to manage symptoms, such as tension, nervousness, insomnia, decreased ability to concentrate, and apathy.
- Refer the patient and his family to the National Alliance for the Mentally Ill for additional educational and supportive resources.

Substance abuse and induced disorders

Substance abuse and dependence causes physical, mental, emotional, or social harm. Examples of abused drugs include opioids, stimulants, depressants, anxiolytics, and hallucinogens. (See *Understanding commonly abused substances*.)

Chronic drug abuse, especially I.V. use, can lead to life-threatening complications, such as cardiac and respiratory arrest, intracranial hemorrhage, acquired immunodeficiency syndrome, tetanus, subacute infective endocarditis, hepatitis, vasculitis, septicemia, thrombophlebitis, pulmonary emboli, gangrene, malnutrition and GI disturbances, respiratory infections, musculoskeletal dysfunction, trauma, depression, increased risk of suicide, and psychosis. Materials used to "cut" street drugs also can cause toxic or allergic reactions.

Psychoactive drug abuse can occur at any age. Experimentation with drugs commonly begins in adolescence or even earlier. In many cases, drug abuse leads to addiction, which may involve physical or psychological dependence or both. The most dangerous form of abuse occurs when users mix several drugs simultaneously—including alcohol.

CAUSES AND INCIDENCE

Psychoactive drug abuse and addiction can result from a combination of personality, environmental, neurobiological, and genetic factors. Substance abuse and addiction commonly occurs with depression, anxiety disorder, antisocial personality disorder, and attention deficit hyperactivity disorder. It's estimated that 30% to 50% of patients with stimulant or opiate addiction also have anxiety or depression disorders. Substance use may begin as curiosity and from peer pressure in adolescence. Taking the drug may give pleasure by relieving tension, abolishing loneliness, causing a temporarily peaceful or euphoric state, or simply relieving boredom. Substance abuse is also linked to poor impulse control and low self-esteem. Repeated substance abuse changes neurobiological processes

(Text continues on page 157)

UNDERSTANDING COMMONLY ABUSED SUBSTANCES

Substance	Signs and symptoms	Interventions

CANNABINOIDS

Marijuana

- *Street names:* pot, grass, weed, Mary Jane, roach, reefer, joint, muggles, Acapulco gold, Texas tea, Yesca, hemp
- *Routes:* ingestion, smoking
- *Dependence:* psychological
- *Duration of effect:* 2 to 3 hours
- *Medical uses:* antiemetic for chemotherapy

- *Of use:* acute psychosis; agitation; amotivational syndrome; anxiety; asthma; bronchitis; conjunctival reddening; decreased muscle strength; delusions; distorted sense of time and self-perception; dry mouth; euphoria; hallucinations; impaired cognition, short-term memory, and mood; incoordination; increased hunger; increased systolic pressure when supine; orthostatic hypotension; paranoia; spontaneous laughter; tachycardia; and vivid visual imagery
- *Of withdrawal:* chills, decreased appetite, increased rapid-eye-movement sleep, insomnia, irritability, nervousness, restlessness, tremors, and weight loss

- Place the patient in a quiet room.
- Monitor his vital signs.
- Give supplemental oxygen for respiratory depression and I.V. fluids for hypotension.
- Give diazepam, as ordered, for extreme agitation and acute psychosis.

DEPRESSANTS

Alcohol

- *Found in:* beer, wine, and distilled spirits; also contained in cough syrup, after-shave, and mouthwash
- *Route:* ingestion
- *Dependence:* physical and psychological

- *Of acute use:* coma, decreased inhibitions, euphoria followed by depression or hostility, impaired judgment, incoordination, respiratory depression, slurred speech, unconsciousness, and vomiting
- *Of withdrawal:* delirium, hallucinations, seizures, and tremors

- Place the patient in a quiet room.
- If alcohol was ingested within 4 hours, induce vomiting or perform gastric lavage; give activated charcoal and a saline cathartic.
- Monitor his vital signs.

(*continued*)

UNDERSTANDING COMMONLY ABUSED SUBSTANCES (continued)

Substance	Signs and symptoms	Interventions

DEPRESSANTS (continued)

▪ *Duration of effect:* varies according to individual and amount ingested; metabolized at rate of 10 ml/hour ▪ *Medical uses:* neurolysis (absolute alcohol); emergency tocolytic; and treatment of ethylene glycol and methanol poisoning		▪ As ordered, give chlor-diazepoxide every 4 hours to prevent withdrawal seizures, tremors, diaphoresis, anxiety, tachycardia, and hypertension. Diazepam may be used if an I.V. route needs to be used. ▪ Institute seizure precautions. ▪ Provide I.V. fluid replacement as well as dextrose, thiamine, B-complex vitamins, and vitamin C to treat dehydration, hypoglycemia, and nutritional deficiencies. ▪ Assess for aspiration pneumonia. ▪ Prepare for dialysis if patient's vital functions are severely depressed.

Barbiturates (amobarbital, phenobarbital, secobarbital)

▪ *Street names:* for barbiturates—barbs and downers; for amobarbital—blue angels and blue devils; for phenobarbital—goofballs and purple hearts; and for secobarbital—reds and red devils ▪ *Routes:* ingestion and injection ▪ *Dependence:* physical and psychological ▪ *Duration:* 1 to 16 hours ▪ *Medical uses:* anesthetic, anticonvulsant, sedative, hypnotic	▪ *Of use:* absent reflexes, blisters or bullous lesions, cyanosis, depressed level of consciousness (LOC) (from confusion to coma), fever, flaccid muscles, hypotension, hypothermia, nystagmus, paradoxical reaction in children and elderly people, poor pupil reaction to light, and respiratory depression ▪ *Of withdrawal:* agitation, anxiety, fever, insomnia, orthostatic hypotension, tachycardia, and tremors ▪ *Of rapid withdrawal:* anorexia, apprehension, hallucinations, orthostatic hypotension, tonic-clonic seizures, tremors, and weakness	▪ If ingestion was recent, induce vomiting or perform gastric lavage. Follow with activated charcoal. ▪ Monitor the patient's vital signs and perform frequent neurologic assessments. ▪ As ordered, give an I.V. fluid bolus for hypotension and alkalinized urine. ▪ Institute seizure precautions. ▪ Relieve withdrawal symptoms as ordered. ▪ Use a hypothermia or hyperthermia blanket for temperature alterations.

UNDERSTANDING COMMONLY ABUSED SUBSTANCES *(continued)*

Substance	Signs and symptoms	Interventions

DEPRESSANTS *(continued)*

Benzodiazepines (alprazolam, chlordiazepoxide, clonazepam, clorazepate, diazepam, flurazepam, halazepam, lorazepam, midazolam, oxazepam, prazepam, quazepam, temazepam, triazolam)

■ *Street names:* dolls and yellow jackets ■ *Routes:* ingestion and injection ■ *Dependence:* physical and psychological ■ *Duration of effect:* 4 to 8 hours ■ Medical uses: anxiolytic, anticonvulsant, sedative, hypnotic	■ *Of use:* ataxia, drowsiness, hypotension, increased self-confidence, relaxation, and slurred speech ■ *Of overdose:* confusion, coma, drowsiness, and respiratory depression ■ *Of withdrawal:* abdominal cramps, agitation, anxiety, diaphoresis, hypertension, tachycardia, tonic-clonic seizures, tremors, and vomiting	■ If the drug was ingested, induce vomiting or perform gastric lavage. Follow with activated charcoal and a cathartic. ■ Monitor the patient's vital signs. ■ Give supplemental oxygen for hypoxia-induced seizures. ■ As ordered, give I.V. fluids for hypertension, and physostigmine salicylate for respiratory or central nervous system (CNS) depression. Flumazenil, a specific benzodiazepine antagonist, can be used in cases of overdose to reverse the effects of the benzodiazepine.

Opiates (codeine, heroin, morphine, meperidine, and opium)

■ *Street names:* for heroin—junk, horse, H, smack, Chinese white, and Mexican mud; for morphine—morph, M, and microdots ■ Routes: for codeine, meperidine, and morphine—ingestion, injection, and smoking; for heroin—ingestion, injection, inhalation, and smoking; for opium—ingestion and smoking	■ *Of use:* anorexia, arrhythmias, clammy skin, constipation, constricted pupils, decreased LOC, detachment from reality, drowsiness, euphoria, hypotension, impaired judgment, increased pigmentation over veins, lack of concern, lethargy, nausea, needle marks, respiratory depression, seizures, shallow or slow respirations, skin lesions or abscesses, slurred speech, swollen or perforated nasal mucosa, thrombotic veins, urine retention, and vomiting	■ If the drug was ingested, induce vomiting or perform gastric lavage. ■ As ordered, give naloxone until CNS effects are reversed. ■ Give I.V. fluids to increase circulatory volume. ■ Use extra blankets for hypothermia; if ineffective, use a hyperthermia blanket. ■ Reorient the patient to time, place, and person. ■ Assess breath sounds to monitor for pulmonary edema.

(continued)

UNDERSTANDING COMMONLY ABUSED SUBSTANCES (*continued*)

Substance	Signs and symptoms	Interventions

DEPRESSANTS (*continued*)

Substance	Signs and symptoms	Interventions
▪ *Dependence:* physical and psychological ▪ *Duration of effect:* 3 to 6 hours ▪ *Medical uses:* for codeine—analgesia and antitussive; for heroin—none; for morphine and meperidine—analgesia; for opium—analgesia and antidiarrheal	▪ *Of withdrawal:* abdominal cramps, anorexia, chills, diaphoresis, dilated pupils, hyperactive bowel sounds, irritability, nausea, panic, piloerection, runny nose, sweating, tremors, watery eyes, and yawning	▪ Monitor for signs and symptoms of withdrawal. ▪ Naltrexone is an opiate antagonist that reverses the effects of the opiate.

HALLUCINOGENS

Lysergic acid diethylamide

Substance	Signs and symptoms	Interventions
▪ *Street names:* LSD, acid, blue dots, cube, D, owsleys, gel tabs, and microdot ▪ *Routes:* ingestion, smoking ▪ *Dependence:* possibly psychological ▪ *Duration of effect:* 8 to 12 hours ▪ *Medical uses:* none	▪ *Of use:* abdominal cramps, arrhythmias, chills, depersonalization, diaphoresis, diarrhea, distorted visual perception and perception of time and space, dizziness, dry mouth, fever, grandiosity, hallucinations, heightened sense of awareness, hyperpnea, hypertension, illusions, increased salivation, muscle aches, mystical experiences, nausea, palpitations, seizures, tachycardia, and vomiting ▪ *Of withdrawal:* none	▪ Place the patient in a quiet room. ▪ If the drug was ingested, induce vomiting or perform gastric lavage. Follow with activated charcoal and a cathartic. ▪ Monitor his vital signs, and give diazepam for seizures as ordered. ▪ Reorient the patient to time, place, and person, and restrain him as needed.

UNDERSTANDING COMMONLY ABUSED SUBSTANCES (continued)

Substance	Signs and symptoms	Interventions

HALLUCINOGENS (continued)

Phencyclidine

- *Street names:* PCP, hog, angel dust, peace pill, dummy mist, aurora, bust bee, guerrilla, rocket fuel
- *Routes:* ingestion, injection, and smoking
- *Dependence:* possibly psychological
- *Duration of effect:* 30 minutes to several days
- *Medical uses:* veterinary anesthetic

- *Of use:* amnesia; blank stare; cardiac arrest; decreased awareness of surroundings; delusions; distorted body image; distorted sense of sight, hearing, and touch; drooling; euphoria; excitation and psychoses; fever; gait ataxia; hallucinations; hyperactivity; hypertensive crisis; individualized unpredictable effects; muscle rigidity; nystagmus; panic; poor perception of time and distance; possible chromosomal damage; psychotic behavior; recurrent coma; renal failure; seizures; sudden behavioral changes; tachycardia; and violent behavior
- *Of withdrawal:* none

- Place the patient in a quiet room.
- If the drug was ingested, induce vomiting or perform gastric lavage. Follow with activated charcoal.
- Add ascorbic acid to I.V. solution to acidify urine.
- Monitor the patient's vital signs and urine output.
- If ordered, give a diuretic; propranolol for hypertension or tachycardia; nitroprusside for severe hypertensive crisis; diazepam for seizures; diazepam or haloperidol for agitation or psychotic behavior; and physostigmine, diazepam, chlordiazepoxide, or chlorpromazine for a "bad trip."

STIMULANTS

Amphetamines

- *Street names:* for amphetamine sulfate—bennies, cartwheels, and grennies; for methamphetamine — speed, meth, and crystal; and for dextroamphetamine sulfate—dexies, hearts, and oranges
- *Routes:* ingestion and injection
- *Dependence:* psychological

- *Of use:* altered mental status (from confusion to paranoia), coma, diaphoresis, dilated reactive pupils, dry mouth, exhaustion, hallucinations, hyperactive deep tendon reflexes, hypertension, hyperthermia, paradoxical reaction in children, psychotic behavior with prolonged use, seizures, shallow respirations, tachycardia, and tremors

- Place the patient in a quiet room.
- If the drug was ingested, induce vomiting or perform gastric lavage; give activated charcoal and a saline or magnesium sulfate cathartic.
- Add ammonium chloride or ascorbic acid to I.V. solution to acidify urine to a pH of 5. Also, administer mannitol to induce diuresis, as ordered.
- Monitor the patent's vital signs.

(continued)

UNDERSTANDING COMMONLY ABUSED SUBSTANCES (continued)

Substance	Signs and symptoms	Interventions
STIMULANTS (continued)		

■ *Duration of effect:* 1 to 4 hours ■ *Medical uses:* hyperkinesis, narcolepsy, and weight control	■ *Of withdrawal:* abdominal tenderness, apathy, depression, disorientation, irritability, long periods of sleep, and muscle aches, or suicide (with sudden withdrawal)	■ As ordered, give a short-acting barbiturate, such as pentobarbital, for seizures; haloperidol for assaultive behavior; phentolamine for hypertension; propranolol for tachyarrhythmias; and lidocaine for ventricular arrhythmias. ■ Restrain the patient if he's experiencing hallucinations or paranoia. ■ Give a tepid sponge bath for fever. ■ Institute suicide precautions.
Cocaine ■ *Street names:* coke, flake, snow, nose candy, hits, gold dust, toot, crack (hardened form), rock, and crank ■ *Routes:* ingestion, injection, sniffing, and smoking ■ *Dependence:* psychological ■ *Duration of effect:* 15 minutes to 2 hours; with crack, rapid high of short duration followed by down feeling ■ *Medical uses:* local anesthetic	■ *Of use:* abdominal pain; alternating euphoria and fear; anorexia; cardiotoxicity, such as ventricular fibrillation or cardiac arrest; coma; confusion; diaphoresis; dilated pupils; excitability; fever; grandiosity; hyperpnea; hypotension or hypertension; insomnia; irritability; nausea and vomiting; pallor or cyanosis; perforated nasal septum with prolonged use; pressured speech; psychotic behavior with large doses; respiratory arrest; seizures; spasms; tachycardia; tachypnea; visual, auditory, and olfactory hallucinations; and weight loss ■ *Of withdrawal:* anxiety, depression, and fatigue	■ Place the patient in a quiet room. ■ If cocaine was ingested, induce vomiting or perform gastric lavage. Follow with activated charcoal and a saline cathartic. ■ If cocaine was sniffed, remove residual drug from mucous membranes. ■ Monitor the patient's vital signs. ■ Give propranolol for tachycardia. ■ Perform cardiopulmonary resuscitation for ventricular fibrillation and cardiac arrest, as indicated. ■ Give a tepid sponge bath for fever. ■ Administer an anticonvulsant, as ordered, for seizures.

in the brain particularly in the frontal cortex. These changes can affect decision making, impulsivity, planning, and memory and may help explain why individuals relapse after addiction treatment. Low levels of serotonin are also linked to increases in impulsivity. Genetic factors may account for 30% to 60% of an individual's total risk of developing an addiction. Genetic factors also determine how various substances affect an individual's receptor sites and how substances are absorbed, distributed, and metabolized. Substance abuse may also occur from taking prescribed medications to relieve physical pain, but this is uncommon.

SIGNS AND SYMPTOMS

The signs and symptoms of acute intoxication vary, depending on the drug. The drug user seldom seeks treatment specifically for his drug problem. Instead, he may seek emergency treatment for drug-related injuries or complications, such as a motor vehicle accident, burns from freebasing, an overdose, physical deterioration from illness or malnutrition, or symptoms of withdrawal. Friends, family members, or law enforcement officials may bring the patient to the hospital because of respiratory depression, unconsciousness, acute injury, or a psychiatric crisis.

Examine the patient for signs and symptoms of drug use or drug-related complications as well as for clues to the type of drug ingested. For example, fever can result from stimulant or hallucinogen intoxication, from withdrawal, or from infection caused by I.V. drug use.

Inspect the eyes for lacrimation from opiate withdrawal, nystagmus from central nervous system (CNS) depressants or phencyclidine intoxication, and drooping eyelids from opiate or CNS depressant use. Constricted pupils occur with opiate use or withdrawal; dilated pupils, with the use of hallucinogens or amphetamines.

Examine the nose for rhinorrhea from opiate withdrawal and the oral and nasal mucosa for signs of drug-induced irritation. Drug sniffing can result in inflammation, atrophy, or perforation of the nasal mucosa. Dental conditions commonly result from the poor oral hygiene associated with chronic drug use. Also inspect under the tongue for evidence of I.V. drug injection.

Inspect the skin. Sweating, a common sign of intoxication with opiates or CNS stimulants, also accompanies most drug withdrawal syndromes. Drug use sometimes induces a sensation of bugs crawling on the skin, known as *formication;* as a result, the patient's skin may be excoriated from scratching. Needle marks or tracks are an obvious sign of I.V. drug abuse. Keep in mind that the patient may attempt to conceal or disguise injection sites with tattoos or by selecting an inconspicuous site such as under the nails. In addition, self-injection can sometimes cause cellulitis or abscesses, especially in the patient who also is a chronic alcoholic. Puffy hands can be a late sign of thrombophlebitis or of fascial infection due to self-injection on the hands or arms.

Auscultation may disclose bilateral crackles and rhonchi caused by smoking and inhaling drugs or by opiate overdose. Other cardiopulmonary signs of overdose include:

- pulmonary edema
- respiratory depression
- aspiration pneumonia
- hypotension
- hypertension or cardiac arrhythmias caused by withdrawal from CNS stimulants and some hallucinogens
- hypotension and cardiac arrhythmias caused by withdrawal from opiates or depressants.

During opiate withdrawal, the patient may report abdominal pain, nausea, or vomiting. He may also complain of hemorrhoids, a consequence of the constipating effects of these drugs. Palpation of an enlarged liver, with or without tenderness, may indicate hepatitis.

Neurologic signs and symptoms of drug abuse include:

- tremors
- hyperreflexia
- hyporeflexia
- seizures
- CNS depression (ranging from lethargy to coma)
- hallucinations

- signs of overstimulation, including euphoria and violent behavior.

Carefully review the patient's medical history. Suspect drug abuse if the individual:

- reports a painful injury or chronic illness but refuses a diagnostic workup
- feigns illnesses, such as migraine headaches, myocardial infarction, and renal colic
- claims an allergy to over-the-counter analgesics
- requests a specific medication
- has a history of prior overdose
- has a high tolerance for potentially addictive drugs
- has a history of hepatitis (may indicate I.V. drug use)
- has a history of human immunodeficiency virus (HIV) infection
- reports a history of amenorrhea.

A patient who abuses drugs may give you a fictitious name and address, be reluctant to discuss previous hospitalizations, or seek treatment at a medical facility across town rather than in his own neighborhood. If possible, obtain the patient's previous medical records, and interview family members to verify his responses.

If the patient admits to drug use, try to determine the extent to which this behavior interferes with his normal functioning. Note whether he expresses a desire to overcome his dependence on drugs. If possible, obtain a drug history consisting of substances ingested, amount, frequency, and last dose. Expect incomplete or inaccurate responses. Drug-induced amnesia, a depressed level of consciousness, or ignorance may distort the patient's recollection of the facts; he also may fabricate answers to avoid arrest or to conceal a suicide attempt.

The abuse of psychoactive substances may cause a need for dosage adjustments to prescribed medications. Cross-tolerance occurs when one drug that has particular properties results in tolerance of another drug. Drugs with similar pharmacologic properties, such as CNS depressants, will cause the need for more of a similar class of drug to get the same response. This may occur, for example, when a patient on an opiate goes to surgery. More anesthesia is needed for this patient than is needed for an opiate-naïve patient.

The hospitalized drug abuser is likely to be:
- uncooperative
- disruptive
- violent.

He may experience:
- mood swings
- anxiety
- impaired memory
- sleep disturbances
- flashbacks
- slurred speech
- depression
- thought disorders.

He may resort to plays on sympathy, bribery, or threats to obtain drugs, or he may try to pit one caregiver against another.

COMPLICATIONS

- Health problems, such as cardiac and respiratory arrest, intracranial hemorrhage, acquired immunodeficiency syndrome, subacute bacterial endocarditis, hepatitis, septicemia, pulmonary emboli, gangrene
- Family and marital relationship problems
- Impaired occupational and school functioning
- Financial problems
- Legal problems from criminal behavior
- Suicide

DIAGNOSTIC CRITERIA

For characteristic findings in patients with this condition, see *Diagnosing substance dependence and related disorders,* page 9.

Various serum or urine toxicology tests can:
- confirm drug use
- determine the amount and type of drug taken
- reveal complications.

Characteristic findings in other tests include:
- elevated serum globulin levels
- hypoglycemia
- leukocytosis
- liver function abnormalities
- positive Venereal Disease Research Laboratory test results
- positive for HIV
- positive rapid plasma reagin test results caused by elevated protein fractions
- elevated mean corpuscular hemoglobin level

- elevated uric acid levels
- reduced blood urea nitrogen levels.

TREATMENT

The patient with acute drug intoxication should receive symptomatic treatment based on the drug ingested. Measures include:

- fluid replacement therapy
- nutritional supplementation
- vitamin supplements
- detoxification with the same drug or a pharmacologically similar drug (exceptions include cocaine, hallucinogens, and marijuana, which aren't used for detoxification)
- sedatives to induce sleep
- anticholinergics and antidiarrheals to relieve GI distress
- anxiolytics for severe agitation (especially in cocaine abusers) and symptomatic treatment of complications.

Depending on the dosage and time elapsed before admission, additional treatment may include:

- gastric lavage
- induced emesis
- activated charcoal
- forced diuresis
- hemoperfusion or hemodialysis.

Treatment of drug dependence commonly involves a triad of care:

- detoxification
- short- and long-term rehabilitation
- aftercare—a lifetime of abstinence, usually aided by participation in Narcotics Anonymous (NA) or a similar self-help group.

Detoxification, the controlled and gradual withdrawal of an abused drug, is achieved through substituting a drug with a similar action. Such gradual replacement of the abused drug controls the effects of withdrawal, thereby reducing the patient's discomfort and associated risks.

Depending on which drug the patient has abused, detoxification may be managed on an inpatient or outpatient basis. For example, withdrawal from depressants can produce hazardous adverse reactions, such as generalized tonic-clonic seizures, status epilepticus, and hypotension. The severity of these reactions determines whether the patient can be safely treated as an outpatient or if he requires hospitalization.

⚠ ALERT

Withdrawal from depressants usually requires detoxification because abrupt or poorly managed withdrawal from barbiturates can cause death.

Opioid withdrawal causes severe physical discomfort and can be life-threatening. To minimize these effects, chronic opioid abusers commonly are detoxified with methadone.

To ease withdrawal from opioids, depressants, and other drugs, useful nonchemical measures may include:

- psychotherapy
- exercise
- relaxation techniques
- nutritional support.

After withdrawal, the patient needs to participate in a rehabilitation program to prevent a recurrence. Rehabilitation programs are available for inpatients and outpatients; they usually last a month or longer and may include individual, group, and family psychotherapy. During and after rehabilitation, participation in a drug-oriented self-help group may be helpful. The largest such group is NA.

Drugs

• Sedatives and tranquilizers may be administered temporarily to help the patient cope with insomnia, anxiety, and depression.
• Buprenorphine with naloxone (Suboxone) is another drug that's being used to lessen craving in opiate-addicted patients. Naloxone is an opiate antagonist; it blocks opiate receptors. A person taking Suboxone won't respond to the effects of other opioids.

SPECIAL CONSIDERATIONS

Focus on restoring the patient's physical health, educating him and his family about drug abuse and dependence, providing support, and encouraging participation in drug treatment programs and self-help groups.

During an acute episode:

⚠ ALERT

Continuously monitor the patient's vital signs, and observe for complications of overdose and withdrawal, such as cardiopulmonary arrest, seizures, and aspiration.

⧉ PREVENTION

Institute seizure precautions.

• Give medications, as ordered, to decrease withdrawal symptoms; monitor and record their effectiveness.
• Maintain a quiet, safe environment during withdrawal from any drug because excessive noise may agitate the patient.
• Remove harmful objects from the patient's room.
• Based on institutional policy, institute appropriate measures to prevent suicide attempts.

After an acute episode:

• Learn to control your reactions to the patient's undesirable behaviors—commonly, psychological dependency, manipulation, anger, frustration, and alienation.
• Set limits for dealing with demanding, manipulative behavior.
• Promote adequate nutrition and monitor the patient's nutritional intake.
• Administer medications carefully to prevent the patient from hoarding. Check the patient's mouth to ensure that he has swallowed the medication. Closely monitor visitors who might supply the patient with drugs.
• Refer the patient for detoxification and rehabilitation, as appropriate. Give him a list of available resources.
• Encourage family members to seek help whether or not the abuser seeks it. You can suggest private therapy or community mental health clinics.

If the patient refuses to participate in a rehabilitation program, teach him how to minimize the risk of drug-related complications, as follows:

PREVENTION

Review measures for preventing HIV infection and hepatitis. Stress that these infections are readily transmitted by sharing needles with other drug users and by having unprotected sexual intercourse.

● Advise the patient to use a new needle for every injection or to clean needles with a solution of one part chlorine bleach with one part water.

PREVENTION

Emphasize the importance of using a condom during intercourse to prevent disease transmission and pregnancy. If necessary, teach the female drug abuser about other methods of birth control. Explain the devastating effects of drugs on the developing fetus.

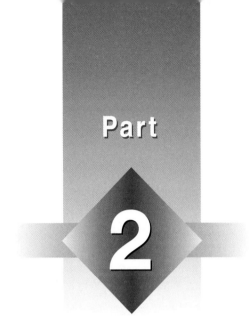

Part

2

Drugs

acamprosate calcium
a-kam-PRO-sate

Campral

Pharmacologic class: synthetic amino acid neurotransmitter analogue
Pregnancy risk category C

AVAILABLE FORMS
Tablets (delayed-release): 333 mg

INDICATIONS & DOSAGES
➤ **Adjunct to management of alcohol abstinence**
Adults: 666 mg P.O. t.i.d.
Adjust-a-dose: In patients with creatinine clearance of 30 to 50 ml/minute, give 333 mg t.i.d.

ADMINISTRATION
P.O.
● Don't crush or break tablets.
● Give drug without regard for food.

ACTION
Restores the balance of neuronal excitation and inhibition, probably by interacting with glutamate and gamma-aminobutyric acid neurotransmitter systems, thus reducing alcohol dependence.

Route	Onset	Peak	Duration
P.O.	Unknown	3–8 hr	Unknown

Half-life: 20 to 33 hours.

ADVERSE REACTIONS
CNS: abnormal thinking, amnesia, anxiety, asthenia, depression, dizziness, headache, insomnia, paresthesia, somnolence, *suicidal thoughts,* syncope, tremor, pain.
CV: hypertension, palpitations, peripheral edema, vasodilation.
EENT: abnormal vision, pharyngitis, rhinitis.
GI: abdominal pain, anorexia, constipation, *diarrhea,* dry mouth, dyspepsia, flatulence, increased appetite, nausea, taste disturbance, vomiting.
GU: impotence.
Metabolic: weight gain.
Musculoskeletal: arthralgia, back pain, chest pain, myalgia.
Respiratory: bronchitis, dyspnea, increased cough.
Skin: increased sweating, pruritus, rash.
Other: accidental injury, chills, decreased libido, flulike symptoms, infection.

INTERACTIONS
None significant.

EFFECTS ON LAB TEST RESULTS
● May increase ALT, AST, bilirubin, blood glucose, and uric acid levels. May decrease hemoglobin level and hematocrit.
● May decrease platelet count.

CONTRAINDICATIONS & CAUTIONS
● Contraindicated in patients allergic to drug or its components and in those whose creatinine clearance is 30 ml/minute or less.
● Use cautiously in pregnant or breast-feeding women, elderly patients, patients with moderate renal impairment, and patients with a history of depression and suicidal thoughts or attempts.

NURSING CONSIDERATIONS
● Use only after the patient successfully becomes abstinent from drinking.
● Drug doesn't eliminate or reduce withdrawal symptoms.
● Monitor patient for development of depression or suicidal thoughts.
● Drug doesn't cause alcohol aversion or a disulfiram-like reaction if used with alcohol.

PATIENT TEACHING
• Tell patient to continue the alcohol abstinence program, including counseling and support.
• Advise patient to notify his prescriber if he develops depression, anxiety, thoughts of suicide, or severe diarrhea.
• Caution patient's family or caregiver to watch for signs of depression or suicidal ideation.
• Tell patient that drug may be taken without regard to meals, but that taking it with meals may help him remember it.
• Tell patient not to crush, break, or chew the tablets but to swallow them whole.
• Advise women to use effective contraception while taking this drug. Tell patient to contact her prescriber if she becomes pregnant or plans to become pregnant.
• Explain that this drug may impair judgment, thinking, or motor skills. Urge patient to use caution when driving or performing hazardous activities until drug's effects are known.
• Tell patient to continue taking acamprosate and to contact his prescriber if he resumes drinking alcohol.

---

activated charcoal
Actidose ◊, Actidose-Aqua ◊, Actidose with Sorbitol ◊, CharcoAid ◊, CharcoAid 2000 ◊, Liqui-Char ◊

charcoal
Charcoal Plus DS ◊, CharcoCaps ◊

Pharmacologic class: adsorbent
Pregnancy risk category C

AVAILABLE FORMS
activated charcoal
Granules: 15 g ◊
Liquid: 12.5 g ◊, 15 g ◊*, 25 g ◊*, 30 g ◊*, 50 g ◊*
Oral suspension: 15 g ◊, 30 g ◊
Powder: 15 g ◊, 30 g ◊, 40 g ◊, 120 g ◊, 240 g ◊
charcoal
Capsules: 260 mg ◊
Tablets: 250 mg ◊

INDICATIONS & DOSAGES
➤ **Flatulence, dyspepsia, diarrhea**
Adults: 500 to 520 mg (charcoal) P.O. after meals or at first sign of discomfort. Repeat as needed, up to 5 g daily.
➤ **Poisoning**
Adults and children: Initially, 1 to 2 g/kg (30 to 100 g) P.O. or 10 times the amount of poison ingested as a suspension in 120 to 240 ml (4 to 8 ounces) of water.

ADMINISTRATION
P.O.
• Give after emesis is complete because activated charcoal absorbs and inactivates ipecac syrup.
• For best effect, give within 30 minutes after poison ingestion.
• Mix powder (most effective form) with tap water to consistency of thick syrup. Add small amount of fruit juice or flavoring to make mix more palatable. Don't mix with ice cream, milk, or sherbet; these decrease adsorptive capacity of activated charcoal.
• Give by large-bore nasogastric tube after lavage, if needed.
• If patient vomits shortly after administration, repeat dose.
• Space doses at least 1 hour apart from other drugs if treatment is for indications other than poisoning.

ACTION
Adheres to many drugs and chemicals, inhibiting their absorption from the GI tract. Also reduces volume of intestinal gas and relieves related discomfort.

Route	Onset	Peak	Duration
P.O.	Immediate	Unknown	Unknown

Half-life: Unknown.

ADVERSE REACTIONS
GI: black stools, **intestinal obstruction,** nausea, constipation.

INTERACTIONS
Drug-drug. *Acetaminophen, barbiturates, carbamazepine, digitoxin, digoxin, furosemide, glutethimide, hydantoins, methotrexate, nizatidine, phenothiazines,*

---

phenylbutazone, propoxyphene, sali-cylates, sulfonamides, sulfonylureas, tetracyclines, theophyllines, tricyclic antidepressants, valproic acid: May reduce absorption of these drugs. Give charcoal at least 2 hours before or 1 hour after other drugs.

Acetylcysteine, ipecac: May inactivate these drugs. Give charcoal after vomiting has been induced by ipecac; remove charcoal by nasogastric tube before giving acetylcysteine.

Drug-food. *Milk, ice cream, sherbet:* May decrease adsorptive capacity of drug. Discourage use together.

EFFECTS ON LAB TEST RESULTS
None reported.

CONTRAINDICATIONS & CAUTIONS
None known.

NURSING CONSIDERATIONS
● Although there are no known contraindications, drug isn't effective for treating all acute poisonings.
● *Alert:* Drug is commonly used for treating poisoning or overdose with acetaminophen, aspirin, atropine, barbiturates, dextropropoxyphene, digoxin, poisonous mushrooms, oxalic acid, parathion, phenol, phenytoin, propantheline, propoxyphene, strychnine, or tricyclic antidepressants. Check with poison control center for use in other types of poisonings or overdoses.
● *Alert:* Don't aspirate or allow patient to aspirate charcoal powder; this may result in death.
● Follow treatment with stool softener or laxative to prevent constipation unless sorbitol is part of product ingredients. Preparations made with sorbitol have a laxative effect that lessens risk of severe constipation or fecal impaction.
● If preparation with sorbitol is used, maintain patient's fluid and electrolyte needs.
● Don't use charcoal with sorbitol in fructose-intolerant patients or in children younger than age 1.
● *Alert:* Drug is ineffective for poisoning or overdose of cyanide, mineral acids, caustic alkalis, and organic solvents; it's not very

effective for overdose of ethanol, lithium, methanol, and iron salts.
● *Look alike–sound alike:* Don't confuse Actidose with Actos.

PATIENT TEACHING
● Explain use and administration of drug to patient (if awake) and family.
● Warn patient that stools will be black until all the charcoal has passed through the body.
● Instruct patient to drink 6 to 8 glasses of liquid per day because drug can cause constipation.

SAFETY ALERT!

alprazolam
al-PRAH-zoe-lam

Apo-Alpraz†, Apo-Alpraz TS†, Niravam, Novo-Alprazol†, Xanax, Xanax XR

Pharmacologic class: benzodiazepine
Pregnancy risk category D
Controlled substance schedule IV

AVAILABLE FORMS
Oral solution: 1 mg/ml (concentrate)
Orally disintegrating tablets (ODTs): 0.25 mg, 0.5 mg, 1 mg, 2 mg
Tablets: 0.25 mg, 0.5 mg, 1 mg, 2 mg
Tablets (extended-release): 0.5 mg, 1 mg, 2 mg, 3 mg

INDICATIONS & DOSAGES
➤ **Anxiety**
Adults: Usual first dose, 0.25 to 0.5 mg P.O. t.i.d. Maximum, 4 mg daily in divided doses.
Elderly patients: Usual first dose, 0.25 mg P.O. b.i.d. or t.i.d. Maximum, 4 mg daily in divided doses.
➤ **Panic disorders**
Adults: 0.5 mg P.O. t.i.d., increased at intervals of 3 to 4 days in increments of no more than 1 mg. Maximum, 10 mg daily in divided doses. If using extended-release tablets, start with 0.5 to 1 mg P.O. once daily. Increase by no more than 1 mg every 3 to 4 days. Maximum daily dose is 10 mg.

Adjust-a-dose: For debilitated patients or those with advanced hepatic disease, usual first dose is 0.25 mg P.O. b.i.d. or t.i.d. Maximum, 4 mg daily in divided doses.

ADMINISTRATION
P.O.
• Don't break or crush extended-release tablets.
• Mix oral solution with liquids or semisolid food, such as water, juices, carbonated beverages, applesauce, and puddings. Use only calibrated dropper provided with this product.
• Use dry hands to remove ODTs from bottle. Discard cotton from inside bottle.
• Discard unused portion if breaking scored ODT.

ACTION
Unknown. Probably potentiates the effects of GABA, depresses the CNS, and suppresses the spread of seizure activity.

Route	Onset	Peak	Duration
P.O.	Unknown	1–2 hr	Unknown
P.O. (extended-release)	Unknown	Unknown	Unknown

Half-life: Immediate-release, 12 to 15 hours; extended-release, 11 to 16 hours.

ADVERSE REACTIONS
CNS: *insomnia, irritability, dizziness, headache, anxiety, confusion, drowsiness, light-headedness, sedation, somnolence, difficulty speaking, impaired coordination, memory impairment, fatigue, depression,* **suicide,** mental impairment, ataxia, paresthesia, dyskinesia, hypoesthesia, lethargy, decreased or increased libido, vertigo, malaise, tremor, nervousness, restlessness, agitation, nightmare, syncope, akathisia, mania.
CV: palpitations, chest pain, hypotension.
EENT: sore throat, allergic rhinitis, blurred vision, nasal congestion.
GI: *diarrhea, dry mouth, constipation,* nausea, increased or decreased appetite, anorexia, vomiting, dyspepsia, abdominal pain.

GU: dysmenorrhea, sexual dysfunction, premenstrual syndrome, difficulty urinating.
Metabolic: increased or decreased weight.
Musculoskeletal: arthralgia, myalgia, arm or leg pain, back pain, muscle rigidity, muscle cramps, muscle twitch.
Respiratory: upper respiratory tract infection, dyspnea, hyperventilation.
Skin: pruritus, increased sweating, dermatitis.
Other: influenza, injury, emergence of anxiety between doses, dependence, feeling warm.

INTERACTIONS
Drug-drug. *Anticonvulsants, antidepressants, antihistamines, barbiturates, benzodiazepines, general anesthetics, narcotics, phenothiazines:* May increase CNS depressant effects. Avoid using together.
Azole antifungals (including fluconazole, itraconazole, ketoconazole, miconazole): May increase and prolong alprazolam level, CNS depression, and psychomotor impairment. Avoid using together.
Carbamazepine, propoxyphene: May induce alprazolam metabolism and may reduce therapeutic effects. May need to increase dose.
Cimetidine, fluoxetine, fluvoxamine, hormonal contraceptives, nefazodone: May increase alprazolam level. Use cautiously together, and consider alprazolam dosage reduction.
Tricyclic antidepressants: May increase levels of these drugs. Monitor patient closely.
Drug-herb. *Kava, valerian root:* May increase sedation. Discourage use together.
St. John's wort: May decrease drug level. Discourage use together.
Drug-food. *Grapefruit juice:* May increase drug level. Discourage use together.
Drug-lifestyle. *Alcohol use:* May cause additive CNS effects. Discourage use together.
Smoking: May decrease effectiveness of drug. Monitor patient closely.

EFFECTS ON LAB TEST RESULTS
• May increase ALT and AST levels.

CONTRAINDICATIONS & CAUTIONS
• Contraindicated in patients hypersensitive to drug or other benzodiazepines and in those with acute angle-closure glaucoma.
• Use cautiously in patients with hepatic, renal, or pulmonary disease.

NURSING CONSIDERATIONS
• The optimum duration of therapy is unknown.
• *Alert:* Don't withdraw drug abruptly; withdrawal symptoms, including seizures, may occur. Abuse or addiction is possible.
• Monitor hepatic, renal, and hematopoietic function periodically in patients receiving repeated or prolonged therapy.
• *Look alike–sound alike:* Don't confuse alprazolam with alprostadil. Don't confuse Xanax with Zantac or Tenex.

PATIENT TEACHING
• Warn patient to avoid hazardous activities that require alertness and good coordination until effects of drug are known.
• Tell patient to avoid use of alcohol while taking drug.
• Advise patient that smoking may decrease drug's effectiveness.
• Warn patient not to stop drug abruptly because withdrawal symptoms or seizures may occur.
• Tell patient to swallow extended-release tablets whole.
• Tell patient using ODT to remove it from bottle using dry hands and to immediately place it on his tongue where it will dissolve and can be swallowed with saliva.
• Tell patient taking half a scored ODT to discard the unused half.
• Advise patient to discard the cotton from the bottle of ODTs and keep it tightly sealed to prevent moisture from dissolving the tablets.

alprostadil
al-PROSS-ta-dil

Caverject, Edex, Muse

Pharmacologic class: prostaglandin
Pregnancy risk category NR

AVAILABLE FORMS
Injection: 5 mcg/ml, 10 mcg/ml, 20 mcg/ml, 40 mcg/ml after reconstitution
Urogenital suppository: 125 mcg, 250 mcg, 500 mcg, 1,000 mcg

INDICATIONS & DOSAGES
➤ **Erectile dysfunction of vasculogenic, psychogenic, or mixed causes**
Injection
Men: Dosages are highly individualized; initially, inject 2.5 mcg intracavernously. If partial response occurs, give second dose of 2.5 mcg; then increase in increments of 5 to 10 mcg until patient achieves erection suitable for intercourse and lasting no longer than 1 hour. If patient doesn't respond to first dose, increase second dose to 7.5 mcg within 1 hour, and then increase further in increments of 5 to 10 mcg until patient achieves suitable erection. Patient must remain in prescriber's office until complete detumescence occurs. Don't repeat procedure for at least 24 hours.
Urogenital suppository
Men: Initially, 125 to 250 mcg, under supervision of prescriber. Adjust dosage as needed until response is sufficient for sexual intercourse. Maximum of two administrations in 24 hours; maximum dose is 1,000 mcg.
➤ **Erectile dysfunction of neurogenic cause (spinal cord injury)**
Men: Dosages are highly individualized; initially, inject 1.25 mcg intracavernously. If partial response occurs, give second dose of 1.25 mcg. Increase in increments of 2.5 mcg, to dose of 5 mcg; then increase in increments of 5 mcg until patient achieves erection suitable for intercourse and lasting no longer than 1 hour. If patient doesn't respond to first dose, give next higher dose within 1 hour. Patient must remain in prescriber's office until complete detumescence occurs. If there is

a response, don't repeat procedure for at least 24 hours.

ADMINISTRATION
• For intracavernous injection, teach patient to follow instructions on package insert.
• Store injection at or below room temperature (77° F [25° C]).
• Vial is designed for a single use. Discard vial if injection solution is discolored or contains precipitate.
• Don't shake injection contents of reconstituted vial.
• Store unopened urogenital suppositories in refrigerator (36° to 46° F [2° to 8° C]).
• Have patient urinate before inserting suppository because moisture makes it easier to insert drug in penis and will help dissolve it.

ACTION
Induces erection by relaxing trabecular smooth muscle and dilating cavernosal arteries. This leads to expansion of lacunar spaces and entrapment of blood by compressing venules against the tunica albuginea, a process referred to as the corporal veno-occlusive mechanism.

Route	Onset	Peak	Duration
Intra-cavernous	5–20 min	5–20 min	1–6 hr
Urogenital	10 min	16 min	1 hr

Half-life: About 5 to 10 minutes.

ADVERSE REACTIONS
CNS: headache, dizziness.
CV: hypertension, hypotension.
EENT: sinusitis, nasal congestion.
GU: *penile pain,* prolonged erection, penile fibrosis, rash, or edema, prostatic disorder.
Musculoskeletal: back pain.
Respiratory: upper respiratory tract infection, cough.
Skin: injection site hematoma or ecchymosis.
Other: localized trauma or pain, flulike syndrome.

INTERACTIONS
Drug-drug. *Anticoagulants:* May increase risk of bleeding from intracavernosal injection site. Monitor patient closely.
Cyclosporine: May decrease cyclosporine level. Monitor cyclosporine level closely.
Vasoactive drugs: Safety and effectiveness haven't been studied. Avoid using together.

EFFECTS ON LAB TEST RESULTS
None reported.

CONTRAINDICATIONS & CAUTIONS
• Contraindicated in patients hypersensitive to drug, in those with conditions predisposing them to priapism (sickle cell anemia or trait, multiple myeloma, leukemia) or penile deformation (angulation, cavernosal fibrosis, Peyronie disease), in men with penile implants or for whom sexual activity is inadvisable or contraindicated, in women or children, and in sexual partners of pregnant women unless condoms are used.

NURSING CONSIDERATIONS
• Stop drug in patients who develop penile angulation, cavernosal fibrosis, or Peyronie disease.

PATIENT TEACHING
• Teach patient how to prepare and give drug before he begins treatment at home. Stress importance of reading and following patient instructions in each package insert. Tell him to store unopened suppositories in refrigerator (36° to 46° F [2° to 8° C]) and store injection at or below room temperature (77° F [25° C]).
• Tell patient not to shake contents of reconstituted vial, and remind him that vial is designed for a single use. Tell him to discard vial if solution is discolored or contains precipitate.
• Instruct patient to urinate before inserting suppository because moisture makes it easier to insert drug in penis and will help dissolve it.
• Review administration and aseptic technique.
• Inform patient that he can expect an erection 5 to 20 minutes after administration, with a preferable duration of no more than 1 hour. If his erection lasts more than

6 hours, tell him to seek medical attention immediately.
● Remind patient to take drug as instructed (generally, no more than three times weekly, with at least 24 hours between each use). Warn him not to change dosage without consulting prescriber.
● Caution patient to use a condom if his sexual partner could be pregnant.
● Review possible adverse reactions. Tell patient to inspect his penis daily and to report redness, swelling, tenderness, curvature, excessive erection (priapism), unusual pain, nodules, or hard tissue.
● Urge patient not to reuse or share needles, syringes, or drug.
● Warn patient that drug doesn't protect against sexually transmitted diseases. Also, caution him that bleeding at injection site can increase risk of transmitting bloodborne diseases to his partner.
● Remind patient to keep regular follow-up appointments so prescriber can evaluate drug effectiveness and safety.

amitriptyline hydrochloride
a-mee-TRIP-ti-leen

Pharmacologic class: tricyclic antidepressant
Pregnancy risk category C

AVAILABLE FORMS
amitriptyline hydrochloride
Injection: 10 mg/ml
Tablets: 10 mg, 25 mg, 50 mg, 75 mg, 100 mg, 150 mg

INDICATIONS & DOSAGES
➤ **Depression**
Adults: Initially, 50 to 100 mg P.O. at bedtime, increasing to 150 mg daily. Maximum, 300 mg daily, if needed. Maintenance, 50 to 100 mg daily. Or, 20 to 30 mg I.M. q.i.d.
Elderly patients and adolescents: 10 mg P.O. t.i.d. and 20 mg at bedtime daily.

ADMINISTRATION
P.O.
● Give drug without regard for food.

I.M.
● *Alert:* Parenteral form of drug is for I.M. administration only. Drug shouldn't be given I.V.

ACTION
Unknown. A tricyclic antidepressant that increases the amount of norepinephrine, serotonin, or both in the CNS by blocking their reuptake by the presynaptic neurons.

Route	Onset	Peak	Duration
P.O., I.M.	Unknown	2–12 hr	Unknown

Half-life: Not established, varies widely.

ADVERSE REACTIONS
CNS: *stroke, seizures, coma,* ataxia, tremor, peripheral neuropathy, anxiety, insomnia, restlessness, drowsiness, dizziness, weakness, fatigue, headache, extrapyramidal reactions, hallucinations, delusions, disorientation.
CV: *orthostatic hypotension, tachycardia, heart block, arrhythmias, MI,* ECG changes, hypertension, edema.
EENT: blurred vision, tinnitus, mydriasis, increased intraocular pressure.
GI: *dry mouth,* nausea, vomiting, anorexia, epigastric pain, diarrhea, constipation, paralytic ileus.
GU: urine retention, altered libido, impotence.
Hematologic: *agranulocytosis, thrombocytopenia, leukopenia,* eosinophilia.
Metabolic: *hypoglycemia,* hyperglycemia.
Skin: rash, urticaria, photosensitivity reactions, diaphoresis.
Other: hypersensitivity reactions.

INTERACTIONS
Drug-drug. *Barbiturates, CNS depressants:* May enhance CNS depression. Avoid using together.
Cimetidine, **fluoxetine, fluvoxamine,** *hormonal contraceptives,* **paroxetine, sertraline:** May increase tricyclic antidepressant level. Monitor drug levels and patient for signs of toxicity.
Clonidine: May cause life-threatening hypertension. Avoid using together.
Epinephrine, norepinephrine: May increase hypertensive effect. Use together cautiously.

MAO inhibitors: May cause severe excitation, hyperpyrexia, or seizures, usually with high doses. Avoid using within 14 days of MAO inhibitor therapy.

Quinolones: May increase the risk of life-threatening arrhythmias. Avoid using together.

Drug-herb. *Evening primrose:* May cause additive or synergistic effect, resulting in lower seizure threshold and increasing the risk of seizures. Discourage use together. *St. John's wort, SAM-e, yohimbe:* May cause serotonin syndrome and decrease amitriptyline level. Discourage use together.

Drug-lifestyle. *Alcohol use:* May enhance CNS depression. Discourage use together. *Smoking:* May lower drug level. Watch for lack of effect. *Sun exposure:* May increase risk of photosensitivity reactions. Advise patient to avoid excessive sunlight exposure.

EFFECTS ON LAB TEST RESULTS
● May increase or decrease glucose level.
● May increase eosinophil count and liver function test values. May decrease granulocyte, platelet, and WBC counts.

CONTRAINDICATIONS & CAUTIONS
● Contraindicated in patients hypersensitive to drug and in those who have received an MAO inhibitor within the past 14 days.
● Contraindicated during acute recovery phase of MI.
● Use cautiously in patients with history of seizures, urine retention, angle-closure glaucoma, or increased intraocular pressure; in those with hyperthyroidism, CV disease, diabetes, or impaired liver function; and in those receiving thyroid drugs.
● Use cautiously in those receiving electroconvulsive therapy.

NURSING CONSIDERATIONS
● *Alert:* Drug may increase the risk of suicidal thinking and behavior in children and adolescents with major depressive disorder or other psychiatric disorder. Don't use in children younger than age 12.
● *Alert:* Drug may increase the risk of suicidal thinking and behavior in young adults ages 18 to 24 during the first 2 months of treatment.

● Amitriptyline has strong anticholinergic effects and is one of the most sedating tricyclic antidepressants. Anticholinergic effects have rapid onset even though therapeutic effect is delayed for weeks.
● Elderly patients may have an increased sensitivity to anticholinergic effects of drug; sedating effects of drug may increase the risk of falls in this population.
● If signs or symptoms of psychosis occur or increase, expect prescriber to reduce dosage. Record mood changes. Monitor patient for suicidal tendencies and allow only minimum supply of drug.
● Because patients using tricyclic antidepressants may suffer hypertensive episodes during surgery, stop drug gradually several days before surgery.
● Monitor glucose level.
● Watch for nausea, headache, and malaise after abrupt withdrawal of long-term therapy; these symptoms don't indicate addiction.
● Don't withdraw drug abruptly.
● *Look alike–sound alike:* Don't confuse amitriptyline with nortriptyline or aminophylline.

PATIENT TEACHING
● Whenever possible, advise patient to take full dose at bedtime, but warn him of possible morning orthostatic hypotension.
● Tell patient to avoid alcohol during drug therapy.
● Advise patient to consult prescriber before taking other drugs.
● Warn patient to avoid activities that require alertness and good psychomotor coordination until CNS effects of drug are known. Drowsiness and dizziness usually subside after a few weeks.
● Inform patient that dry mouth may be relieved with sugarless hard candy or gum. Saliva substitutes may be useful.
● To prevent photosensitivity reactions, advise patient to use a sunblock, wear protective clothing, and avoid prolonged exposure to strong sunlight.
● Warn patient not to stop drug abruptly.
● Advise patient that it may take as long as 30 days to achieve full therapeutic effect.

aripiprazole
air-eh-PIP-rah-zole

Abilify, Abilify Discmelt

Pharmacologic class: quinolone
derivative
Pregnancy risk category C

AVAILABLE FORMS
Injection: 9.75 mg/1.3 ml (7.5 mg/ml)
single-dose vial
Oral solution: 1 mg/ml
Orally disintegrating tablets (ODTs):
10 mg, 15 mg, 20 mg, 30 mg
Tablets: 2 mg, 5 mg, 10 mg, 15 mg, 20 mg,
30 mg

INDICATIONS & DOSAGES
✴ *NEW INDICATION:* **Schizophrenia**
Adults: Initially, 10 to 15 mg P.O. daily;
increase to maximum daily dose of 30 mg
if needed, after at least 2 weeks.
Adolescents age 13 to 17: Initially, 2 mg
P.O. daily; increase to 5 mg after 2 days,
then to recommended dose of 10 mg in
2 more days. May titrate to maximum daily
dose of 30 mg in 5-mg increments.
Adjust-a-dose: When using with CYP3A4
inhibitors such as ketoconazole or
CYP2D6 inhibitors, such as quinidine,
fluoxetine, or paroxetine, give half the aripiprazole dose. When using with CYP3A4
inducers such as carbamazepine, double
the aripiprazole dose. Return to original
dosing after the other drugs are stopped.
➤ **Bipolar mania, including manic
and mixed episodes**
Adults: Initially, 30 mg P.O. once daily.
May reduce dose to 15 mg daily based on
patient tolerance. Safety of doses greater
than 30 mg daily and treatment lasting
beyond 6 weeks hasn't been established.
➤ **Agitation associated with
schizophrenia or bipolar 1 disorder, mixed or manic**
Adults: 5.25 to 15 mg by deep I.M. injection. Recommended dose is 9.75 mg. May
give a second dose after 2 hours, if needed.
Safety of giving more frequently than every 2 hours or a total daily dose more than
30 mg isn't known. Switch to oral form as
soon as possible.

ADMINISTRATION
P.O.
● Give drug without regard for food.
● Substitute the oral solution on a
milligram-by-milligram basis for the 5-,
10-, 15-, or 20-mg tablets, up to 25 mg.
Give patients taking 30-mg tablets 25 mg
of solution.
● Keep ODTs in blister package until
ready to use. Use dry hands to carefully
peel open the foil package and remove the
tablet. Don't split tablet.
● Store oral solution in refrigerator; it can
be used up to 6 months after opening.
I.M.
● Inject slowly and deep into the muscle
mass.
● Don't give I.V. or subcutaneously.

ACTION
Thought to exert partial agonist activity at
D2 and serotonin 1A receptors and antago-
nist activity at serotonin 2A receptors.

Route	Onset	Peak	Duration
P.O.	Unknown	3–5 hr	Unknown
I.M.	Unknown	1–3 hr	Unknown

Half-life: About 75 hours in patients with
normal metabolism; about 6 days in those
who can't metabolize the drug through
CYP2D6.

ADVERSE REACTIONS
CNS: *headache, anxiety, insomnia, light-
headedness, somnolence, akathisia, increased suicide risk, neuroleptic malignant syndrome, seizures, suicidal
thoughts,* tremor, asthenia, depression,
fatigue, dizziness, nervousness, hostility,
manic behavior, confusion, abnormal gait,
cogwheel rigidity, fever, tardive dyskinesia.
CV: peripheral edema, chest pain, hypertension, tachycardia, orthostatic hypotension, *bradycardia.*
EENT: rhinitis, blurred vision, increased
salivation, conjunctivitis, ear pain.
GI: *nausea, vomiting, constipation,*
anorexia, dry mouth, dyspepsia, diarrhea,
abdominal pain, esophageal dysmotility.
GU: urinary incontinence.
Hematologic: ecchymosis, anemia.

Metabolic: weight gain, weight loss, hyperglycemia, hypercholesterolemia.
Musculoskeletal: neck pain, neck stiffness, muscle cramps.
Respiratory: dyspnea, pneumonia, cough.
Skin: rash, dry skin, pruritus, sweating, ulcer.
Other: flulike syndrome.

INTERACTIONS
Drug-drug. *Antihypertensives:* May enhance antihypertensive effects. Monitor blood pressure.
Carbamazepine and other CYP3A4 inducers: May decrease levels and effectiveness of aripiprazole. Double the usual dose of aripiprazole, and monitor the patient closely.
Ketoconazole and other CYP3A4 inhibitors: May increase risk of serious toxic effects. Start treatment with half the usual dose of aripiprazole, and monitor patient closely.
Potential CYP2D6 inhibitors (fluoxetine, paroxetine, quinidine): May increase levels and toxicity of aripiprazole. Give half the usual dose of aripiprazole.
Drug-food. *Grapefruit juice:* May increase drug level. Tell patient not to take drug with grapefruit juice.
Drug-lifestyle. *Alcohol use:* May increase CNS effects. Discourage use together.

EFFECTS ON LAB TEST RESULTS
• May increase CK and glucose levels.

CONTRAINDICATIONS & CAUTIONS
• Contraindicated in patients hypersensitive to drug.
• Use cautiously in patients with CV disease, cerebrovascular disease, or conditions that could predispose the patient to hypotension, such as dehydration or hypovolemia.
• Use cautiously in patients with history of seizures or with conditions that lower the seizure threshold.
• Use cautiously in patients who engage in strenuous exercise, are exposed to extreme heat, take anticholinergics, or are susceptible to dehydration.
• Use cautiously in patients at risk for aspiration pneumonia, such as those with Alzheimer disease.

• Use cautiously in pregnant and breast-feeding women.

NURSING CONSIDERATIONS
• *Alert:* Neuroleptic malignant syndrome may occur. Monitor patient for hyperpyrexia, muscle rigidity, altered mental status, irregular pulse or blood pressure, tachycardia, diaphoresis, and cardiac dysrhythmias.
• If signs and symptoms of neuroleptic malignant syndrome occur, immediately stop drug and notify prescriber.
• Monitor patient for signs and symptoms of tardive dyskinesia. Elderly patients, especially women, are at highest risk of developing this adverse effect.
• *Alert:* Fatal cerebrovascular adverse events (stroke, transient ischemic attack) may occur in elderly patients with dementia. Drug isn't safe or effective in these patients.
• *Alert:* Hyperglycemia may occur. Monitor patient with diabetes regularly. Patient with risk factors for diabetes should undergo fasting blood glucose testing at baseline and periodically. Monitor all patients for symptoms of hyperglycemia including increased hunger, thirst, frequent urination, and weakness. Hyperglycemia may resolve when patient stops taking drug.
• *Alert:* Monitor patient for symptoms of metabolic syndrome (significant weight gain and increased body mass index, hypertension, hyperglycemia, hypercholesterolemia, and hypertriglyceridemia).
• Treat patient with the smallest dose for the shortest time and periodically reevaluate for need to continue.
• Give prescriptions only for small quantities of drug, to reduce risk of overdose.
• Don't give I.V. or subcutaneously.

PATIENT TEACHING
• Tell patient to use caution while driving or operating hazardous machinery because psychoactive drugs may impair judgment, thinking, or motor skills.
• Tell patient that drug may be taken without regard to meals.
• Advise patients that grapefruit juice may interact with aripiprazole and to limit or avoid its use.

Reactions may be *common*, uncommon, *life-threatening*, or COMMON AND LIFE-THREATENING.
Interaction may have a *rapid onset* or **delayed onset**.

• Advise patient that gradual improvement in symptoms should occur over several weeks rather than immediately.
• Tell patients to avoid alcohol use while taking drug.
• Advise patients to limit strenuous activity while taking drug to avoid dehydration.
• Tell patient to keep ODT in blister package until ready to use. Using dry hands, he should carefully peel open the foil backing and place tablet on the tongue. Tell him not to split tablet.
• Tell patient to store oral solution in refrigerator, and that the solution can be used for up to 6 months after opening.

---

aspirin
(acetylsalicylic acid, ASA)
ASS-pir-in

Aspergum ◊, Bayer ◊, Ecotrin ◊, Empirin ◊, Halfprin, Heartline ◊, Norwich ◊, Novasen† ◊, St Joseph's ◊, ZORprin ◊

Pharmacologic class: salicylate
Pregnancy risk category D

AVAILABLE FORMS
Chewing gum: 227.5 mg ◊
Suppositories: 120 mg ◊, 200 mg ◊, 300 mg ◊, 600 mg ◊
Tablets: 325 mg ◊, 500 mg ◊
Tablets (chewable): 81 mg ◊
Tablets (controlled-release): 800 mg
Tablets (enteric-coated): 81 mg ◊, 165 mg ◊, 325 mg ◊, 500 mg ◊, 650 mg ◊, 975 mg
Tablets (extended-release): 650 mg ◊

INDICATIONS & DOSAGES
➤ **Rheumatoid arthritis, osteoarthritis, or other polyarthritic or inflammatory conditions**
Adults: Initially, 2.4 to 3.6 g P.O. daily in divided doses. Maintenance dosage is 3.2 to 6 g P.O. daily in divided doses.
➤ **Juvenile rheumatoid arthritis**
Children who weigh more than 25 kg (55 lb): 2.4 to 3.6 g P.O. daily in divided doses.
Children who weigh 25 kg or less: 60 to 130 mg/kg daily P.O. in divided doses.

Increase by 10 mg/kg daily at no more than weekly intervals. Maintenance dosages usually range from 80 to 100 mg/kg daily; up to 130 mg/kg daily.
➤ **Mild pain or fever**
Adults and children older than age 11: 325 to 650 mg P.O. or P.R. every 4 hours p.r.n.
Children ages 2 to 11: 10 to 15 mg/kg/dose P.O. or P.R. every 4 hours up to 80 mg/kg daily.
➤ **To prevent thrombosis**
Adults: 1.3 g P.O. daily, divided b.i.d. to q.i.d.
➤ **To reduce risk of MI in patients with previous MI or unstable angina**
Adults: 75 to 325 mg P.O. daily.
➤ **Kawasaki syndrome (mucocutaneous lymph node syndrome)**
Children: 80 to 100 mg/kg P.O. daily, divided q.i.d. with immune globulin I.V. After the fever subsides, reduce dosage to 3 to 5 mg/kg once daily. Aspirin therapy usually continues for 6 to 8 weeks.
➤ **Acute rheumatic fever**
Adults: 5 to 8 g P.O. daily.
Children: 100 mg/kg daily P.O. for 2 weeks; then 75 mg/kg daily P.O. for 4 to 6 weeks.
➤ **To reduce risk of recurrent transient ischemic attacks and stroke or death in patients at risk**
Adults: 50 to 325 mg P.O. daily.
➤ **Acute ischemic stroke**
Adults: 160 to 325 mg P.O. daily, started within 48 hours of stroke onset and continued for up to 2 to 4 weeks.
➤ **Acute pericarditis after MI**
Adults: 160 to 325 mg P.O. daily. Higher doses (650 mg P.O. every 4 to 6 hours) may be needed.

ADMINISTRATION
P.O.
• For patient with swallowing difficulties, crush non–enteric-coated aspirin and dissolve in soft food or liquid. Give liquid immediately after mixing because drug will break down rapidly.
• Give drug with food, milk, antacid, or large glass of water to reduce GI effects.
• Give sustained-release or enteric-coated forms whole; don't crush or break these tablets.

Rectal
● Refrigerate suppositories.

ACTION
Thought to produce analgesia and exert its anti-inflammatory effect by inhibiting prostaglandin and other substances that sensitize pain receptors. Drug may relieve fever through central action in the hypothalamic heat-regulating center. In low doses, drug also appears to interfere with clotting by keeping a platelet-aggregating substance from forming.

Route	Onset	Peak	Duration
P.O. (buffered)	5–30 min	1–2 hr	1–4 hr
P.O. (enteric-coated)	5–30 min	Variable	1-4 hr
P.O. (extended-release)	5–30 min	1–4 hr	1–4 hr
P.O. (solution)	5–30 min	15–40 min	1–4 hr
P.O. (tablet)	5–30 min	25–40 min	1–4 hr
P.R.	Unknown	3–4 hr	Unknown

Half-life: 15 to 20 minutes.

ADVERSE REACTIONS
EENT: *tinnitus, hearing loss.*
GI: *nausea, **GI bleeding,** dyspepsia,* GI distress, occult bleeding.
Hematologic: *prolonged bleeding time, leukopenia, thrombocytopenia.*
Hepatic: *hepatitis.*
Skin: *rash,* bruising, urticaria.
Other: *angioedema, Reye syndrome,* hypersensitivity reactions.

INTERACTIONS
Drug-drug. *ACE inhibitors:* May decrease antihypertensive effects. Monitor blood pressure closely.
Ammonium chloride and other urine acidifiers: May increase levels of aspirin products. Watch for aspirin toxicity.
Antacids in high doses and other urine alkalinizers: May decrease levels of aspirin products. Watch for decreased aspirin effect.

Anticoagulants: May increase risk of bleeding. Use with extreme caution if must be used together.
Beta blockers: May decrease antihypertensive effect. Avoid long-term aspirin use if patient is taking antihypertensives.
Corticosteroids: May enhance salicylate elimination and decrease drug level. Watch for decreased aspirin effect.
Heparin: May increase risk of bleeding. Monitor coagulation studies and patient closely if used together.
Ibuprofen, other NSAIDs: May negate the antiplatelet effect of low-dose aspirin therapy. Patients using immediate-release aspirin (not enteric-coated) should take ibuprofen at least 30 minutes after or more than 8 hours before aspirin. Occasional use of ibuprofen is unlikely to have a negative effect.
Methotrexate: May increase risk of methotrexate toxicity. Avoid using together.
Nizatidine: May increase risk of salicylate toxicity in patients receiving high doses of aspirin. Monitor patient closely.
Oral antidiabetics: May increase hypoglycemic effect. Monitor patient closely.
Probenecid, sulfinpyrazone: May decrease uricosuric effect. Avoid using together.
Valproic acid: May increase valproic acid level. Avoid using together.
Drug-herb. *Dong quai, feverfew, ginkgo, horse chestnut, kelpware, red clover:* May increase risk of bleeding. Monitor patient closely for increased effects. Discourage use together.
White willow: May increase risk of adverse effects. Discourage use together.
Drug-food. *Caffeine:* May increase drug absorption. Watch for increased effects.
Drug-lifestyle. *Alcohol use:* May increase risk of GI bleeding. Discourage use together.

EFFECTS ON LAB TEST RESULTS
● May increase liver function test values. May decrease platelet and WBC counts.
● May falsely increase protein-bound iodine level. May interfere with urine glucose analysis with Diastix, Chemstrip uG, Clinitest, and Benedict solution; with urinary 5-hydroxyindoleacetic acid

and vanillylmandelic acid tests; and with Gerhardt test for urine acetoacetic acid.

CONTRAINDICATIONS & CAUTIONS

• Contraindicated in patients hypersensitive to drug and in those with NSAID-induced sensitivity reactions, G6PD deficiency, or bleeding disorders, such as hemophilia, von Willebrand disease, or telangiectasia.

• Use cautiously in patients with GI lesions, impaired renal function, hypoprothrombinemia, vitamin K deficiency, thrombocytopenia, thrombotic thrombocytopenic purpura, or severe hepatic impairment.

• *Alert:* Oral and rectal OTC products containing aspirin and nonaspirin salicylates shouldn't be given to children or teenagers who have or are recovering from chickenpox or flulike symptoms because of the risk of Reye syndrome.

NURSING CONSIDERATIONS

• For inflammatory conditions, rheumatic fever, and thrombosis, give aspirin on a schedule rather than as needed.

• Because enteric-coated and sustained-release tablets are slowly absorbed, they aren't suitable for rapid relief of acute pain, fever, or inflammation. They cause less GI bleeding and may be better suited for long-term therapy, such as for arthritis.

• For patients who can't tolerate oral drugs, ask prescriber about using aspirin rectal suppositories. Watch for rectal mucosal irritation or bleeding.

• Febrile, dehydrated children can develop toxicity rapidly.

• Monitor elderly patients closely because they may be more susceptible to aspirin's toxic effects.

• Monitor salicylate level. Therapeutic salicylate level for arthritis is 150 to 300 mcg/ml. Tinnitus may occur at levels above 200 mcg/ml, but this isn't a reliable indicator of toxicity, especially in very young patients and those older than age 60. With long-term therapy, severe toxic effects may occur with levels exceeding 400 mcg/ml.

• During prolonged therapy, assess hematocrit, hemoglobin level, PT, INR, and renal function periodically.

• Drug irreversibly inhibits platelet aggregation. Stop drug 5 to 7 days before elective surgery to allow time for production and release of new platelets.

• Monitor patient for hypersensitivity reactions, such as anaphylaxis and asthma.

• *Look alike–sound alike:* Don't confuse aspirin with Asendin or Afrin.

PATIENT TEACHING

• Tell patient who's allergic to tartrazine to avoid aspirin.

• Advise patient on a low-salt diet that 1 tablet of buffered aspirin contains 553 mg of sodium.

• Advise patient to take drug with food, milk, antacid, or large glass of water to reduce GI reactions.

• Tell patient not to crush or chew sustained-release or enteric-coated forms but to swallow them whole.

• Instruct patient to discard aspirin tablets that have a strong vinegar-like odor.

• Tell patient to consult prescriber if giving drug to children for longer than 5 days or adults for longer than 10 days.

• Advise patient receiving prolonged treatment with large doses of aspirin to watch for small, round, red pinprick spots, bleeding gums, and signs of GI bleeding, and to drink plenty of fluids. Encourage use of a soft-bristled toothbrush.

• Because of the many drug interactions with aspirin, warn patient taking prescription drugs to check with prescriber or pharmacist before taking aspirin or OTC products containing aspirin.

• Ibuprofen can interfere with the antiplatelet effect of low-dose aspirin therapy, negating its effect. Tell patient how to safely use ibuprofen in relation to aspirin therapy.

• Urge pregnant woman to avoid aspirin during last trimester of pregnancy unless specifically directed by prescriber.

• Drug is a leading cause of poisoning in children. Caution parents to keep drug out of reach of children. Encourage use of child-resistant containers.

---

atomoxetine hydrochloride
at-oh-MOX-ah-teen

Strattera

Pharmacologic class: selective
norepinephrine reuptake inhibitor
Pregnancy risk category C

AVAILABLE FORMS
Capsules: 10 mg, 18 mg, 25 mg, 40 mg,
60 mg, 80 mg, 100 mg

INDICATIONS & DOSAGES
➤ **Attention-deficit hyperactivity
disorder (ADHD)**
*Adults, children, and adolescents who
weigh more than 70 kg (154 lb):* Initially,
40 mg P.O. daily; increase after at least
3 days to a total of 80 mg/day P.O., as a
single dose in the morning or two evenly
divided doses in the morning and late
afternoon or early evening. After 2 to
4 weeks, increase total dose to a maximum
of 100 mg, if needed.
Children who weigh 70 kg or less: Initially,
0.5 mg/kg P.O. daily; increase after a
minimum of 3 days to a target total daily
dose of 1.2 mg/kg P.O. as a single dose
in the morning or two evenly divided
doses in the morning and late afternoon or
early evening. Don't exceed 1.4 mg/kg or
100 mg daily, whichever is less.
Adjust-a-dose: In patients with moderate
hepatic impairment, reduce to 50% of the
normal dose; in those with severe hepatic
impairment, reduce to 25% of the normal
dose. Poor metabolizers of CYP2D6 may
require a reduced dose. In children who
weigh less than 70 kg, adjust dosage to
0.5 mg/kg daily and increase to 1.2 mg/kg
daily if symptoms don't improve after
4 weeks and if first dose is tolerated. In
children and adults who weigh more than
70 kg, start at 40 mg daily and increase to
80 mg daily if symptoms don't improve
after 4 weeks and if first dose is tolerated.

ADMINISTRATION
P.O.
• Give drug without regard for meals.
• Capsules should be swallowed whole and
not opened.

ACTION
May be related to selective inhibition of
the presynaptic norepinephrine transporter.

Route	Onset	Peak	Duration
P.O.	Rapid	1–2 hr	Unknown

Half-life: 21½ hours.

ADVERSE REACTIONS
CNS: *headache, insomnia,* dizziness, somnolence, crying, irritability, mood swings,
pyrexia, fatigue, sedation, depression,
tremor, early-morning awakening, paresthesia, abnormal dreams, sleep disorder.
CV: orthostatic hypotension, tachycardia,
hypertension, palpitations, hot flashes.
EENT: ear infection, rhinorrhea, sore
throat, nasal congestion, nasopharyngitis,
sinus congestion, mydriasis, sinusitis.
GI: *abdominal pain, constipation,* dyspepsia, *nausea, vomiting, decreased appetite,*
gastroenteritis, *dry mouth,* flatulence.
GU: urinary retention, urinary hesitation,
ejaculatory problems, difficulty in micturi-
tion, dysmenorrhea, erectile disturbance,
impotence, delayed menses, menstrual
disorder, prostatitis.
Metabolic: weight loss.
Musculoskeletal: arthralgia, myalgia.
Respiratory: *cough,* upper respiratory
tract infection.
Skin: *dermatitis, pruritus, increased
sweating.*
Other: influenza, decreased libido, rigors.

INTERACTIONS
Drug-drug. *Albuterol:* May increase CV
effects. Use together cautiously.
MAO inhibitors: May cause hyperthermia,
rigidity, myoclonus, autonomic instability
with possible rapid fluctuations of vital
signs, and mental status changes. Avoid
use within 2 weeks of MAO inhibitor.
Pressor agents: May increase blood pressure. Use together cautiously.
*Strong CYP2D6 inhibitors (fluoxetine,
paroxetine, quinidine):* May increase atomoxetine level. Reduce first dose.

EFFECTS ON LAB TEST RESULTS
None reported.

Reactions may be *common,* uncommon, ***life-threatening,*** or COMMON AND LIFE-THREATENING.
Interaction may have a *rapid onset* or ***delayed onset.***

CONTRAINDICATIONS & CAUTIONS
• Contraindicated in patients hypersensitive to atomoxetine or to components of drug, in those who have taken an MAO inhibitor within the past 2 weeks, and in those with angle-closure glaucoma.
• Use cautiously in patients with hypertension, tachycardia, or CV or cerebrovascular disease, and in pregnant or breast-feeding women.
• Safety and efficacy haven't been established in patients younger than age 6.

NURSING CONSIDERATIONS
• Use drug as part of a total treatment program for ADHD, including psychological, educational, and social intervention.
• *Alert:* Monitor children and adolescents closely for worsening of condition, agitation, irritability, suicidal thinking or behaviors, and unusual changes in behavior, especially the first few months of therapy or when the dosage is increased or decreased.
• Patients taking drug for extended periods must be reevaluated periodically to determine drug's usefulness.
• Monitor growth during treatment. If growth or weight gain is unsatisfactory, consider interrupting therapy.
• *Alert:* Severe liver injury may occur and progress to liver failure. Notify prescriber of any sign of liver injury: yellowing of the skin or the sclera of the eyes, pruritus, dark urine, upper right-sided tenderness, or unexplained flulike syndrome.
• Monitor blood pressure and pulse at baseline, after each dose increase, and during treatment periodically.
• Monitor for urinary hesitancy or retention and sexual dysfunction.
• Patient can stop drug without tapering off.

PATIENT TEACHING
• *Alert:* Advise parents to call prescriber immediately about unusual behavior or suicidal thoughts.
• Tell pregnant women, women planning to become pregnant, and breast-feeding women to consult prescriber before taking atomoxetine.
• Tell patient to use caution when operating a vehicle or machinery until the effects of drug are known.

---

bupropion hydrochloride
byoo-PROE-pee-on

Budeprion SR, Wellbutrin, Wellbutrin SR, Wellbutrin XL, Zyban

Pharmacologic class: aminoketone
Pregnancy risk category B

AVAILABLE FORMS
Tablets (extended-release): 150 mg, 300 mg
Tablets (immediate-release): 75 mg, 100 mg
Tablets (sustained-release): 100 mg, 150 mg, 200 mg

INDICATIONS & DOSAGES
➤ **Seasonal affective disorder**
Adults: Start treatment in autumn before depressive symptoms appear. Initially, 150 mg extended-release P.O. once daily in the morning. After 1 week, increase to 300 mg once daily, if tolerated. Continue 300 mg daily during the autumn and winter and taper to 150 mg daily for 2 weeks before stopping the drug in the early spring.
➤ **Depression**
Adults: For immediate-release, initially, 100 mg P.O. b.i.d.; increase after 3 days to 100 mg P.O. t.i.d., if needed. If patient doesn't improve after several weeks of therapy, increase dosage to 150 mg t.i.d. No single dose should exceed 150 mg. Allow at least 6 hours between successive doses. Maximum dose is 450 mg daily. For sustained-release, initially, 150 mg P.O. every morning; increase to target dose of 150 mg P.O. b.i.d., as tolerated, as early as day 4 of dosing. Allow at least 8 hours between successive doses. Maximum dose is 400 mg daily. For extended-release, initially, 150 mg P.O. every morning; increase to target dosage of 300 mg P.O. daily, as tolerated, as early as day 4 of dosing. Allow at least 24 hours between successive doses. Maximum is 450 mg daily.

➤ **Aid to smoking-cessation treatment**

Adults: 150 mg Zyban P.O. daily for 3 days; increased to maximum of 300 mg daily in two divided doses at least 8 hours apart.

Adjust-a-dose: In patients with mild to moderate hepatic cirrhosis or renal impairment, reduce frequency and dose. In patients with severe hepatic cirrhosis, don't exceed 75 mg immediate-release P.O. daily, 100 mg sustained-release P.O. daily, 150 mg (sustained-release) P.O. every other day, or 150 mg extended-release P.O. every other day.

ADMINISTRATION
P.O.
- Don't crush or split tablets.
- When switching patients from regular or sustained-release tablets to extended-release tablets, give the same total daily dose (when possible) as the once-daily dosage provided.

ACTION
Unknown. Drug doesn't inhibit MAO, but it weakly inhibits norepinephrine, dopamine, and serotonin reuptake. Noradrenergic or dopaminergic mechanisms, or both, may cause drug's effect.

Route	Onset	Peak	Duration
P.O. (extended-release)	Unknown	5 hr	Unknown
P.O. (immediate-release)	Unknown	2 hr	Unknown
P.O. (sustained-release)	Unknown	3 hr	Unknown

Half-life: 8 to 24 hours.

ADVERSE REACTIONS
CNS: *abnormal dreams, insomnia, headache, sedation, tremor, agitation, dizziness, seizures, suicidal behavior,* anxiety, confusion, delusions, euphoria, fever, hostility, impaired concentration, impaired sleep quality, akinesia, akathisia, fatigue, syncope.

CV: *tachycardia, arrhythmias,* hypertension, hypotension, palpitations, chest pain.

EENT: *blurred vision, rhinitis,* auditory disturbances, epistaxis, pharyngitis, sinusitis.

GI: *constipation, nausea, vomiting, anorexia, dry mouth,* taste disturbance, dyspepsia, diarrhea, abdominal pain.

GU: impotence, menstrual complaints, urinary frequency, urine retention.

Metabolic: increased appetite, *weight loss, weight gain.*

Musculoskeletal: arthritis, myalgia, arthralgia, muscle spasm or twitch.

Respiratory: upper respiratory complaints, increase in coughing.

Skin: *excessive sweating,* pruritus, rash, cutaneous temperature disturbance, urticaria.

Other: fever and chills, decreased libido, accidental injury.

INTERACTIONS
Drug-drug. *Amantadine, levodopa:* May increase risk of adverse reactions. If used together, give small first doses of bupropion and increase dosage gradually.
Antidepressants, antipsychotics, systemic corticosteroids, theophylline: May lower seizure threshold. Use cautiously together.
Beta blockers, class IC antiarrhythmics: May increase levels of these drugs and adverse reactions. Use a reduced dose if used with bupropion.
Carbamazepine, phenobarbital, phenytoin: May enhance metabolism of bupropion and decrease its effect. Monitor patient closely.
MAO inhibitors: May increase the risk of bupropion toxicity. Don't use drugs within 14 days of each other.
Nicotine replacement agents: May cause hypertension. Monitor blood pressure.
Ritonavir: May increase bupropion level. Monitor patient closely for adverse reactions.
Drug-lifestyle. *Alcohol use:* May alter seizure threshold. Discourage use together.
Sun exposure: May increase risk of photosensitivity reactions. Advise patient to avoid excessive sunlight exposure.

EFFECTS ON LAB TEST RESULTS
• May increase liver function test values.

CONTRAINDICATIONS & CAUTIONS
• Contraindicated in patients hypersensitive to drug, in those who have taken MAO inhibitors within previous 14 days, and in those with seizure disorders or history of bulimia or anorexia nervosa because of a higher risk of seizures.
• Contraindicated in patients abruptly stopping use of alcohol or sedatives (including benzodiazepines).
• Don't use with other drugs containing bupropion.
• Use cautiously in patients with recent history of MI, unstable heart disease, renal or hepatic impairment, a history of seizures, head trauma, or other predisposition to seizures, and in those being treated with drugs that lower seizure threshold.

NURSING CONSIDERATIONS
• Many patients experience a period of increased restlessness, including agitation, insomnia, and anxiety, especially at start of therapy.
• *Alert:* To minimize the risk of seizures, don't exceed maximum recommended dose.
• *Alert:* Patient with major depressive disorder may experience a worsening of depression and suicidal thoughts. Carefully monitor patient for worsening depression or suicidal thoughts, especially at the beginning of therapy and during dosage changes.
• *Alert:* Drug may increase the risk of suicidal thinking and behavior in children and adolescents with major depressive disorder or other psychiatric disorder.
• *Alert:* Drug may increase the risk of suicidal thinking and behavior in young adults ages 18 to 24 during the first 2 months of treatment.
• Closely monitor patient with history of bipolar disorder. Antidepressants can cause manic episodes during the depressed phase of bipolar disorder. This may be less likely to occur with bupropion than with other antidepressants.
• Begin smoking-cessation treatment while patient is still smoking; about 1 week is needed to achieve steady-state drug levels.

• Stop smoking-cessation treatment if patient hasn't progressed toward abstinence by week 7. Treatment usually lasts up to 12 weeks. Patient can stop taking drug without tapering off.
• *Look alike–sound alike:* Don't confuse bupropion with buspirone or Wellbutrin with Wellcovorin.

PATIENT TEACHING
• *Alert:* Explain that excessive use of alcohol, abrupt withdrawal from alcohol or other sedatives, and addiction to cocaine, opiates, or stimulants during therapy may increase risk of seizures. Seizure risk is also increased in those using OTC stimulants, in anorectics, and in diabetic patients using oral antidiabetics or insulin.
• Tell patient not to chew, crush, or divide tablets.
• Advise patient to consult prescriber before taking other prescription or OTC drugs.
• Advise patient to avoid hazardous activities that require alertness and good psychomotor coordination until effects of drug are known.
• *Alert:* Advise patient that Zyban and Wellbutrin contain the same active ingredient and shouldn't be used together.
• Tell patient that it may take 4 weeks to reach full antidepressant effect.
• *Alert:* Advise patient to report mood swings or suicidal thoughts immediately.
• Inform patient that tablets may have an odor.

buspirone hydrochloride
byoo-SPYE-rone

BuSpar

Pharmacologic class: azaspirodecanedione derivative
Pregnancy risk category B

AVAILABLE FORMS
Tablets: 5 mg, 10 mg, 15 mg, 30 mg

INDICATIONS & DOSAGES
➤ **Anxiety disorders**
Adults: Initially, 7.5 mg P.O. b.i.d. Increase dosage by 5 mg daily at 2- to 3-day

intervals. Usual maintenance dosage is 20 to 30 mg daily in divided doses. Don't exceed 60 mg daily.

ADMINISTRATION
P.O.
• Don't give drug with grapefruit juice.
• Give drug at the same times each day, and always with or always without food.

ACTION
May inhibit neuronal firing and reduce serotonin turnover in cortical, amygdaloid, and septohippocampal tissue.

Route	Onset	Peak	Duration
P.O.	Unknown	40–90 min	Unknown

Half-life: 2 to 3 hours.

ADVERSE REACTIONS
CNS: *dizziness, drowsiness, headache,* nervousness, insomnia, light-headedness, fatigue, numbness.
CV: tachycardia, nonspecific chest pain.
EENT: blurred vision.
GI: dry mouth, nausea, diarrhea, abdominal distress.

INTERACTIONS
Drug-drug. *Azole antifungals:* May inhibit first-pass metabolism of buspirone. Monitor patient closely for adverse effects; adjust dosage as needed.
CNS depressants: May increase CNS depression. Use together cautiously.
Drugs metabolized by CYP3A4 (erythromycin, nefazodone): May increase buspirone level. Monitor patient; decrease buspirone dosage and adjust carefully.
MAO inhibitors: May elevate blood pressure. Avoid using together.
Drug-food. *Grapefruit juice:* May increase drug level, increasing adverse effects. Give with liquid other than grapefruit juice.
Drug-lifestyle. *Alcohol use:* May increase CNS depression. Discourage use together.

EFFECTS ON LAB TEST RESULTS
None reported.

CONTRAINDICATIONS & CAUTIONS
• Contraindicated in patients hypersensitive to drug and within 14 days of MAO inhibitor therapy.
• Drug isn't recommended for patients with severe hepatic or renal impairment.

NURSING CONSIDERATIONS
• Monitor patient closely for adverse CNS reactions. Drug is less sedating than other anxiolytics, but CNS effects may be unpredictable.
• *Alert:* Before starting therapy, don't stop a previous benzodiazepine regimen abruptly because a withdrawal reaction may occur.
• Drug shows no potential for abuse and isn't classified as a controlled substance.
• *Look alike–sound alike:* Don't confuse buspirone with bupropion.

PATIENT TEACHING
• Warn patient to avoid hazardous activities that require alertness and good coordination until effects of drug are known.
• Remind patient that drug effects may not be noticeable for several weeks.
• Warn patient not to abruptly stop a benzodiazepine because of risk of withdrawal symptoms.
• Tell patient to avoid use of alcohol during therapy.

---

carbamazepine
kar-ba-MAZ-e-peen

Carbatrol, Epitol, Equetro, Novo-Carbamaz†, Tegretol, Tegretol CR†, Tegretol-XR, Teril

Pharmacologic class: iminostilbene derivative
Pregnancy risk category D

AVAILABLE FORMS
Capsules (extended-release): 100 mg, 200 mg, 300 mg
Oral suspension: 100 mg/5 ml
Tablets: 200 mg
Tablets (chewable): 100 mg, 200 mg
Tablets (extended-release): 100 mg, 200 mg, 300 mg, 400 mg†

INDICATIONS & DOSAGES
➤ **Generalized tonic-clonic and complex partial seizures, mixed seizure patterns**
Adults and children older than age 12:
Initially, 200 mg P.O. b.i.d. (conventional or extended-release tablets), or 100 mg P.O. q.i.d. of suspension with meals. May be increased weekly by 200 mg P.O. daily in divided doses at 12-hour intervals for extended-release tablets or 6- to 8-hour intervals for conventional tablets or suspension, adjusted to minimum effective level. Maximum, 1,000 mg daily in children ages 12 to 15, and 1,200 mg daily in patients older than age 15. Usual maintenance dosage is 800 to 1,200 mg daily.
Children ages 6 to 12: Initially, 100 mg P.O. b.i.d. (conventional or extended-release tablets) or 50 mg of suspension P.O. q.i.d. with meals, increased at weekly intervals by up to 100 mg P.O. divided in three to four doses daily (divided b.i.d. for extended-release form). Maximum, 1,000 mg daily. Usual maintenance dosage is 400 to 800 mg daily; or, 20 to 30 mg/kg in divided doses three to four times daily.
Children younger than age 6: 10 to 20 mg/kg in two to three divided doses (conventional tablets) or four divided doses (suspension). Maximum dosage is 35 mg/kg in 24 hours.
➤ **Acute manic and mixed episodes associated with bipolar I disorder**
Adults: Initially, 200 mg Equetro P.O. b.i.d. Increase by 200 mg daily to achieve therapeutic response. Doses higher than 1,600 mg daily haven't been studied.
➤ **Trigeminal neuralgia**
Adults: Initially, 100 mg P.O. b.i.d. (conventional or extended-release tablets) or 50 mg of suspension q.i.d. with meals, increased by 100 mg every 12 hours for tablets or 50 mg of suspension q.i.d. until pain is relieved. Maximum, 1,200 mg daily. Maintenance dosage is usually 200 to 400 mg P.O. b.i.d.
➤ **Restless legs syndrome ♦**
Adults: 100 to 300 mg P.O. at bedtime.
➤ **Nonneuritic pain syndromes (painful neuromas, phantom limb pain) ♦**

Adults: Initially, 100 mg P.O. b.i.d. Maintenance dose is 600 to 1,400 mg daily.

ADMINISTRATION
P.O.
● Shake oral suspension well before measuring dose.
● Contents of extended-release capsules may be sprinkled over applesauce if patient has difficulty swallowing capsules. Capsules and tablets shouldn't be crushed or chewed, unless labeled as chewable form.
● When giving by nasogastric tube, mix dose with an equal volume of water, normal saline solution, or D_5W. Flush tube with 100 ml of diluent after giving dose.
● Don't crush or split extended-release form or give broken or chipped tablets.

ACTION
Thought to stabilize neuronal membranes and limit seizure activity by either increasing efflux or decreasing influx of sodium ions across cell membranes in the motor cortex during generation of nerve impulses.

Route	Onset	Peak	Duration
P.O.	Unknown	1½–12 hr	Unknown
P.O. (extended-release)	Unknown	4–8 hr	Unknown

Half-life: 25 to 65 hours with single dose; 8 to 29 hours with long-term use.

ADVERSE REACTIONS
CNS: *ataxia, dizziness, drowsiness, vertigo, **worsening of seizures,** confusion, fatigue, fever, headache, syncope.
CV: *arrhythmias, AV block, heart failure,* aggravation of coronary artery disease, hypertension, hypotension.
EENT: blurred vision, conjunctivitis, diplopia, dry pharynx, nystagmus.
GI: *nausea, vomiting,* abdominal pain, anorexia, diarrhea, dry mouth, glossitis, stomatitis.
GU: albuminuria, glycosuria, impotence, urinary frequency, urine retention.
Hematologic: *agranulocytosis, aplastic anemia, thrombocytopenia,* eosinophilia, leukocytosis.
Hepatic: *hepatitis.*
Metabolic: hyponatremia, SIADH.

Respiratory: pulmonary hypersensitivity.
Skin: *erythema multiforme, Stevens-Johnson syndrome,* excessive diaphoresis, rash, urticaria.
Other: chills.

INTERACTIONS
Drug-drug. *Atracurium, cisatracurium, pancuronium, rocuronium, vecuronium:* May decrease the effects of nondepolarizing muscle relaxant, causing it to be less effective. May need to increase the dose of the nondepolarizing muscle relaxant.
Cimetidine, danazol, diltiazem, fluoxetine, fluvoxamine, isoniazid, macrolides, propoxyphene, valproic acid, verapamil: May increase carbamazepine level. Use together cautiously.
Clarithromycin, erythromycin, troleandomycin: May inhibit metabolism of carbamazepine, increasing carbamazepine level and risk of toxicity. Avoid using together.
Doxycycline, felbamate, haloperidol, hormonal contraceptives, phenytoin, theophylline, tiagabine, topiramate, valproate, warfarin: May decrease levels of these drugs. Watch for decreased effect.
Lamotrigine: May decrease lamotrigine level and increase carbamazepine level. Monitor patient for clinical effects and toxicity.
Lithium: May increase CNS toxicity of lithium. Avoid using together.
MAO inhibitors: May increase depressant and anticholinergic effects. Avoid using together.
Phenobarbital, phenytoin, primidone: May decrease carbamazepine level. Watch for decreased effect.
Nefazodone: May increase carbamazepine levels and toxicity while reducing nefazodone levels and therapeutic benefits. Use together is contraindicated.
Drug-herb. *Plantains (psyllium seed):* May inhibit GI absorption of drug. Discourage use together.

EFFECTS ON LAB TEST RESULTS
• May increase BUN level. May decrease hemoglobin level and hematocrit.
• May increase liver function test values and eosinophil and WBC counts. May decrease thyroid function test values and granulocyte and platelet counts.
• May cause false pregnancy test results.

CONTRAINDICATIONS & CAUTIONS
• Contraindicated in patients hypersensitive to this drug or tricyclic antidepressants and in those with a history of bone marrow suppression; also contraindicated in those who have taken an MAO inhibitor within 14 days.
• Use cautiously in patients with mixed seizure disorders because they may experience an increased risk of seizures. Also, use with caution in patients with hepatic dysfunction.

NURSING CONSIDERATIONS
• Watch for worsening of seizures, especially in patients with mixed seizure disorders, including atypical absence seizures.
• Obtain baseline determinations of urinalysis, BUN and iron levels, liver function, CBC, and platelet and reticulocyte counts. Monitor these values periodically thereafter.
• Never stop drug suddenly when treating seizures. Notify prescriber immediately if adverse reactions occur.
• Adverse reactions may be minimized by gradually increasing dosage.
• Therapeutic level is 4 to 12 mcg/ml. Monitor level and effects closely. Ask patient when last dose was taken to better evaluate drug level.
• When managing seizures, take appropriate precautions.
• *Alert:* Watch for signs of anorexia or subtle appetite changes, which may indicate excessive drug level.
• *Look alike–sound alike:* Don't confuse Tegretol or Tegretol-XR with Topamax, Toprol-XL, or Toradol. Don't confuse Carbatrol with carvedilol.

PATIENT TEACHING
• Instruct patient to take drug with food to minimize GI distress. Tell patient taking suspension form to shake container well before measuring dose.
• Tell patient not to crush or chew extended-release form and not to take broken or chipped tablets.

• Tell patient that Tegretol-XR tablet coating may appear in stool because it isn't absorbed.

• Advise patient to keep tablets in the original container and to keep the container tightly closed and away from moisture. Some formulations may harden when exposed to excessive moisture, so that less is available in the body, decreasing seizure control.

• Inform patient that when drug is used for trigeminal neuralgia, an attempt to decrease dosage or withdraw drug is usually made every 3 months.

• Advise patient to notify prescriber immediately if fever, sore throat, mouth ulcers, or easy bruising or bleeding occurs.

• Tell patient that drug may cause mild to moderate dizziness and drowsiness when first taken. Advise him to avoid hazardous activities until effects disappear, usually within 3 to 4 days.

• Advise patient that periodic eye examinations are recommended.

• Advise woman of risks to fetus if pregnancy occurs while taking carbamazepine.

• Advise woman that breast-feeding isn't recommended during therapy.

SAFETY ALERT!

chloral hydrate
KLOR-al HYE-drate

Aquachloral Supprettes, Somnote

Pharmacologic class: CNS depressant
Pregnancy risk category C
Controlled substance schedule IV

AVAILABLE FORMS
Capsules: 500 mg
Suppositories: 325 mg, 500 mg, 650 mg
Syrup: 250 mg/5 ml, 500 mg/5 ml

INDICATIONS & DOSAGES
➤ **Sedation**
Adults: 250 mg P.O. or P.R. t.i.d. after meals. Maximum single or daily dose is 2 g.

Children: 8 mg/kg P.O. t.i.d. Maximum dosage is 500 mg t.i.d.
➤ **Insomnia**
Adults: 500 mg to 1 g P.O. or P.R. 15 to 30 minutes before bedtime. Maximum daily dose is 2 g.
Children: 50 mg/kg P.O. or P.R. 15 to 30 minutes before bedtime. Maximum single dose is 1 g.
➤ **Preoperatively to produce sedation and relieve anxiety**
Adults: 500 mg to 1 g P.O. or P.R. 30 minutes before surgery.
➤ **Alcohol withdrawal**
Adults: 500 mg to 1 g P.R. every 6 hours p.r.n.
➤ **Premedication for EEG**
Children: 20 to 25 mg/kg P.O. or P.R. up to 500 mg/single dose. May give divided doses.

ADMINISTRATION
P.O.
• Give drug after meals.
• Give capsule with full glass of water or juice, and have patient swallow capsule whole.
• To minimize unpleasant taste and stomach irritation, dilute syrup or give with liquid such as $1/2$ glass water, fruit juice, or ginger ale.
• Store capsules or liquid in dark container.
Rectal
• Refrigerate suppositories at least 2 hours before intended use.
• Store suppositories in refrigerator.

ACTION
Unknown. Sedative effects may be caused by drug's main metabolite, trichloroethanol.

Route	Onset	Peak	Duration
P.O.	30 min	Unknown	4–8 hr
P.R.	Unknown	Unknown	4–8 hr

Half-life: 8 to 10 hours for trichloroethanol.

ADVERSE REACTIONS
CNS: drowsiness, nightmares, dizziness, ataxia, paradoxical excitement, hangover, somnolence, disorientation, delirium, light-headedness, hallucinations,

confusion, somnambulism, vertigo, malaise, physical and psychological dependence.
GI: *nausea, vomiting, diarrhea,* flatulence.
Hematologic: eosinophilia, *leukopenia.*
Other: hypersensitivity reactions.

INTERACTIONS
Drug-drug. *CNS depressants including opioid analgesics:* May cause excessive CNS depression or vasodilation reaction. Use together cautiously.
Furosemide I.V: May cause sweating, flushes, variable blood pressure, nausea, and uneasiness. Use together cautiously or use a different hypnotic drug.
Oral anticoagulants: May increase risk of bleeding. Monitor patient closely.
Phenytoin: May decrease phenytoin level. Monitor patient closely.
Drug-lifestyle. *Alcohol use:* May react synergistically, increasing CNS depression, or, rarely, may produce a disulfiram-like reaction. Strongly discourage alcohol use with these drugs.

EFFECTS ON LAB TEST RESULTS
● May increase eosinophil count. May decrease WBC count.
● May cause false-positive results in urine glucose tests that use cupric sulfate, such as Benedict's reagent, and in phentolamine tests.

CONTRAINDICATIONS & CAUTIONS
● Contraindicated in patients hypersensitive to drug and in those with hepatic or renal impairment.
● Oral administration is contraindicated in patients with gastric disorders.
● Use with caution in patients with severe cardiac disease.
● Use cautiously in patients with mental depression, suicidal tendencies, or history of drug abuse.
● Some products may contain tartrazine; use cautiously in patients with aspirin sensitivity.

NURSING CONSIDERATIONS
● *Alert:* Note two strengths of oral liquid form. Double-check dose, especially when giving to children. Fatal overdoses have occurred.

● Take precautions to prevent hoarding or overdosing by patients who are depressed, suicidal, or drug dependent or who have history of drug abuse.
● Long-term use isn't recommended; drug loses its effectiveness in promoting sleep after 14 days of continued use. Long-term use may cause drug dependence, and patient may experience withdrawal symptoms if drug is suddenly stopped.
● Monitor BUN level; large doses may raise BUN level.
● Don't give drug for 48 hours before fluorometric test.

PATIENT TEACHING
● Instruct patient to take capsule with a full glass of water or juice and to swallow capsule whole.
● Tell patient to avoid alcohol during drug therapy.
● Caution patient to avoid performing activities that require mental alertness or physical coordination.
● Advise patient to store drug in dark container and to store suppositories in refrigerator.

SAFETY ALERT!

chlordiazepoxide hydrochloride
klor-dye-az-e-POX-ide

Librium

Pharmacologic class: benzodiazepine
Pregnancy risk category D
Controlled substance schedule IV

AVAILABLE FORMS
Capsules: 5 mg, 10 mg, 25 mg
Powder for injection: 100-mg ampule

INDICATIONS & DOSAGES
➤ **Mild to moderate anxiety**
Adults: 5 to 10 mg P.O. t.i.d. or q.i.d.
Children older than age 6: 5 mg P.O. b.i.d. to q.i.d. Maximum, 10 mg P.O. b.i.d. or t.i.d.

➤ **Severe anxiety**
Adults: 20 to 25 mg P.O. t.i.d. or q.i.d.
Elderly patients: 5 mg P.O. b.i.d. to q.i.d.
Adjust-a-dose: For debilitated patients,
5 mg P.O. b.i.d. to q.i.d.
➤ **Withdrawal symptoms of acute alcoholism**
Adults: 50 to 100 mg P.O., I.V., or I.M. Repeat in 2 to 4 hours, as needed. Maximum, 300 mg daily.
➤ **Preoperative apprehension and anxiety**
Adults: 5 to 10 mg P.O. t.i.d. or q.i.d. on day before surgery; or 50 to 100 mg I.M. 1 hour before surgery.

ADMINISTRATION
P.O.
● *Alert:* 5-mg and 25-mg capsules may look similar in color through the packaging. Verify contents and read label carefully.
I.V.
● Parenteral form isn't recommended for children younger than age 12.
● Make sure equipment and staff needed for emergency airway management are available. Monitor respirations every 5 to 15 minutes and before each I.V. dose.
● Keep powder refrigerated and away from light; mix just before use and discard remainder.
● Injectable form comes in two ampules—diluent and powdered drug. Read directions carefully.
● Don't give prepackaged diluent I.V. because air bubbles may form.
● Use 5 ml of normal saline solution or sterile water for injection as diluent for an ampule containing 100 mg of drug.
● Give over 1 minute.
● **Incompatibilities:** Other I.V. drugs.
I.M.
● For I.M. use, add 2 ml of diluent to powder and agitate gently until clear. Don't use the supplied diluent for I.V. use. Use immediately.
● I.M. form may be absorbed erratically.

ACTION
A benzodiazepine that may potentiate the effects of GABA, depress the CNS, and suppress the spread of seizure activity.

Route	Onset	Peak	Duration
P.O.	Unknown	½–4 hr	Unknown
I.V.	1–5 min	Unknown	15–60 min
I.M.	Unknown	Unknown	Unknown

Half-life: 5 to 30 hours.

ADVERSE REACTIONS
CNS: *drowsiness, lethargy,* ataxia, confusion, extrapyramidal reactions, minor changes in EEG patterns.
CV: edema.
GI: nausea, constipation.
GU: menstrual irregularities.
Hematologic: *agranulocytosis.*
Hepatic: jaundice.
Skin: *swelling and pain at injection site,* skin eruptions.
Other: altered libido.

INTERACTIONS
Drug-drug. *Cimetidine:* May decrease chlordiazepoxide clearance and increase risk of adverse reactions. Monitor patient carefully.
CNS depressants: May increase CNS depression. Use together cautiously.
Digoxin: May increase digoxin level and risk of toxicity. Monitor patient and digoxin level closely.
Disulfiram: May decrease clearance and increase half-life of chlordiazepoxide. Monitor patient for enhanced effects. Consider dosage adjustment.
Fluconazole, itraconazole, ketoconazole, miconazole: May increase and prolong chlordiazepoxide levels, CNS depression, and psychomotor impairment. Avoid using together.
Levodopa: May decrease control of parkinsonian symptoms in patients with Parkinson disease. Use together cautiously.
Drug-herb. *Kava:* May increase sedation. Discourage use together.
Drug-lifestyle. *Alcohol use:* May cause additive CNS effects. Discourage use together.
Smoking: May decrease effectiveness of drug. Monitor patient closely.

EFFECTS ON LAB TEST RESULTS
● May increase liver function test values. May decrease granulocyte count.

• May cause a false-positive pregnancy test result. May alter urinary 17-ketosteroid (Zimmerman reaction), urine alkaloid (Frings thin-layer chromatography method), and urinary glucose determinations (with Chemstrip uG and Diastix).

CONTRAINDICATIONS & CAUTIONS
• Contraindicated in patients hypersensitive to drug and in pregnant women, especially in first trimester.
• Use cautiously in patients with mental depression, porphyria, or hepatic or renal disease.

NURSING CONSIDERATIONS
• In patients receiving repeated or prolonged therapy, monitor hepatic, renal, and hematopoietic function periodically.
• *Alert:* Use of this drug may lead to abuse and addiction. Don't withdraw drug abruptly after long-term use because withdrawal symptoms may occur.

PATIENT TEACHING
• Warn patient to avoid hazardous activities that require alertness and coordination until effects of drug are known.
• Tell patient to avoid use of alcohol while taking drug.
• Notify patient that smoking may decrease drug's effectiveness.
• Warn patient not to abruptly stop the drug because withdrawal symptoms may occur.
• Warn woman to avoid use during pregnancy.

---

chlorpromazine hydrochloride
klor-PROE-ma-zeen

Thorazine

Pharmacologic class: phenothiazine
Pregnancy risk category C

AVAILABLE FORMS
Capsules (extended-release): 200 mg, 300 mg
Injection: 25 mg/ml
Oral concentrate: 30 mg/ml, 100 mg/ml
Suppositories: 25 mg, 100 mg
Syrup: 10 mg/5 ml

Tablets: 10 mg, 25 mg, 50 mg, 100 mg, 200 mg

INDICATIONS & DOSAGES
➤ **Psychosis, mania**
Adults: For hospitalized patients with acute disease, 25 mg I.M.; may give an additional 25 to 50 mg I.M. in 1 hour if needed. Increase over several days to 400 mg every 4 to 6 hours. Switch to oral therapy as soon as possible. Or, 25 mg P.O. t.i.d. initially; then gradually increase to 400 mg daily in divided doses. For outpatients, 30 to 75 mg daily in two to four divided doses. Increase dosage by 20 to 50 mg twice weekly until symptoms are controlled.
Children age 6 months and older: 0.55 mg/kg P.O. every 4 to 6 hours or I.M. every 6 to 8 hours. Or, 1.1 mg/kg P.R. every 6 to 8 hours. Maximum I.M. dose in children younger than age 5 or who weigh less than 22.7 kg (50 lb) is 40 mg. Maximum I.M. dose in children ages 5 to 12 or who weigh 22.7 to 45.4 kg (50 to 100 lb) is 75 mg.
➤ **Nausea and vomiting**
Adults: 10 to 25 mg P.O. every 4 to 6 hours, p.r.n. Or, 50 to 100 mg P.R. every 6 to 8 hours, p.r.n. Or, 25 mg I.M. initially. If no hypotension occurs, 25 to 50 mg I.M. every 3 to 4 hours may be given, p.r.n., until vomiting stops.
Children age 6 months and older: 0.55 mg/kg P.O. every 4 to 6 hours or I.M. every 6 to 8 hours. Or, 1.1 mg/kg P.R. every 6 to 8 hours. Maximum I.M. dose in children younger than age 5 or who weigh less than 22.7 kg (50 lb) is 40 mg. Maximum I.M. dose in children ages 5 to 12 or who weigh 22.7 to 45.4 kg (50 to 100 lb) is 75 mg.
➤ **Acute intermittent porphyria, intractable hiccups**
Adults: 25 to 50 mg P.O. t.i.d. or q.i.d. If symptoms persist for 2 to 3 days, 25 to 50 mg I.M. For hiccups, if symptoms still persist, 25 to 50 mg diluted in 500 to 1,000 ml of normal saline solution and infused slowly with patient in supine position.
➤ **Tetanus**
Adults: 25 to 50 mg I.V. or I.M. t.i.d. or q.i.d.

Reactions may be *common,* uncommon, *life-threatening,* or COMMON AND LIFE-THREATENING.
Interaction may have a *rapid onset* or *delayed onset.*

Children age 6 months and older:
0.55 mg/kg I.M. or I.V. every 6 to 8 hours.
Maximum parenteral dosage in children
who weigh less than 22.7 kg (50 lb) is
40 mg daily; for children who weigh 22.7
to 45.4 kg (50 to 100 lb), 75 mg, except
in severe cases. If giving I.V., dilute to
1 mg/ml with normal saline and give at a
rate of 0.5 mg/minute.

➤ **Surgery**
Adults: Preoperatively, 25 to 50 mg P.O.
2 to 3 hours before surgery or 12.5 to
25 mg I.M. 1 to 2 hours before surgery;
during surgery, 12.5 mg I.M., repeated
in 30 minutes, if needed, or fractional
2-mg doses I.V. at 2-minute intervals to
maximum dose of 25 mg; postoperatively,
10 to 25 mg P.O. every 4 to 6 hours or
12.5 to 25 mg I.M., repeated in 1 hour, if
needed.
Children age 6 months and older: Preoperatively, 0.55 mg/kg P.O. 2 to 3 hours
before surgery or I.M. 1 to 2 hours before
surgery. During surgery, 0.275 mg/kg
I.M., repeated in 30 minutes if needed,
or fractional 1-mg doses I.V. at 2-minute
intervals to maximum of 0.275 mg/kg.
May repeat fractional I.V. regimen in
30 minutes if needed. Postoperatively,
0.55 mg/kg P.O. or I.M. every 4 to 6 hours
(oral dose) or 1 hour (I.M. dose), if needed
and if hypotension doesn't occur.
Elderly patients: Lower dosages are sufficient; dosage increments should be more
gradual than in adults.

ADMINISTRATION
P.O.
● Wear gloves when preparing solutions
and avoid contact with skin and clothing. Oral liquid forms can cause contact
dermatitis.
● Slight yellowing of concentrate is common and doesn't affect potency. Discard
markedly discolored solutions.
● Protect liquid concentrate from light.
Dilute with fruit juice, milk, or semisolid
food just before giving.
● Don't crush or break extended-release
capsules.
I.V.
● Wear gloves when preparing solutions
and avoid contact with skin and cloth-

ing. Parenteral forms can cause contact
dermatitis.
● Drug is compatible with most common
I.V. solutions, including D_5W, Ringer's
injection, lactated Ringer's injection, and
normal saline solution for injection.
● For direct injection, dilute with normal
saline solution for injection and give into
a large vein or through the tubing of a
free-flowing I.V. solution.
● Don't exceed 1 mg/minute for adults or
0.5 mg/minute for children.
● For intermittent infusion, dilute with 50
or 100 ml of a compatible solution.
● Infuse over 30 minutes.
● **Incompatibilities:** Aminophylline, amphotericin B, ampicillin, chloramphenicol
sodium succinate, chlorothiazide, cimetidine, dimenhydrinate, furosemide, heparin
sodium, linezolid, melphalan, methohexital, paclitaxel, penicillin, pentobarbital,
phenobarbital, solutions with a pH of 4 to
5, thiopental.
I.M.
● Wear gloves when preparing solutions and avoid contact with skin and
clothing. Parenteral forms can cause contact dermatitis.
● Slight yellowing of injection is common and doesn't affect potency. Discard
markedly discolored solutions.
● Monitor blood pressure before and after
I.M. administration; keep patient supine
for 1 hour afterward and have him get up
slowly.
● Give deep I.M. only in upper outer
quadrant of buttocks. Consider giving
injection by Z-track method. Massage
slowly afterward to prevent sterile abscess.
Injection stings. Rotate injection sites.
Rectal
● Store suppositories in well-closed containers between 15° and 30° C (59° and
86° F).

ACTION
A piperidine phenothiazine that may block
postsynaptic dopamine receptors in the
brain.

Route	Onset	Peak	Duration
P.O.	30–60 min	Unknown	4–6 hr
P.O. (extended)	30–60 min	Unknown	10–12 hr
I.V., I.M.	Unknown	Unknown	Unknown
P.R.	> 1 hr	Unknown	3–4 hr

Half-life: 20 to 24 hours.

ADVERSE REACTIONS

CNS: *extrapyramidal reactions, sedation, tardive dyskinesia, pseudoparkinsonism,* **neuroleptic malignant syndrome, seizures,** dizziness, drowsiness.
CV: *orthostatic hypotension,* tachycardia, quinidine-like ECG effects.
EENT: ocular changes, blurred vision, nasal congestion.
GI: *dry mouth, constipation,* nausea.
GU: *urine retention,* menstrual irregularities, inhibited ejaculation, priapism.
Hematologic: *leukopenia, agranulocytosis, aplastic anemia, thrombocytopenia,* eosinophilia, hemolytic anemia.
Hepatic: jaundice.
Skin: *mild photosensitivity reactions, pain at I.M. injection site,* allergic reactions, sterile abscess, skin pigmentation changes.
Other: gynecomastia, lactation, galactorrhea.

INTERACTIONS

Drug-drug. *Antacids:* May inhibit absorption of oral phenothiazines. Separate antacid and phenothiazine doses by at least 2 hours.
Anticholinergics such as tricyclic antidepressants, antiparkinsonians: May increase anticholinergic activity, aggravated parkinsonian symptoms. Use together cautiously.
Anticonvulsants: May lower seizure threshold. Monitor patient closely.
Barbiturates, lithium: May decrease phenothiazine effect. Monitor patient.
Centrally acting antihypertensives: May decrease antihypertensive effect. Monitor blood pressure.
CNS depressants: May increase CNS depression. Use together cautiously.
Electroconvulsive therapy, insulin: May cause severe reactions. Monitor patient closely.

Lithium: May increase neurologic effects. Monitor patient closely.
Meperidine: May cause excessive sedation and hypotension. Don't use together.
Propranolol: May increase levels of both propranolol and chlorpromazine. Monitor patient closely.
Warfarin: May decrease effect of oral anticoagulants. Monitor PT and INR.
Drug-herb. *St. John's wort:* May cause photosensitivity reactions. Advise patient to avoid excessive sunlight exposure.
Drug-lifestyle. *Alcohol use:* May increase CNS depression, particularly psychomotor skills. Strongly discourage alcohol use.
Sun exposure: May increase risk of photosensitivity reactions. Advise patient to avoid excessive sunlight exposure.

EFFECTS ON LAB TEST RESULTS

● May decrease hemoglobin level and hematocrit.
● May increase liver function test values and eosinophil count. May decrease granulocyte, platelet, and WBC counts.
● May cause false-positive results for urinary porphyrin, urobilinogen, amylase, and 5-hydroxyindoleacetic acid tests and for urine pregnancy tests that use human chorionic gonadotropin.

CONTRAINDICATIONS & CAUTIONS

● Contraindicated in patients hypersensitive to drug; in those with CNS depression, bone marrow suppression, or subcortical damage, and in those in coma.
● Use cautiously in elderly or debilitated patients and in patients with hepatic or renal disease, severe CV disease (may suddenly decrease blood pressure), respiratory disorders, hypocalcemia, glaucoma, or prostatic hyperplasia. Also use cautiously in those exposed to extreme heat or cold (including antipyretic therapy) or organophosphate insecticides.
● Use cautiously in acutely ill or dehydrated children.

NURSING CONSIDERATIONS

● Obtain baseline blood pressure measurements before therapy, and monitor regularly. Watch for orthostatic hypotension, especially with parenteral administration.

Reactions may be *common,* uncommon, *life-threatening,* or COMMON AND LIFE-THREATENING.
Interaction may have a *rapid onset* or *delayed onset.*

• Monitor patient for tardive dyskinesia, which may occur after prolonged use. It may not appear until months or years later and may disappear spontaneously or persist for life, despite stopping drug.
• After abrupt withdrawal of long-term therapy, gastritis, nausea, vomiting, dizziness, or tremor may occur.
• *Alert:* Watch for evidence of neuroleptic malignant syndrome (extrapyramidal effects, hyperthermia, autonomic disturbance), which is rare but usually fatal. It may not be related to length of drug use or type of neuroleptic; more than 60% of affected patients are men.
• If jaundice, symptoms of blood dyscrasia (fever, sore throat, infection, cellulitis, weakness), or persistent extrapyramidal reactions (longer than a few hours) develop, or if such reactions occur in children or pregnant women, withhold dose and notify prescriber.
• Don't withdraw drug abruptly unless required by severe adverse reactions.
• *Look alike–sound alike:* Don't confuse chlorpromazine with clomipramine or with chlorpropamide, a hypoglycemic.

PATIENT TEACHING
• Warn patient to avoid activities that require alertness or good coordination until effects of drug are known. Drowsiness and dizziness usually subside after first few weeks.
• *Alert:* Advise patient not to crush, chew, or break extended-release capsule before swallowing.
• Tell patient to avoid alcohol while taking drug.
• Have patient report signs of urine retention or constipation.
• Tell patient to use sunblock and to wear protective clothing to avoid oversensitivity to the sun. This drug is more likely to cause sun sensitivity than other drugs in its class.
• Tell patient to relieve dry mouth with sugarless gum or hard candy.
• Advise patient receiving drug by any method other than by mouth to remain lying down for 1 hour afterward and to rise slowly.

---

citalopram hydrobromide
si-TAL-oh-pram

Celexa

Pharmacologic class: SSRI
Pregnancy risk category C

AVAILABLE FORMS
Solution: 10 mg/5 ml
Tablets: 10 mg, 20 mg, 40 mg
Tablets (orally disintegrating): 10 mg, 20 mg, 40 mg

INDICATIONS & DOSAGES
➤ **Depression**
Adults: Initially, 20 mg P.O. once daily, increasing to 40 mg daily after no less than 1 week. Maximum recommended dose is 40 mg daily.
Elderly patients: 20 mg daily P.O. with adjustment to 40 mg daily only for unresponsive patients.
Adjust-a-dose: For patients with hepatic impairment, use 20 mg daily P.O. with adjustment to 40 mg daily only for unresponsive patients.

ADMINISTRATION
P.O.
• Allow orally disintegrating tablet (ODT) to dissolve on the patient's tongue, then be swallowed, with or without water.
• Don't cut, break, or crush ODTs.
• Give drug without regard for food.

ACTION
Probably linked to potentiation of serotonergic activity in the CNS resulting from inhibition of neuronal reuptake of serotonin.

Route	Onset	Peak	Duration
P.O.	Unknown	4 hr	Unknown

Half-life: 35 hours.

ADVERSE REACTIONS
CNS: *somnolence, insomnia,* **suicide attempt,** anxiety, agitation, dizziness, paresthesia, migraine, impaired concentration, amnesia, depression, apathy, tremor, confusion, fatigue, fever.

CV: tachycardia, orthostatic hypotension, hypotension.
EENT: rhinitis, sinusitis, abnormal accommodation.
GI: *dry mouth, nausea,* diarrhea, anorexia, dyspepsia, vomiting, abdominal pain, taste perversion, increased saliva, flatulence, increased appetite.
GU: dysmenorrhea, amenorrhea, ejaculation disorder, impotence, anorgasmia, polyuria.
Metabolic: decreased or increased weight.
Musculoskeletal: arthralgia, myalgia.
Respiratory: upper respiratory tract infection, coughing.
Skin: rash, pruritus.
Other: *increased sweating,* yawning, decreased libido.

INTERACTIONS

Drug-drug. *Amphetamines, buspirone, dextromethorphan, dihydroergotamine, meperidine, other SSRIs or SSNRIs (duloxetine, venlafaxine),* **tramadol***, trazodone, tricyclic antidepressants, tryptophan:* May increase the risk of serotonin syndrome. Avoid other drugs that increase the availability of serotonin in the CNS; monitor patient closely if used together.
Carbamazepine: May increase citalopram clearance. Monitor patient for effects.
CNS drugs: May cause additive effects. Use together cautiously.
Drugs that inhibit cytochrome P-450 isoenzymes 3A4 and 2C19: May cause decreased clearance of citalopram. Monitor patient for increased adverse effects.
Imipramine, other tricyclic antidepressants: May increase level of imipramine metabolite desipramine by about 50%. Use together cautiously.
Lithium: May enhance serotonergic effect of citalopram. Use together cautiously, and monitor lithium level.
MAO inhibitors (phenelzine, selegiline, tranylcypromine): May cause serotonin syndrome. Avoid using within 14 days of MAO inhibitor therapy.
Sumatriptan: May cause weakness, hyperreflexia, and incoordination. Monitor patient closely.
Drug-herb. *St. John's wort:* May increase the risk of serotonin syndrome. Discourage use together.

Drug-lifestyle. *Alcohol use:* May increase CNS effects. Discourage use together.

EFFECTS ON LAB TEST RESULTS
None reported.

CONTRAINDICATIONS & CAUTIONS
● Contraindicated in patients hypersensitive to drug or its inactive components, within 14 days of MAO inhibitor therapy, and in patients taking pimozide.
● Use cautiously in patients with history of mania, seizures, suicidal thoughts, or hepatic or renal impairment.
● Use in third trimester of pregnancy may be linked to neonatal complications at birth. Consider the risk versus benefit of treatment during this time.
● Safety and efficacy of drug haven't been established in children.

NURSING CONSIDERATIONS
● Although drug hasn't been shown to impair psychomotor performance, any psychoactive drug has the potential to impair judgment, thinking, or motor skills.
● The possibility of a suicide attempt is inherent in depression and may persist until significant remission occurs. Closely supervise high-risk patients at start of drug therapy. Reduce risk of overdose by limiting amount of drug available per refill.
● *Alert:* Drug may increase the risk of suicidal thinking and behavior in children and adolescents with major depressive disorder or other psychiatric disorders.
● *Alert:* Drug may increase the risk of suicidal thinking and behavior in young adults ages 18 to 24 during the first 2 months of treatment.
● At least 14 days should elapse between MAO inhibitor therapy and citalopram therapy.
● *Alert:* Combining triptans with an SSRI or an SSNRI may cause serotonin syndrome. Signs and symptoms may include restlessness, hallucinations, loss of coordination, fast heartbeat, rapid changes in blood pressure, increased body temperature, overactive reflexes, nausea, vomiting, and diarrhea. Serotonin syndrome may be more likely to occur when starting or increasing the dose of triptan, SSRI, or SNRI.

• **Look alike–sound alike:** Don't confuse Celexa with Celebrex or Cerebyx.

PATIENT TEACHING
• Caution patient against use of MAO inhibitors while taking citalopram.
• Inform patient that, although improvement may take 1 to 4 weeks, he should continue therapy as prescribed.
• Advise patient not to stop drug abruptly.
• Tell patient that drug may be taken in the morning or evening without regard to meals. If drowsiness occurs, he should take drug in evening.
• Tell patient to allow orally disintegrating tablet to dissolve on his tongue then swallow, with or without water. Tell him not to cut, crush, or chew.
• Instruct patient to exercise caution when driving or operating hazardous machinery; drug may impair judgment, thinking, and motor skills.
• Advise patient to consult prescriber before taking other prescription or OTC drugs.
• Advise woman of childbearing age to consult prescriber before breast-feeding.
• Warn patient to avoid alcohol during drug therapy.
• Instruct woman of childbearing age to use contraceptives during drug therapy and to notify prescriber immediately if pregnancy is suspected.

---

clomipramine hydrochloride
kloe-MI-pra-meen

Anafranil

Pharmacologic class: tricyclic antidepressant (TCA)
Pregnancy risk category C

AVAILABLE FORMS
Capsules: 25 mg, 50 mg, 75 mg

INDICATIONS & DOSAGES
➤ **Obsessive-compulsive disorder**
Adults: Initially, 25 mg P.O. daily with meals, gradually increased to 100 mg daily in divided doses during first 2 weeks. Thereafter, increase to maximum dose of 250 mg daily in divided doses with meals,

as needed. After adjustment, give total daily dose at bedtime.
Children and adolescents: Initially, 25 mg P.O. daily with meals, gradually increased over first 2 weeks to daily maximum of 3 mg/kg or 100 mg P.O. in divided doses, whichever is smaller. Maximum daily dose is 3 mg/kg or 200 mg, whichever is smaller; give at bedtime after adjustment. Reassess and adjust dosage periodically.
➤ **To manage panic disorder with or without agoraphobia**
Adults: 12.5 to 150 mg P.O. daily (maximum 200 mg).
➤ **Depression, chronic pain ♦**
Adults: 100 to 250 mg P.O. daily.
➤ **Cataplexy and related narcolepsy ♦**
Adults: 25 to 200 mg P.O. daily.

ADMINISTRATION
P.O.
• Give drug without regard for food.

ACTION
Unknown. Inhibits reuptake of serotonin and norepinephrine at the presynaptic neuron.

Route	Onset	Peak	Duration
P.O.	Unknown	2–6 hr	Unknown

Half-life: Parent compound, 32 hours; active metabolite, 69 hours.

ADVERSE REACTIONS
CNS: *somnolence, tremor, dizziness, headache, insomnia, nervousness, myoclonus, fatigue,* **seizures,** EEG changes.
CV: orthostatic hypotension, palpitations, tachycardia.
EENT: *pharyngitis, rhinitis, visual changes.*
GI: *dry mouth, constipation, nausea, dyspepsia, increased appetite, anorexia, abdominal pain,* diarrhea.
GU: *urinary hesitancy,* UTI, *dysmenorrhea, ejaculation failure, impotence.*
Hematologic: purpura.
Metabolic: *weight gain.*
Musculoskeletal: *myalgia.*
Skin: *diaphoresis,* rash, pruritus, dry skin.
Other: *altered libido.*

INTERACTIONS

Drug-drug. *Barbiturates:* May decrease TCA level. Watch for decreased antidepressant effect.

Cimetidine, fluoxetine, fluvoxamine, paroxetine, sertraline: May increase TCA level. Monitor drug level and patient for signs of toxicity.

Clonidine: May cause life-threatening hypertension. Avoid using together.

CNS depressants: May enhance CNS depression. Avoid using together.

Epinephrine, norepinephrine: May increase hypertensive effect. Use together cautiously.

MAO inhibitors: May cause hyperpyretic crisis, seizures, coma, or death. Avoid using within 14 days of MAO inhibitor therapy.

Quinolones: May increase the risk of life-threatening arrhythmias. Avoid using together.

Drug-herb. *Evening primrose oil:* May cause additive or synergistic effect, resulting in lower seizure threshold and increasing the risk of seizure. Discourage use together.

St. John's wort, SAM-e, yohimbe: May cause serotonin syndrome. Discourage use together.

Drug-lifestyle. *Alcohol use:* May enhance CNS depression. Discourage use together.

Sun exposure: May increase risk of photosensitivity reactions. Advise patient to avoid excessive sunlight exposure.

EFFECTS ON LAB TEST RESULTS
None reported.

CONTRAINDICATIONS & CAUTIONS
• Contraindicated in patients hypersensitive to drug or other tricyclic antidepressants, in those who have taken MAO inhibitors within previous 14 days, and in patients in acute recovery period after MI.
• Use cautiously in patients with history of seizure disorders or with brain damage of varying cause; in patients receiving other seizure threshold–lowering drugs; in patients at risk for suicide; in patients with history of urine retention or angle-closure glaucoma, increased intraocular pressure, CV disease, impaired hepatic or renal function, or hyperthyroidism;

in patients with tumors of the adrenal medulla; in patients receiving thyroid drug or electroconvulsive therapy; and in those undergoing elective surgery.

NURSING CONSIDERATIONS
• Monitor mood and watch for suicidal tendencies. Allow patient to have only the minimum amount of drug.
• *Alert:* Drug may increase risk of suicidal thinking and behavior in children, adolescents, and young adults ages 18 to 24 during the first 2 months of treatment, especially in those with major depressive disorder or other psychiatric disorder.
• Don't withdraw drug abruptly.
• Because patients may suffer hypertensive episodes during surgery, stop drug gradually several days before surgery.
• Relieve dry mouth with sugarless candy or gum. Saliva substitutes may be needed.
• *Look alike–sound alike:* Don't confuse clomipramine with chlorpromazine or clomiphene, or Anafranil with enalapril, nafarelin, or alfentanil.

PATIENT TEACHING
• Warn patient to avoid hazardous activities requiring alertness and good coordination, especially during adjustment. Daytime sedation and dizziness may occur.
• Tell patient to avoid alcohol during drug therapy.
• Warn patient not to stop drug suddenly.
• Advise patient to use sunblock, wear protective clothing, and avoid prolonged exposure to strong sunlight to prevent oversensitivity to the sun.

SAFETY ALERT!

clonazepam
kloe-NAZ-e-pam

Klonopin, Klonopin wafers

Pharmacologic class: benzodiazepine
Pregnancy risk category D
Controlled substance schedule IV

AVAILABLE FORMS
Tablets: 0.5 mg, 1 mg, 2 mg

Tablets (orally disintegrating): 0.125 mg, 0.25 mg, 0.5 mg, 1 mg, 2 mg

INDICATIONS & DOSAGES

➤ **Lennox-Gastaut syndrome, atypical absence seizures, akinetic and myoclonic seizures**
Adults: Initially, no more than 1.5 mg P.O. daily in three divided doses. May be increased by 0.5 to 1 mg every 3 days until seizures are controlled. If given in unequal doses, give largest dose at bedtime. Maximum recommended daily dose is 20 mg.
Children up to age 10 or 30 kg (66 lb): Initially, 0.01 to 0.03 mg/kg P.O. daily (not to exceed 0.05 mg/kg daily) in two or three divided doses. Increase by 0.25 to 0.5 mg every third day to maximum maintenance dose of 0.1 to 0.2 mg/kg daily, as needed.
➤ **Panic disorder**
Adults: Initially, 0.25 mg P.O. b.i.d.; increase to target dose of 1 mg daily after 3 days. Some patients may benefit from dosages up to maximum of 4 mg daily. To achieve 4 mg daily, increase dosage in increments of 0.125 to 0.25 mg b.i.d. every 3 days, as tolerated, until panic disorder is controlled. Taper drug with decrease of 0.125 mg b.i.d. every 3 days until drug is stopped.
➤ **Acute manic episodes of bipolar disorder ◆**
Adults: 0.75 to 16 mg daily P.O.
➤ **Adjunct treatment for schizophrenia ◆**
Adults: 0.5 to 2 mg daily P.O.
➤ **Periodic leg movements during sleep ◆**
Adults: 0.5 to 2 mg P.O. at bedtime.
➤ **Parkinsonian (hypokinetic) dysarthria ◆**
Adults: 0.25 to 0.5 mg daily P.O.
➤ **Multifocal tic disorders ◆**
Adults: 1.5 to 12 mg daily P.O.
➤ **Neuralgias (deafferentation pain syndromes) ◆**
Adults: 2 to 4 mg daily P.O.

ADMINISTRATION
P.O.
● Peel back the foil of the orally disintegrating tablet (ODT) pouch carefully. Don't push ODT through foil.

● Give ODT to patient with or without water.

ACTION
Unknown. Probably acts by facilitating the effects of the inhibitory neurotransmitter GABA.

Route	Onset	Peak	Duration
P.O.	Unknown	1–2 hr	Unknown

Half-life: 18 to 50 hours.

ADVERSE REACTIONS
CNS: *drowsiness,* agitation, ataxia, behavioral disturbances, confusion, depression, slurred speech, tremor.
CV: palpitations.
EENT: abnormal eye movements, nystagmus.
GI: anorexia, change in appetite, constipation, diarrhea, gastritis, nausea, sore gums, vomiting.
GU: dysuria, enuresis, nocturia, urine retention.
Hematologic: *leukopenia, thrombocytopenia,* eosinophilia.
Respiratory: *respiratory depression,* chest congestion, shortness of breath.
Skin: rash.

INTERACTIONS
Drug-drug. *Carbamazepine, phenobarbital, phenytoin:* May lower clonazepam levels. Monitor patient closely.
CNS depressants: May increase CNS depression. Avoid using together.
Fluconazole, itraconazole, ketoconazole, miconazole: May increase and prolong drug levels, CNS depression, and psychomotor impairment. Avoid using together.
Drug-lifestyle. *Alcohol use:* May cause additive CNS effects. Discourage use together.
Smoking: May increase clearance of clonazepam. Monitor patient for decreased drug effects.

EFFECTS ON LAB TEST RESULTS
● May increase liver function test values and eosinophil count. May decrease platelet and WBC counts.

CONTRAINDICATIONS & CAUTIONS

• Contraindicated in patients hypersensitive to benzodiazepines and in those with significant hepatic disease or acute angle-closure glaucoma.
• Use cautiously in patients with mixed-type seizures because drug may cause generalized tonic-clonic seizures.
• Use cautiously in children and in patients with chronic respiratory disease, open-angle glaucoma, or a history of drug or alcohol addiction.

NURSING CONSIDERATIONS

• Watch for behavioral disturbances, especially in children.
• Don't stop drug abruptly because this may worsen seizures. Call prescriber at once if adverse reactions develop.
• Assess elderly patient's response closely. Elderly patients are more sensitive to drug's CNS effects.
• Monitor patient for oversedation.
• Monitor CBC and liver function tests.
• Withdrawal symptoms are similar to those of barbiturates.
• To reduce inconvenience of somnolence when drug is used for panic disorder, giving one dose at bedtime may be desirable.

PATIENT TEACHING

• Advise patient to avoid driving and other hazardous activities that require mental alertness until drug's CNS effects are known.
• Instruct parent to monitor child's school performance because drug may interfere with attentiveness.
• Warn patient and parents not to stop drug abruptly because seizures may occur.
• Advise patient that drug isn't for use during pregnancy or breast-feeding.
• Tell patients to open pouch of ODTs and peel back the foil. He shouldn't push the tablet *through* the foil.
• Tell patient to use dry hands when removing the ODT.
• Tell patient that ODTs can be taken with or without water.

clorazepate dipotassium
klor-AZ-e-pate

Gen-Xene, Novo-Clopate†, Tranxene, Tranxene-SD

Pharmacologic class: benzo-diazepine
Pregnancy risk category D
Controlled substance schedule IV

AVAILABLE FORMS

Capsules: 3.75 mg, 7.5 mg, 15 mg
Tablets: 3.75 mg, 7.5 mg, 15 mg
Tablets (extended-release): 11.25 mg, 22.5 mg

INDICATIONS & DOSAGES

➤ **Acute alcohol withdrawal**
Adults: Day 1, give 30 mg P.O. initially; then 30 to 60 mg P.O. in divided doses. Day 2, give 45 to 90 mg P.O. in divided doses. Day 3, give 22.5 to 45 mg P.O. in divided doses. Day 4, give 15 to 30 mg P.O. in divided doses. Then gradually reduce dosage to 7.5 to 15 mg daily. Maximum dosage is 90 mg daily.
➤ **Anxiety**
Adults: 15 to 60 mg P.O. daily.
Elderly patients: Initially, 7.5 to 15 mg daily in divided doses or as a single dose at bedtime.
Adjust-a-dose: For debilitated patients, initially, 7.5 to 15 mg daily in divided doses or as a single dose at bedtime.
➤ **Adjunctive treatment for partial seizure disorder**
Adults and children older than age 12: Maximum first dose is 7.5 mg P.O. t.i.d. Dosage increases shouldn't exceed 7.5 mg weekly. Maximum daily dose is 90 mg.
Children ages 9 to 12: Maximum first dose is 7.5 mg P.O. b.i.d. Dosage increases shouldn't exceed 7.5 mg weekly. Maximum daily dose is 60 mg.

ADMINISTRATION

P.O.
• Don't crush or break extended-release tablets.

ACTION

Unknown. Probably potentiates the effects of GABA, depresses the CNS, and suppresses the spread of seizure activity.

Route	Onset	Peak	Duration
P.O.	Unknown	30 min–1 hr	Unknown

Half-life: 1 to 9 days.

ADVERSE REACTIONS

CNS: *drowsiness, dizziness,* nervousness, confusion, headache, insomnia, depression, irritability, tremor, minor changes in EEG patterns.
CV: hypotension.
EENT: blurred vision, diplopia.
GI: nausea, vomiting, abdominal discomfort, dry mouth.
GU: urine retention, incontinence.
Skin: rash.

INTERACTIONS

Drug-drug. *Cimetidine:* May decrease clorazepate clearance and increase risk of adverse reactions. Monitor patient carefully.
CNS depressants: May increase CNS depression. Use together cautiously.
Digoxin: May increase digoxin level and risk of toxicity. Monitor patient and digoxin level closely.
Levodopa: May decrease effectiveness of levodopa. Monitor patient closely.
Drug-herb. *Kava:* May increase sedation. Discourage use together.
Drug-lifestyle. *Alcohol use:* May cause additive CNS effects. Discourage use together.
Smoking: May decrease benzodiazepine effectiveness. Urge patient to quit smoking, and monitor patient closely.

EFFECTS ON LAB TEST RESULTS

• May increase liver function test values.

CONTRAINDICATIONS & CAUTIONS

• Contraindicated in patients hypersensitive to drug and in those with acute angle-closure glaucoma.
• Use cautiously in patients with suicidal tendencies, renal or hepatic impairment, pulmonary disease, or history of drug abuse.

• Don't give drug to pregnant women, especially during first trimester.
• Drug isn't recommended for children younger than age 9.

NURSING CONSIDERATIONS

• *Alert:* Monitor hepatic, renal, and hematopoietic function periodically in patients receiving repeated or prolonged therapy.
• *Alert:* Use of this drug may lead to abuse and addiction. Don't withdraw drug abruptly after prolonged use because withdrawal symptoms may occur.
• *Look alike–sound alike:* Don't confuse clorazepate with clofibrate.

PATIENT TEACHING

• Warn patient to avoid activities that require alertness and good coordination until effects of drug are known.
• *Alert:* Advise patient to swallow Tranxene-SD whole and not to crush, break, or chew.
• Tell patient to avoid alcohol while taking drug.
• Advise patient that smoking may decrease drug's effectiveness.
• Warn patient not to stop drug abruptly because withdrawal symptoms may occur.
• Warn woman of childbearing age to avoid use during pregnancy.
• Inform patient that sugarless chewing gum or hard candy can relieve dry mouth.

SAFETY ALERT!

clozapine
KLOE-za-peen

Clozaril, FazaClo

Pharmacologic class: dibenzapine derivative
Pregnancy risk category B

AVAILABLE FORMS

Orally disintegrating tablets (ODTs): 12.5 mg, 25 mg, 100 mg
Tablets: 25 mg, 100 mg, 200 mg

INDICATIONS & DOSAGES

➤ **Schizophrenia in severely ill patients unresponsive to other therapies; to reduce risk of recurrent suicidal behavior in schizophrenia or schizoaffective disorders**

Adults: Initially, 12.5 mg P.O. once daily or b.i.d. If using the ODT, cut in half and discard the unused half. Adjust dose upward by 25 to 50 mg daily (if tolerated) to 300 to 450 mg daily by end of 2 weeks. Individual dosage is based on clinical response, patient tolerance, and adverse reactions. Subsequent dosage shouldn't be increased more than once or twice weekly and shouldn't exceed 50- to 100-mg increments. Many patients respond to dosages of 200 to 600 mg daily, but some may need as much as 900 mg daily. Don't exceed 900 mg daily.

ADMINISTRATION

P.O.
- Peel the foil from the ODT blister and gently remove the tablet immediately before giving.
- Give ODT with or without water.

ACTION

Unknown. Binds selectively to dopaminergic receptors in the CNS and may interfere with adrenergic, cholinergic, histaminergic, and serotonergic receptors.

Route	Onset	Peak	Duration
P.O.	Unknown	2½ hr	4–12 hr

Half-life: Proportional to dose; may range from 8 to 12 hours.

ADVERSE REACTIONS

CNS: *drowsiness, sedation, dizziness, vertigo, headache, seizures,* syncope, tremor, disturbed sleep or nightmares, restlessness, hypokinesia or akinesia, agitation, rigidity, akathisia, confusion, fatigue, insomnia, hyperkinesia, weakness, lethargy, ataxia, slurred speech, depression, myoclonus, anxiety, fever.
CV: tachycardia, *cardiomyopathy, myocarditis, pulmonary embolism, cardiac arrest,* hypotension, hypertension, chest pain, ECG changes, orthostatic hypotension.

EENT: visual disturbances.
GI: *constipation, excessive salivation,* dry mouth, nausea, vomiting, heartburn, diarrhea.
GU: urinary frequency or urgency, urine retention, incontinence, abnormal ejaculation.
Hematologic: *leukopenia, agranulocytosis, granulocytopenia,* eosinophilia.
Metabolic: *hyperglycemia,* weight gain, hypercholesterolemia, hypertriglyceridemia.
Musculoskeletal: muscle pain or spasm, muscle weakness.
Respiratory: *respiratory arrest.*
Skin: rash, diaphoresis.

INTERACTIONS

Drug-drug. *Anticholinergics:* May potentiate anticholinergic effects of clozapine. Use together cautiously.
Antihypertensives: May potentiate hypotensive effects. Monitor blood pressure.
Benzodiazepines: May increase risk of sedation and CV and respiratory arrest. Use together cautiously.
Bone marrow suppressants: May increase bone marrow toxicity. Avoid using together.
Citalopram, *fluoroquinolones,* **fluoxetine, fluvoxamine,** *paroxetine,* **sertraline:** May increase clozapine levels and toxicity. Adjust clozapine dose as needed.
Digoxin, other highly protein-bound drugs, warfarin: May increase levels of these drugs. Monitor patient closely for adverse reactions.
Phenytoin: May decrease clozapine level and cause breakthrough psychosis. Monitor patient for psychosis and adjust clozapine dosage.
Psychoactive drugs: May cause additive effects. Use together cautiously.
Ritonavir: May increase clozapine levels and toxicity. Avoid using together.
Drug-herb. *St. John's wort:* May decrease drug level. Discourage use together.
Drug-lifestyle. *Alcohol use:* May increase CNS depression. Discourage use together.
Smoking: May decrease drug level. Urge patient to quit smoking. Monitor patient for effectiveness and adjust dosage.

EFFECTS ON LAB TEST RESULTS
● May increase glucose, cholesterol, and triglyceride levels.
● May increase eosinophil count. May decrease granulocyte and WBC counts.

CONTRAINDICATIONS & CAUTIONS
● Contraindicated in patients with un-controlled epilepsy, history of clozapine-induced agranulocytosis, WBC count below 3,500/mm^3, severe CNS depression or coma, paralytic ileus, and myelosuppressive disorders.
● Contraindicated in patients taking other drugs that suppress bone marrow function.
● Use cautiously in patients with prostatic hyperplasia or angle-closure glaucoma because drug has potent anticholinergic effects.

NURSING CONSIDERATIONS
● ODTs contain phenylalanine.
● *Alert:* Drug carries significant risk of agranulocytosis. If possible, give patient at least two trials of standard antipsychotic before starting clozapine. Obtain baseline WBC and differential counts before clozapine therapy. Baseline WBC count must be at least 3,500/mm^3 and baseline antineutrophil cytoplasmic antibody (ANCA) at least 2,000/mm^3. Monitor WBC and ANCA values weekly for at least 4 weeks after stopping drug, regardless of how often you were monitoring when therapy stopped.
● During the first 6 months of therapy, monitor patient weekly and dispense no more than a 1-week supply of drug. If acceptable WBC and ANCA values [WBC 3,500/mm^3 or higher and ANCA 2,000/mm^3 or higher] are maintained during the first 6 months of continuous therapy, reduce monitoring to every other week. After 6 months of every-other-week monitoring without interruption by leukopenia, reduce frequency of monitoring WBC and ANCA to monthly.
● If WBC count drops below 3,500/mm^3 after therapy begins or if it drops substantially from baseline, monitor patient closely for signs and symptoms of infection. If WBC count is 3,000 to 3,500/mm^3 and granulocyte count is above

1,500/mm^3, perform WBC and differential count twice weekly. If WBC count drops to 2,000/mm^3 to 3,000/mm^3 or granulocyte count drops to 1,000/mm^3 to 1,500/mm^3, interrupt therapy and notify prescriber. Monitor WBC and differential daily until WBC exceeds 3,000/mm^3 and ANCA exceeds 1,500/mm^3, and monitor patient for signs and symptoms of infection. Continue monitoring WBC and differential counts twice weekly until WBC count exceeds 3,500/mm^3 and ANCA exceeds 2,000/mm^3. Then, restart therapy with weekly monitoring for 1 year before returning to the usual monitoring schedule of every 2 weeks for 6 months and then every 4 weeks.
● If WBC count drops below 2,000/mm^3 and granulocyte count drops below 1,000/mm^3, patient may need protective isolation. Bone marrow aspiration may be needed to assess bone marrow function. Future clozapine therapy is contraindicated in these patients.
● *Alert:* Drug increases the risk of fatal myocarditis, especially during, but not limited to, the first month of therapy. In patients in whom myocarditis is suspected (unexplained fatigue, dyspnea, tachypnea, chest pain, tachycardia, fever, palpitations, and other signs or symptoms of heart failure or ECG abnormalities, such as ST-T wave abnormalities or arrhythmias), stop therapy immediately and don't restart.
● *Alert:* Drug may cause hyperglycemia. Monitor patients with diabetes regularly. In patients with risk factors for diabetes, obtain fasting blood glucose test results at baseline and periodically.
● *Alert:* Monitor patient for metabolic syndrome, including significant weight gain and increased body mass index, hypertension, hyperglycemia, hypercholesterolemia, and hypertriglyceridemia.
● Monitor patient for signs and symptoms of cardiomyopathy.
● Seizures may occur, especially in patients receiving high doses.
● Some patients experience transient fever with temperature higher than 100.4° F (38° C), especially in the first 3 weeks of therapy. Monitor these patients closely.

• *Alert:* Drug isn't indicated for use in elderly patients with dementia-related psychoses because of an increased risk for death from CV disease or infection.
• After abrupt withdrawal of long-term therapy, abrupt recurrence of psychosis is possible.
• If therapy must be stopped, withdraw drug gradually over 1 or 2 weeks. If changes in patient's medical condition (including development of leukopenia) require that drug be stopped immediately, monitor patient closely for recurrence of psychosis.
• If therapy is reinstated in patients withdrawn from drug, follow usual guidelines for dosage increase. Reexposure of patient to drug may increase severity and risk of adverse reactions. If therapy was stopped because WBC counts were below 2,000/mm^3 or granulocyte counts were below 1,000/mm^3, don't restart.
• *Look alike–sound alike:* Don't confuse clozapine with clonidine, clofazimine, or Klonopin.

PATIENT TEACHING
• Tell patient about need for weekly blood tests to check for blood-cell deficiency. Advise him to report flulike symptoms, fever, sore throat, lethargy, malaise, or other signs of infection.
• Warn patient to avoid hazardous activities that require alertness and good coordination while taking drug.
• Tell patient to check with prescriber before taking alcohol or OTC drugs.
• Advise patient that smoking may decrease drug effectiveness.
• Tell patient to rise slowly to avoid dizziness.
• Tell patient to keep ODTs in the blister package until ready to take it.
• Inform patient that ice chips or sugarless candy or gum may help relieve dry mouth.

dantrolene sodium
DAN-troe-leen

Dantrium, Dantrium Intravenous

Pharmacologic class: hydantoin derivative
Pregnancy risk category C

AVAILABLE FORMS
Capsules: 25 mg, 50 mg, 100 mg
Injection: 20 mg/vial

INDICATIONS & DOSAGES
➤ **Spasticity and sequelae from severe chronic disorders, such as multiple sclerosis, cerebral palsy, spinal cord injury, stroke**
Adults: 25 mg P.O. daily. Increase by 25-mg increments, up to 100 mg t.i.d. to q.i.d. Maintain each dosage level for 7 days to determine response. Maximum, 400 mg daily.
Children: Initially, 0.5 mg/kg P.O. daily for 7 days; then 0.5 mg/kg t.i.d. for 7 days, 1 mg/kg t.i.d. for 7 days, and finally, 2 mg/kg, t.i.d. for 7 days. May increase up to 3 mg/kg b.i.d. to q.i.d. if necessary. Maximum, 100 mg q.i.d.
➤ **To manage malignant hyperthermic crisis**
Adults and children: Initially, 1 mg/kg I.V. push. Repeat, as needed, up to cumulative dose of 10 mg/kg.
➤ **To prevent or attenuate malignant hyperthermic crisis in susceptible patients who need surgery**
Adults and children: 4 to 8 mg/kg P.O. daily in three or four divided doses for 1 or 2 days before procedure. Give final dose 3 or 4 hours before procedure. Or, 2.5 mg/kg I.V. about 1 hour before anesthesia; infuse over 1 hour.
➤ **To prevent recurrence of malignant hyperthermic crisis**
Adults: 4 to 8 mg/kg P.O. daily in four divided doses for up to 3 days after hyperthermic crisis.

ADMINISTRATION
P.O.
- Give drug with food or milk.
- Prepare oral suspension for single dose by dissolving capsule contents in juice or other liquid. For multiple doses, use acid vehicle and refrigerate. Use within several days.

I.V.
- Reconstitute drug by adding 60 ml of sterile water for injection and shaking vial until clear. Don't use a diluent that contains a bacteriostatic drug.
- Protect solution from light, and use within 6 hours.
- **Incompatibilities:** D_5W, normal saline solution, other I.V. drugs mixed in a syringe.

ACTION
Acts directly on skeletal muscle to decrease excitation and contraction coupling and reduce muscle strength by interfering with intracellular calcium movement.

Route	Onset	Peak	Duration
P.O.	Unknown	5 hr	Unknown
I.V.	Unknown	Unknown	3 hr after infusion

Half-life: P.O., 9 hours; I.V., 4 to 8 hours.

ADVERSE REACTIONS
CNS: *drowsiness, dizziness, malaise, fatigue,* **seizures,** headache, light-headedness, confusion, nervousness, insomnia, fever, depression.
CV: tachycardia, blood pressure changes, phlebitis, thrombophlebitis, heart failure.
EENT: excessive lacrimation, speech disturbance, diplopia, visual disturbances.
GI: anorexia, constipation, cramping, dysphagia, metallic taste, severe diarrhea, GI bleeding, vomiting.
GU: urinary frequency, hematuria, incontinence, nocturia, dysuria, crystalluria, difficult erection, urine retention.
Hematologic: *leukopenia, thrombocytopenia, lymphocytic lymphoma,* anemia.
Hepatic: *hepatitis.*
Musculoskeletal: *muscle weakness,* myalgia, back pain.
Respiratory: pleural effusion with pericarditis, *pulmonary edema.*

Skin: eczematous eruption, pruritus, urticaria, abnormal hair growth, diaphoresis, photosensitivity.
Other: chills.

INTERACTIONS
Drug-drug. *Clofibrate, warfarin:* May decrease protein binding of dantrolene. Use together cautiously.
CNS depressants: May increase CNS depression. Avoid using together.
Estrogens: May increase risk of hepatotoxicity. Use together cautiously.
I.V. verapamil and other calcium channel blockers: May cause hyperkalemia, ventricular fibrillation, and myocardial depression. Stop verapamil before giving I.V. dantrolene.
Vecuronium: May increase neuromuscular blockade effect. Use together cautiously.
Drug-lifestyle. *Alcohol use:* May increase CNS depression. Discourage use together.
Sun exposure: May cause photosensitivity reactions. Advise patient to avoid excessive sunlight exposure.

EFFECTS ON LAB TEST RESULTS
- May increase ALT, AST, alkaline phosphatase, LDH, bilirubin, and BUN levels.

CONTRAINDICATIONS & CAUTIONS
- Contraindicated for spasms in rheumatic disorders and when spasticity is used to maintain motor function.
- Contraindicated in breast-feeding patients and patients with upper motor neuron disorders or active hepatic disease.
- Use cautiously in women, patients older than age 35, and patients with hepatic disease (such as cirrhosis or hepatitis) or severely impaired cardiac or pulmonary function.

NURSING CONSIDERATIONS
- Start therapy as soon as malignant hyperthermia reaction is recognized.
- Liver damage may occur with long-term use. If benefits don't occur within 45 days, stop therapy.
- Obtain liver function test results at start of therapy.
- *Alert:* Watch for fever, jaundice, severe diarrhea, weakness, and sensitivity

reactions, including skin eruptions. With-hold dose and notify prescriber.
• *Look alike–sound alike:* Don't confuse Dantrium with Daraprim.

PATIENT TEACHING
• Instruct patient to take drug with meals or milk in four divided doses.
• Tell patient to eat carefully to avoid choking. Some patients may have trouble swallowing during therapy.
• Warn patient to avoid driving and other hazardous activities until CNS effects of drug are known.
• Advise patient to avoid combining drug with alcohol or other CNS depressants.
• Advise patient to notify prescriber if skin or eyes turn yellow, skin itches, or fever develops.
• Tell patient to avoid photosensitivity reactions by using sunblock and wearing protective clothing, to report abdominal discomfort or GI problems immediately, and to follow prescriber's orders regarding rest and physical therapy.

---

desipramine hydrochloride
dess-IP-ra-meen

Norpramin

Pharmacologic class: tricyclic antidepressant (TCA)
Pregnancy risk category NR

AVAILABLE FORMS
Tablets: 10 mg, 25 mg, 50 mg, 75 mg, 100 mg, 150 mg

INDICATIONS & DOSAGES
➤ **Depression**
Adults: 100 to 200 mg P.O. daily in divided doses; increase to maximum of 300 mg daily. Or, give entire dose at bedtime.
Adolescents and elderly patients: 25 to 100 mg P.O. daily in divided doses; increase gradually to maximum of 150 mg daily, if needed.

ADMINISTRATION
P.O.
• Give drug without regard for food.

ACTION
Unknown. Increases the amount of nor-epinephrine, serotonin, or both in the CNS by blocking their reuptake by the presynaptic neurons.

Route	Onset	Peak	Duration
P.O.	Unknown	4–6 hr	Unknown

Half-life: Unknown.

ADVERSE REACTIONS
CNS: *drowsiness, dizziness, seizures,* excitation, tremor, weakness, confusion, anxiety, restlessness, agitation, headache, nervousness, EEG changes, extrapyramidal reactions.
CV: *tachycardia,* orthostatic hypotension, ECG changes, hypertension.
EENT: *blurred vision,* tinnitus, mydriasis.
GI: *dry mouth,* constipation, nausea, vomiting, anorexia, paralytic ileus.
GU: urine retention.
Metabolic: *hypoglycemia,* hyperglycemia.
Skin: rash, urticaria, photosensitivity reactions, diaphoresis.
Other: *sudden death in children,* hypersensitivity reactions.

INTERACTIONS
Drug-drug. *Barbiturates, CNS depressants:* May enhance CNS depression. Avoid using together.
Cimetidine, fluoxetine, fluvoxamine, paroxetine, sertraline: May increase desipramine level. Monitor drug levels and patient for signs of toxicity.
Clonidine: May cause life-threatening blood pressure elevations. Avoid using together.
Epinephrine, norepinephrine: May increase hypertensive effect. Use together cautiously.
MAO inhibitors: May cause severe excitation, hyperpyrexia, or seizures, usually with high doses. Avoid using within 14 days of MAO inhibitor therapy.
Quinolones: May increase the risk of life-threatening arrhythmias. Avoid using together.
Drug-herb. *Evening primrose oil:* May cause additive or synergistic effect, resulting in lower seizure threshold and

---

increasing the risk of seizure. Discourage use together.

St. John's wort, SAM-e, yohimbe: May cause serotonin syndrome. Discourage use together.

Drug-lifestyle. *Alcohol use:* May enhance CNS depression. Discourage use together.

Smoking: May lower drug level. Monitor patient for lack of effect.

Sun exposure: May increase risk of photosensitivity reactions. Advise patient to avoid excessive sunlight exposure.

EFFECTS ON LAB TEST RESULTS
● May increase or decrease glucose level.
● May increase liver function test values.

CONTRAINDICATIONS & CAUTIONS
● Contraindicated in patients hypersensitive to drug and in those who have taken MAO inhibitors within previous 14 days.
● Contraindicated during acute recovery phase after MI.
● Use with extreme caution in patients with CV disease; in those with history of urine retention, glaucoma, seizure disorders, or thyroid disease; and in those taking thyroid drug.

NURSING CONSIDERATIONS
● Monitor patient for nausea, headache, and malaise after abrupt withdrawal of long-term therapy; these symptoms don't indicate addiction.
● Don't withdraw drug abruptly.
● Because patients may suffer hypertensive episodes during surgery, stop drug gradually several days before surgery.
● If signs or symptoms of psychosis occur or increase, notify prescriber. Record mood changes. Monitor patient for suicidal tendencies.
● *Alert:* Drug may increase risk of suicidal thinking and behavior in children, adolescents, and young adults ages 18 to 24 during the first 2 months of treatment, especially in those with major depressive disorder or other psychiatric disorder.
● Because drug produces fewer anticholinergic effects than other TCAs, it's often prescribed for cardiac patients.
● Recommend sugarless hard candy or gum to relieve dry mouth. Saliva substitutes may be needed.

● *Alert:* Norpramin may contain tartrazine.
● *Look alike–sound alike:* Don't confuse desipramine with disopyramide or imipramine.

PATIENT TEACHING
● Advise patient to take full dose at bedtime to avoid daytime sedation; if insomnia occurs, tell him to take drug in the morning.
● Warn patient to avoid hazardous activities that require alertness and good coordination until effects of drug are known. Drowsiness and dizziness usually subside after a few weeks.
● Advise patient to call prescriber if fever and sore throat occur. Blood counts may need to be obtained.
● Tell patient to avoid alcohol during therapy because it may antagonize effects of drug.
● Tell patient to consult prescriber before taking other prescription or OTC drugs.
● Warn patient not to stop drug suddenly.
● To prevent sensitivity to the sun, advise patient to use sunblock, wear protective clothing, and avoid prolonged exposure to strong sunlight.

---

dexmethylphenidate hydrochloride
decks-meth-ill-FEN-i-date

Focalin, Focalin XR

Pharmacologic class: methylphenidate derivative
Pregnancy risk category C
Controlled substance schedule II

AVAILABLE FORMS
Capsules (extended-release): 5 mg, 10 mg, 20 mg
Tablets: 2.5 mg, 5 mg, 10 mg

INDICATIONS & DOSAGES
➤ **Attention deficit hyperactivity disorder (ADHD)**
immediate-release tablets
Adults and children age 6 and older:
For patients who aren't now taking methylphenidate, initially, 2.5 mg P.O. b.i.d., given at least 4 hours apart. Increase

weekly by 2.5 to 5 mg daily, up to a maximum of 20 mg daily in divided doses.

For patients who are now taking methylphenidate, initially give half the current methylphenidate dosage, up to a maximum of 20 mg P.O. daily in divided doses.

extended-release capsules
Adults: For patients who aren't now taking dexmethylphenidate or methylphenidate, or who are on stimulants other than methylphenidate, give 10 mg P.O. once daily in the morning. May adjust in weekly increments of 10 mg to a maximum dose of 20 mg daily.

For patients who are now taking methylphenidate, initially give half the total daily dose of methylphenidate. Patients who are now taking the immediate-release form of dexmethylphenidate may be switched to the same daily dose of extended-release form. Maximum daily dose is 20 mg.
Children ages 6 and older: For patients who aren't now taking dexmethylphenidate or methylphenidate, or who are on stimulants other than methylphenidate, give 5 mg P.O. once daily in the morning. May adjust in weekly increments of 5 mg to a maximum daily dose of 20 mg.

For patients who are now taking methylphenidate, initially give half the total daily dose of methylphenidate. Patients who are now taking the immediate-release form of dexmethylphenidate may be switched to the same daily dose of extended-release form. Maximum daily dose is 20 mg.

ADMINISTRATION
P.O.
• Capsules may be swallowed whole or the contents sprinkled on a small amount of applesauce and eaten immediately.
• Don't crush or divide the capsule or its contents.

ACTION
Blocks presynaptic reuptake of norepinephrine and dopamine and increases their release, increasing concentration in the synapse.

Route	Onset	Peak	Duration
P.O. (immediate-release)	Unknown	1–1½ hr	Unknown
P.O. (extended-release)	Unknown	1–4 hr; 4½–7 hr	Unknown

Half-life: 2 to 3 hours.

ADVERSE REACTIONS
CNS: *headache, anxiety, feeling jittery,* nervousness, insomnia, fever, dizziness.
CV: tachycardia.
EENT: throat pain.
GI: *anorexia, abdominal pain,* nausea, dyspepsia, dry mouth.
Musculoskeletal: twitching (motor or vocal tics).
Other: hypersensitivity reactions.

INTERACTIONS
Drug-drug. *Antacids, acid suppressants:* May alter the release of extended-release form. Avoid using together.
Anticoagulants, phenobarbital, phenytoin, primidone, tricyclic antidepressants: May inhibit metabolism of these drugs. May need to decrease dosage of these drugs; monitor drug levels.
Antihypertensives: May decrease effectiveness of these drugs. Use together cautiously; monitor blood pressure.
Clonidine, other centrally acting alpha agonists: May cause serious adverse effects. Use together cautiously.
MAO inhibitors: May increase risk of hypertensive crisis. Using together within 14 days of MAO inhibitor therapy is contraindicated.

EFFECTS ON LAB TEST RESULTS
None reported.

CONTRAINDICATIONS & CAUTIONS
• Contraindicated in patients hypersensitive to methylphenidate or other components.
• Contraindicated in patients with severe anxiety, tension, or agitation; glaucoma; or motor tics or a family history or diagnosis of Tourette syndrome, or within 14 days of MAO inhibitor therapy.

• Use cautiously in patients with a psychiatric illness, bipolar disorder, depression, or family history of suicide; seizures, hypertension, hyperthyroidism, heart failure, recent MI, or a history of drug or alcohol abuse.

• Use in pregnant women only if the benefits outweigh the risks; drug may delay skeletal ossification, suppress weight gain, and impair organ development in the fetus.

• Use cautiously in breast-feeding women. It's unknown if drug appears in breast milk.

• Don't use in children or adolescents with structural cardiac abnormalities or other serious heart problems.

NURSING CONSIDERATIONS

• Diagnosis of ADHD must be based on complete history and evaluation of the patient by psychological and educational experts.

• Obtain a detailed patient history, including a family history for mental disorders, family suicide, ventricular arrhythmias, or sudden death.

• Refer patient for psychological, educational, and social support.

• Periodically reevaluate the long-term usefulness of the drug.

• Monitor CBC and differential and platelet counts during prolonged therapy.

• Don't use for severe depression or normal fatigue states.

• Stop treatment or reduce dosage if symptoms worsen or adverse reactions occur.

• Long-term stimulant use may temporarily suppress growth. Monitor children for growth and weight gain. If growth slows or weight gain is lower than expected, stop drug.

• Routinely monitor blood pressure and pulse.

• Monitor patient for signs of drug dependence or abuse.

• If seizures occur, stop drug.

PATIENT TEACHING

• Stress the importance of taking the correct dose of drug at the same time every day. Report accidental overdose immediately.

• *Alert:* Warn patient the misuse of amphetamines can have serious effects including sudden death.

• Advise patients unable to swallow capsules to empty the contents of the capsule onto a spoonful of applesauce and eat immediately.

• *Alert:* Tell patient not to cut, crush, or chew the contents of the extended-release beaded capsule.

• Advise parents to monitor child for medication abuse or sharing. Also inform parents to watch for increased aggression or hostility and to report worsening behavior.

• Advise parents to monitor child's height and weight and to tell the prescriber if they suspect growth is slowing.

• Caution patient to expect blurred vision or difficulty with accommodation and to exercise caution while performing activities that require a clear visual field. Advise patient to report blurred vision to the prescriber.

---

dextroamphetamine sulfate
dex-troe-am-FET-a-meen

Dexedrine*, Dexedrine Spansule, Dextroam, DextroStat

Pharmacologic class: amphetamine
Pregnancy risk category C
Controlled substance schedule II

AVAILABLE FORMS
Capsules (extended-release): 5 mg, 10 mg, 15 mg
Tablets: 5 mg, 10 mg

INDICATIONS & DOSAGES
➤ **Narcolepsy**
Adults: 5 to 60 mg P.O. daily in divided doses.
Children ages 6 to 12: Give 5 mg P.O. daily. Increase by 5 mg at weekly intervals as needed.
Children age 12 and older: 10 mg P.O. daily. Increase by 10 mg at weekly intervals, as needed. Give first dose on awakening; additional doses (one or two) given at intervals of 4 to 6 hours.

➤ **Attention deficit hyperactivity disorder (ADHD)**
Children age 6 and older: 5 mg P.O. once daily or b.i.d. Increase by 5 mg at weekly intervals, as needed. It's rarely necessary to exceed 40 mg/day.
Children ages 3 to 5: Give 2.5 mg P.O. daily. Increase by 2.5 mg at weekly intervals, as needed.

➤ **Short-term adjunct in exogenous obesity ◆**
Adults and children age 12 and older: 5 to 30 mg P.O. daily 30 to 60 minutes before meals in divided doses of 5 to 10 mg. Or, 10- or 15-mg extended-release capsule daily in the morning.

ADMINISTRATION
P.O.
• Give drug 30 to 60 minutes before meals if used for weight reduction and at least 6 hours before bedtime to avoid sleep interference.
• Certain formulations may contain tartrazine.

ACTION
Unknown. Probably promotes nerve impulse transmission by releasing stored dopamine and norepinephrine from nerve terminals in the brain. Main sites of activity appear to be the cerebral cortex and the reticular activating system.

Route	Onset	Peak	Duration
P.O.	30–60 min	2 hr	4 hr
P.O. (extended)	60 min	2 hr	8 hr

Half-life: 10 to 12 hours.

ADVERSE REACTIONS
CNS: *insomnia, nervousness, restlessness,* tremor, dizziness, headache, chills, overstimulation, dysphoria, euphoria.
CV: *tachycardia, palpitations, **arrhythmias,*** hypertension.
GI: dry mouth, taste perversion, diarrhea, constipation, anorexia, other GI disturbances.
GU: impotence.
Metabolic: weight loss.
Skin: urticaria.
Other: increased libido.

INTERACTIONS
Drug-drug. *Acetazolamide, alkalizing drugs, antacids, sodium bicarbonate:* May increase renal reabsorption. Monitor patient for enhanced amphetamine effects.
Acidifying drugs, ammonium chloride, ascorbic acid: May decrease level and increase renal clearance of dextroamphetamine. Monitor patient for decreased amphetamine effects.
Adrenergic blockers: May inhibit adrenergic blocking effects. Avoid using together.
Chlorpromazine: May inhibit central stimulant effects of amphetamines. May use to treat amphetamine poisoning.
Insulin, oral antidiabetics: May decrease antidiabetic requirements. Monitor glucose level.
MAO inhibitors: May cause severe hypertension or hypertensive crisis. Avoid using within 14 days of MAO inhibitor therapy.
Meperidine: May potentiate analgesic effect. Use together cautiously.
Methenamine: May increase urinary excretion of amphetamines and reduce effectiveness. Monitor drug effects.
Norepinephrine: May enhance adrenergic effect of norepinephrine. Monitor patient.
Phenobarbital, phenytoin: May delay absorption of these drugs. Monitor patient closely.
Drug-food. *Caffeine:* May increase amphetamine and related amine effects. Urge caution.

EFFECTS ON LAB TEST RESULTS
• May increase corticosteroid level.

CONTRAINDICATIONS & CAUTIONS
• Contraindicated in patients hypersensitive to or with idiosyncratic reactions to sympathomimetic amines and in those with hyperthyroidism, moderate to severe hypertension, symptomatic CV disease, glaucoma, advanced arteriosclerosis, or history of drug abuse.
• Contraindicated as first-line treatment for obesity or within 14 days of MAO inhibitor therapy.
• Use cautiously in agitated patients and patients with motor tics, phonic tics, or Tourette syndrome. Also use cautiously in patients whose underlying condition may be worsened by an increase in blood

pressure or heart rate (preexisting hypertension, heart failure, recent MI); patients with a psychiatric illness, bipolar disorder, depression, or family history of suicide; those with a seizure disorder.
• Don't use in children or adolescents with structural cardiac abnormalities or other serious heart problems.

NURSING CONSIDERATIONS
• Obtain a detailed patient history, including a family history for mental disorders, family suicide, ventricular arrhythmias, or sudden death.
• Drug shouldn't be used to prevent fatigue.
• Obese patients should follow a weight-reduction program.
• Drug has a high abuse potential and may cause dependence.
• *Alert:* Overdose may cause seizures.
• If tolerance to anorexigenic effect develops, stop drug and notify prescriber.
• Monitor for growth retardation in children.
• *Look alike–sound alike:* Don't confuse Dexedrine with dextran or Excedrin.

PATIENT TEACHING
• *Alert:* Warn patient the misuse of amphetamines can cause serious CV adverse events including sudden death.
• Tell patient to take drug 30 to 60 minutes before meals if used for weight reduction and at least 6 hours before bedtime to avoid sleep interference.
• Warn patient to avoid activities that require alertness, a clear visual field, or good coordination until CNS effects of drug are known.
• Tell patient he may get tired as drug effects wear off.
• Ask patient to report signs and symptoms of excessive stimulation.
• Inform parents that children may show increased aggression or hostility and to report worsening of behavior.
• Advise patient to consume caffeine-containing products cautiously.
• Warn patient with a seizure disorder that drug may decrease seizure threshold. Instruct him to notify prescriber if seizures occur.

diazepam
dye-AZ-e-pam

Diastat, Diazemuls†, Diazepam Intensol, Novo-Dipam†, Valium

Pharmacologic class: benzo-diazepine
Pregnancy risk category D
Controlled substance schedule IV

AVAILABLE FORMS
Injection: 5 mg/ml
Oral solution: 5 mg/5 ml, 5 mg/ml
Rectal gel twin packs: 2.5 mg (pediatric), 5 mg (pediatric), 10 mg, 15 mg (adult), 20 mg (adult)
Tablets: 2 mg, 5 mg, 10 mg

INDICATIONS & DOSAGES
➤ **Anxiety**
Adults: Depending on severity, 2 to 10 mg P.O. b.i.d. to q.i.d. Or, 2 to 10 mg I.M. or I.V. every 3 to 4 hours, as needed.
Children age 6 months and older: 1 to 2.5 mg P.O. t.i.d. or q.i.d., increase gradually, as needed and tolerated.
Elderly patients: Initially, 2 to 2.5 mg once daily or b.i.d.; increase gradually.
➤ **Acute alcohol withdrawal**
Adults: 10 mg P.O. t.i.d. or q.i.d. first 24 hours; reduce to 5 mg P.O. t.i.d. or q.i.d., as needed. Or, initially, 10 mg I.V. or I.M. Then, 5 to 10 mg I.V. or I.M. every 3 to 4 hours, as needed.
➤ **Before endoscopic procedures**
Adults: Adjust I.V. dose to desired sedative response (up to 20 mg). Or, 5 to 10 mg I.M. 30 minutes before procedure.
➤ **Muscle spasm**
Adults: 2 to 10 mg P.O. b.i.d. to q.i.d. Or, 5 to 10 mg I.V. or I.M. initially; then 5 to 10 mg I.V. or I.M. every 3 to 4 hours, as needed. For tetanus, larger doses up to 20 mg every 2 to 8 hours may be needed.
Children age 5 and older: 5 to 10 mg I.V. or I.M. every 3 to 4 hours, as needed.
Children ages 1 month to 5 years: 1 to 2 mg I.V. or I.M. slowly; repeat every 3 to 4 hours, as needed.

➤ **Preoperative sedation**
Adults: 10 mg I.M. (preferred) or I.V. before surgery.

➤ **Cardioversion**
Adults: 5 to 15 mg I.V. within 5 to 10 minutes before procedure.

➤ **Adjunct treatment for seizure disorders**
Adults: 2 to 10 mg P.O. b.i.d. to q.i.d.
Children age 6 months and older: 1 to 2.5 mg P.O. t.i.d. or q.i.d. initially; increase as needed and as tolerated.

➤ **Status epilepticus, severe recurrent seizures**
Adults: 5 to 10 mg I.V. or I.M. initially. Use I.M. route only if I.V. access is unavailable. Repeat every 10 to 15 minutes, as needed, up to maximum dose of 30 mg. Repeat every 2 to 4 hours, if needed.
Children age 5 and older: 1 mg I.V. every 2 to 5 minutes to maximum of 10 mg. Repeat every 2 to 4 hours, if needed.
Children ages 1 month to 5 years: 0.2 to 0.5 mg I.V. slowly every 2 to 5 minutes up to maximum of 5 mg. Repeat every 2 to 4 hours, if needed.

➤ **Patients on stable regimens of antiepileptic drugs who need diazepam intermittently to control bouts of increased seizure activity**
Adults and children age 12 and older: 0.2 mg/kg P.R., rounding up to the nearest available dose form. A second dose may be given 4 to 12 hours later.
Children ages 6 to 11: 0.3 mg/kg P.R., rounding up to the nearest available dose form. A second dose may be given 4 to 12 hours later.
Children ages 2 to 5: 0.5 mg/kg P.R., rounding up to the nearest available dose form. A second dose may be given 4 to 12 hours later.
Adjust-a-dose: For elderly and debilitated patients, reduce dosage to decrease the likelihood of ataxia and oversedation.

ADMINISTRATION
P.O.
● When using oral solution, dilute dose just before giving.
I.V.
● I.V. route is the more reliable parenteral route; I.M. route isn't recommended be-
cause absorption is variable and injection is painful.
● Keep emergency resuscitation equipment and oxygen at bedside.
● Avoid infusion sets or containers made from polyvinyl chloride.
● If possible, inject directly into a large vein. If not, inject slowly through infusion tubing as near to the insertion site as possible. Give at no more than 5 mg/minute. Watch closely for phlebitis at injection site.
● Monitor respirations every 5 to 15 minutes and before each dose.
● Don't store parenteral solution in plastic syringes.
● **Incompatibilities:** All other I.V. drugs, most I.V. solutions.
I.M.
● Use the I.M. route if I.V. administration is impossible.
Rectal
● Use Diastat rectal gel to treat no more than five episodes per month and no more than one episode every 5 days because tolerance may develop.
● *Alert:* Only caregivers who can distinguish the distinct cluster of seizures or events from the patient's ordinary seizure activity, who have been instructed and can give the treatment competently, who understand which seizures may be treated with Diastat, and who can monitor the clinical response and recognize when immediate professional medical evaluation is needed should give Diastat rectal gel.

ACTION
A benzodiazepine that probably potentiates the effects of GABA, depresses the CNS, and suppresses the spread of seizure activity.

Route	Onset	Peak	Duration
P.O.	30 min	2 hr	20–80 hr
I.V.	1–5 min	1–5 min	15–60 min
I.M.	Unknown	2 hr	Unknown
P.R.	Unknown	90 min	Unknown

Half-life: About 1 to 12 days.

ADVERSE REACTIONS
CNS: *drowsiness,* dysarthria, slurred speech, tremor, transient amnesia, fatigue, ataxia, headache, insomnia, paradoxical

anxiety, hallucinations, minor changes in EEG patterns, *pain.*
CV: *CV collapse, bradycardia,* hypotension.
EENT: diplopia, blurred vision, nystagmus.
GI: nausea, constipation, diarrhea with rectal form.
GU: incontinence, urine retention.
Hematologic: *neutropenia.*
Hepatic: jaundice.
Respiratory: *respiratory depression, apnea.*
Skin: rash, *phlebitis at injection site.*
Other: altered libido, physical or psychological dependence.

INTERACTIONS
Drug-drug. *Cimetidine, disulfiram, fluoxetine, fluvoxamine, hormonal contraceptives, isoniazid, metoprolol, propoxyphene, propranolol, valproic acid:* May decrease clearance of diazepam and increase risk of adverse effects. Monitor patient for excessive sedation and impaired psychomotor function.
CNS depressants: May increase CNS depression. Use together cautiously.
Digoxin: May increase digoxin level and risk of toxicity. Monitor patient and digoxin level closely.
Diltiazem: May increase CNS depression and prolong effects of diazepam. Reduce dose of diazepam.
Fluconazole, itraconazole, ketoconazole, miconazole: May increase and prolong diazepam level, CNS depression, and psychomotor impairment. Avoid using together.
Levodopa: May decrease levodopa effectiveness. Monitor patient.
Phenobarbital: May increase effects of both drugs. Use together cautiously.
Drug-herb. *Kava:* May increase sedation. Discourage use together.
Drug-lifestyle. *Alcohol use:* May cause additive CNS effects. Discourage use together.
Smoking: May decrease effectiveness of drug. Monitor patient closely.

EFFECTS ON LAB TEST RESULTS
● May increase liver function test values. May decrease neutrophil count.

CONTRAINDICATIONS & CAUTIONS
● Contraindicated in patients hypersensitive to drug or soy protein; in patients experiencing shock, coma, or acute alcohol intoxication (parenteral form); in pregnant women, especially in first trimester; and in infants younger than age 6 months (oral form).
● Diastat rectal gel is contraindicated in patients with acute angle-closure glaucoma.
● Use cautiously in patients with liver or renal impairment, depression, or chronic open-angle glaucoma. Use cautiously in elderly and debilitated patients.

NURSING CONSIDERATIONS
● Monitor periodic hepatic, renal, and hematopoietic function studies in patients receiving repeated or prolonged therapy.
● Monitor elderly patients for dizziness, ataxia, mental status changes. Patients are at an increased risk for falls.
● *Alert:* Use of drug may lead to abuse and addiction. Don't withdraw drug abruptly after long-term use; withdrawal symptoms may occur.
● *Look alike–sound alike:* Don't confuse diazepam with diazoxide.

PATIENT TEACHING
● Warn patient to avoid activities that require alertness and good coordination until effects of drug are known.
● Tell patient to avoid alcohol while taking drug.
● Notify patient that smoking may decrease drug's effectiveness.
● Warn patient not to abruptly stop drug because withdrawal symptoms may occur.
● Warn woman to avoid use during pregnancy.
● Instruct patient's caregiver on the proper use of Diastat rectal gel.

diphenhydramine hydrochloride
dye-fen-HYE-drah-meen

Allerdryl † ◊, AllerMax ◊*, Aller-Max Caplets ◊, Allernix† ◊, Altaryl Children's Allergy† ◊, Banophen ◊, Benadryl ◊, Benadryl Allergy ◊, Children's Pedia Care Nightime Cough† ◊, Compoz ◊, Diphen Cough ◊, Diphenhist ◊, Diphenhist Captabs ◊, Dytan ◊, Genahist ◊, Hydramine Cough ◊*, Siladryl ◊*, Silphen ◊*, Sominex ◊, Triaminic MultiSymptom ◊*, Tusstat ◊*, Twilite Caplets ◊

Pharmacologic class: ethanolamine
Pregnancy risk category B

AVAILABLE FORMS
Capsules: 25 mg ◊, 50 mg ◊
Elixir: 12.5 mg/5 ml ◊*
Injection: 50 mg/ml
Strips (orally disintegrating): 12.5 mg ◊*, 25 mg ◊
Syrup: 12.5 mg/5 ml ◊*
Tablets: 25 mg ◊, 50 mg ◊
Tablets (chewable): 12.5 mg ◊

INDICATIONS & DOSAGES
➤ **Rhinitis, allergy symptoms, motion sickness, Parkinson's disease**
Adults and children age 12 and older: 25 to 50 mg P.O. every 4 to 6 hours. Maximum, 300 mg P.O. daily. Or, 10 to 50 mg I.V. or deep I.M. Maximum I.V. or I.M. dosage, 400 mg daily.
Children ages 6 to 11: 12.5 to 25 mg P.O. every 4 to 6 hours. Maximum dose is 150 mg daily. Or, 5 mg/kg day divided into four doses P.O., deep I.M., or I.V. Maximum dose is 300 mg daily.
Children ages 2 to 5: 6.25 mg every 4 to 6 hours. Maximum dose is 37.5 mg daily. Or, 5 mg/kg day divided into four doses P.O., deep I.M., or I.V. Maximum dose is 300 mg daily.
Children weighing less than 9.1 kg (20 lb): 5 mg/kg day divided into four doses P.O., deep I.M., or I.V. Maximum dose is 300 mg daily.

➤ **Sedation**
Adults: 25 to 50 mg P.O. or deep I.M. as needed.
➤ **Nighttime sleep aid**
Adults: 25 to 50 mg P.O. at bedtime.
➤ **Nonproductive cough**
Adults and children age 12 and older: 25 mg (syrup) P.O. every 4 hours. Don't exceed 150 mg daily. Or, 25 to 50 mg (liquid) every 4 hours. Don't exceed 300 mg daily.
Children ages 6 to 11: 12.5 mg (syrup) P.O. every 4 hours. Don't exceed 75 mg daily. Or, 12.5 to 25 mg (liquid) every 4 hours. Don't exceed 150 mg daily.
Children ages 2 to 5: 6.25 mg (syrup) P.O. every 4 hours. Don't exceed 25 mg daily.
➤ **Antipsychotic-induced dystonia ♦**
Adults: 50 mg I.M. or I.V.

ADMINISTRATION
P.O.
• Give drug with food or milk to reduce GI distress.
I.V.
• Don't exceed 25 mg/minute.
• **Incompatibilities:** Allopurinol, amobarbital, amphotericin B, cefepime, dexamethasone, foscarnet, haloperidol lactate, pentobarbital, phenobarbital, phenytoin, thiopental.
I.M.
• Give I.M. injection deep into large muscle.
• Alternate injection sites to prevent irritation.

ACTION
Competes with histamine for H_1-receptor sites. Prevents, but doesn't reverse, histamine-mediated responses, particularly those of the bronchial tubes, GI tract, uterus, and blood vessels. Structurally related to local anesthetics, drug provides local anesthesia and suppresses cough reflex.

Route	Onset	Peak	Duration
P.O.	15 min	1–4 hr	6–8 hr
I.V.	Immediate	1–4 hr	6–8 hr
I.M.	Unknown	1–4 hr	6–8 hr

Half-life: 2.4 to 9.3 hours.

ADVERSE REACTIONS
CNS: *drowsiness, sedation, sleepiness, dizziness, incoordination, **seizures,*** confusion, insomnia, headache, vertigo, fatigue, restlessness, tremor, nervousness.
CV: palpitations, hypotension, tachycardia.
EENT: diplopia, blurred vision, nasal congestion, tinnitus.
GI: *dry mouth, nausea, epigastric distress,* vomiting, diarrhea, constipation, anorexia.
GU: dysuria, urine retention, urinary frequency.
Hematologic: *thrombocytopenia, agranulocytosis,* hemolytic anemia.
Respiratory: *thickening of bronchial secretions.*
Skin: urticaria, photosensitivity, rash.
Other: *anaphylactic shock.*

INTERACTIONS
Drug-drug. *CNS depressants:* May increase sedation. Use together cautiously.
MAO inhibitors: May increase anticholinergic effects. Avoid using together.
Other products that contain diphenhydramine (including topical therapy): May increase risk of adverse reactions. Avoid using together.
Drug-lifestyle. *Alcohol use:* May increase CNS depression. Discourage use together.
Sun exposure: May cause photosensitivity reactions. Advise patient to avoid extensive sunlight exposure.

EFFECTS ON LAB TEST RESULTS
● May decrease hemoglobin level and hematocrit.
● May decrease granulocyte and platelet counts.
● May prevent, reduce, or mask positive result in diagnostic skin test.

CONTRAINDICATIONS & CAUTIONS
● Contraindicated in patients hypersensitive to drug; newborns; premature neonates; breast-feeding women; patients with angle-closure glaucoma, stenosing peptic ulcer, symptomatic prostatic hyperplasia, bladder neck obstruction, or pyloroduodenal obstruction; and those having an acute asthmatic attack.

● Avoid use in patients taking MAO inhibitors.
● Use with caution in patients with prostatic hyperplasia, asthma, COPD, increased intraocular pressure, hyperthyroidism, CV disease, and hypertension.
● Children younger than age 12 should use drug only as directed by prescriber.

NURSING CONSIDERATIONS
● Stop drug 4 days before diagnostic skin testing.
● Dizziness, excessive sedation, syncope, toxicity, paradoxical stimulation, and hypotension are more likely to occur in elderly patients.
● ***Look alike–sound alike:*** Don't confuse diphenhydramine with dimenhydrinate; don't confuse Benadryl with Bentyl or benazepril.

PATIENT TEACHING
● Warn patient not to take this drug with any other products that contain diphenhydramine (including topical therapy) because of increased adverse reactions.
● Instruct patient to take drug 30 minutes before travel to prevent motion sickness.
● Tell patient to take diphenhydramine with food or milk to reduce GI distress.
● Warn patient to avoid alcohol and hazardous activities that require alertness until CNS effects of drug are known.
● Inform patient that sugarless gum, hard candy, or ice chips may relieve dry mouth.
● Tell patient to notify prescriber if tolerance develops because a different antihistamine may need to be prescribed.
● Drug is in many OTC sleep and cold products. Advise patient to consult prescriber before using these products.
● Warn patient of possible photosensitivity reactions. Advise use of a sunblock.

disulfiram
dye-SUL-fi-ram

Antabuse

Pharmacologic class: aldehyde
dehydrogenase inhibitor
Pregnancy risk category NR

AVAILABLE FORMS
Tablets: 250 mg, 500 mg

INDICATIONS & DOSAGES
➤ **Adjunct to management of alcohol abstinence**
Adults: 250 to 500 mg P.O. as single dose in morning for 1 to 2 weeks or in evening if drowsiness occurs. Maintenance dosage is 125 to 500 mg P.O. daily (average 250 mg) until permanent self-control is established. Treatment may continue for months or years.

ADMINISTRATION
P.O.
● Never give until patient has abstained from alcohol for at least 12 hours. He should clearly understand consequences of drug and give permission for its use. Use drug only in patients who are cooperative, well motivated, and receiving supportive psychiatric therapy.

ACTION
Blocks oxidation of alcohol at the acetaldehyde stage. Excess acetaldehyde produces a highly unpleasant reaction in the presence of even small amounts of alcohol.

Route	Onset	Peak	Duration
P.O.	1–2 hr	Unknown	14 days

Half-life: Unknown.

ADVERSE REACTIONS
CNS: drowsiness, headache, fatigue, delirium, depression, neuritis, peripheral neuritis, polyneuritis, restlessness, psychotic reactions.
EENT: optic neuritis.
GI: metallic or garlicky aftertaste.
GU: impotence.

Skin: acneiform or allergic dermatitis, occasional eruptions.
Other: *disulfiram reaction precipitated by alcohol use.*

INTERACTIONS
Drug-drug. *Barbiturates:* May prolong duration of barbiturate effect. Closely monitor patient.
CNS depressants: May increase CNS depression. Use together cautiously.
Coumarin anticoagulants: May increase anticoagulant effect. Adjust dosage of anticoagulant.
Isoniazid: May cause ataxia or marked change in behavior. Avoid using together.
Metronidazole: May cause psychotic reaction. Avoid using together.
Midazolam: May increase midazolam level. Use together cautiously.
Paraldehyde: May cause toxic level of acetaldehyde. Avoid using together.
Phenytoin: May increase toxic effect of phenytoin. Monitor phenytoin level closely, and adjust dose as necessary.
Tricyclic antidepressants, especially amitriptyline: May cause transient delirium. Closely monitor patient.
Drug-herb. *Herbal preparations containing alcohol:* May cause disulfiram reaction. Warn patient against using together. Alcohol reaction may occur as long as 2 weeks after single drug dose.
Drug-food. *Caffeine:* May increase elimination half-life of caffeine. Tell patient to watch for effects.
Drug-lifestyle. *Alcohol use:* May cause disulfiram reaction including flushing, tachycardia, bronchospasm, sweating, nausea and vomiting, or death. Warn patient not to use products containing alcohol, including back rub preparations, cough syrups, liniments, and shaving lotion, or to drink alcoholic beverages.

EFFECTS ON LAB TEST RESULTS
● May increase cholesterol level.

CONTRAINDICATIONS & CAUTIONS
● Contraindicated in patients hypersensitive to drug or other thiram derivatives used in pesticides and rubber vulcanization; in those with psychoses, myocardial disease, or coronary occlusion; in those

---

Reactions may be *common,* uncommon, *life-threatening,* or COMMON AND LIFE-THREATENING.
Interaction may have a *rapid onset* or **delayed onset**.

receiving metronidazole, paraldehyde, alcohol, or alcohol-containing products; and in those experiencing alcohol intoxication or who have ingested alcohol in preceding 12 hours.
• Don't give drug during pregnancy.
• Use with caution in patients also receiving phenytoin therapy and in those with diabetes mellitus, hypothyroidism, seizure disorder, cerebral damage, nephritis, or hepatic cirrhosis or insufficiency.

NURSING CONSIDERATIONS
• Perform complete physical examination and laboratory studies, including CBC, SMA-12, and transaminase level, before therapy and repeat regularly.
• Disulfiram reaction may result from alcohol use, with flushing, throbbing headache, dyspnea, nausea, copious vomiting, diaphoresis, thirst, chest pain, palpitations, hyperventilation, hypotension, syncope, anxiety, weakness, blurred vision, confusion, and arthropathy.
• *Alert:* A severe disulfiram reaction can cause respiratory depression, CV collapse, arrhythmias, MI, acute heart failure, seizures, unconsciousness, and death.
• The longer the patient remains on the drug, the more sensitive he becomes to alcohol.
• *Look alike–sound alike:* Don't confuse Antabuse with Anturane.

PATIENT TEACHING
• *Alert:* Caution patient's family that drug should never be given to patient without his knowledge; severe reaction or death could result if patient drinks alcohol.
• Tell patient to carry medical identification that identifies him as a disulfiram user.
• Mild reactions may occur in sensitive patient with blood alcohol levels of 5 to 10 mg/dl; symptoms are fully developed at 50 mg/dl; unconsciousness typically occurs at 125 to 150 mg/dl level. Reaction may last from 30 minutes to several hours or as long as alcohol remains in blood.
• Reassure patient that drug-induced adverse reactions (unrelated to alcohol use), such as drowsiness, fatigue, impotence, headache, peripheral neuritis, and metallic

or garlic taste, subside after about 2 weeks of therapy.
• Advise patient not to drink alcoholic beverages or use products containing alcohol, including topical preparations and mouthwash.
• Have patient verify content of OTC products with pharmacist before use.

---

donepezil hydrochloride
doe-NEP-ah-zill

Aricept, Aricept ODT

Pharmacologic class: cholinesterase inhibitor
Pregnancy risk category C

AVAILABLE FORMS
Orally disintegrating tablets (ODTs):
5 mg, 10 mg
Tablets: 5 mg, 10 mg

INDICATIONS & DOSAGES
➤ **Mild to severe Alzheimer dementia**
Adults: Initially, 5 mg P.O. daily at bedtime. After 4 to 6 weeks, increase to 10 mg daily, if needed.

ADMINISTRATION
P.O.
• Allow ODT to dissolve on tongue; then follow with water.
• Give drug at bedtime, without regard for food.

ACTION
Thought to increase acetylcholine level by inhibiting cholinesterase enzyme, which causes acetylcholine hydrolysis.

Route	Onset	Peak	Duration
P.O.	Unknown	3–4 hr	Unknown

Half-life: 70 hours.

ADVERSE REACTIONS
CNS: *headache, insomnia, seizures,* dizziness, fatigue, depression, abnormal dreams, somnolence, tremor, irritability, paresthesia, aggression, vertigo, ataxia,

---

restlessness, abnormal crying, nervousness, aphasia, syncope, pain.
CV: chest pain, hypertension, vasodilation, atrial fibrillation, hot flashes, hypotension.
EENT: cataract, blurred vision, eye irritation, sore throat.
GI: *nausea, diarrhea,* vomiting, anorexia, fecal incontinence, ***GI bleeding,*** bloating, epigastric pain.
GU: urinary frequency.
Metabolic: weight loss, dehydration.
Musculoskeletal: muscle cramps, arthritis, bone fracture.
Respiratory: dyspnea, bronchitis.
Skin: pruritus, urticaria, diaphoresis, ecchymoses.
Other: toothache, influenza, increased libido.

INTERACTIONS
Drug-drug. *Anticholinergics:* May decrease donepezil effects. Avoid using together.
Anticholinesterases, cholinomimetics: May have synergistic effect. Monitor patient closely.
Bethanechol, succinylcholine: May have additive effects. Monitor patient closely.
Carbamazepine, dexamethasone, phenobarbital, phenytoin, rifampin: May increase rate of donepezil elimination. Monitor patient.

EFFECTS ON LAB TEST RESULTS
None reported.

CONTRAINDICATIONS & CAUTIONS
• Contraindicated in patients hypersensitive to drug or piperidine derivatives and in breast-feeding women.
• Use cautiously in pregnant women and in patients who take NSAIDs or have CV disease, asthma, obstructive pulmonary disease, urinary outflow impairment, or history of ulcer disease.

NURSING CONSIDERATIONS
• Monitor patient for evidence of active or occult GI bleeding.
• ***Look alike–sound alike:*** Don't confuse Aricept with Ascriptin.

PATIENT TEACHING
• Stress that drug doesn't alter underlying degenerative disease but can temporarily stabilize or relieve symptoms. Effectiveness depends on taking drug at regular intervals.
• Tell caregiver to give drug just before patient's bedtime.
• ODTs may be taken with or without food. Have patient allow tablet to dissolve on his tongue, then swallow with a sip of water.
• Advise patient and caregiver to report immediately significant adverse effects or changes in overall health status and to inform health care team that patient is taking drug before he receives anesthesia.
• Tell patient to avoid OTC cold or sleep remedies because of risk of increased anticholinergic effects.

---

doxapram hydrochloride
DOCKS-a-pram

Dopram

Pharmacologic class: analeptic
Pregnancy risk category B

AVAILABLE FORMS
Injection: 20 mg/ml (benzyl alcohol 0.9%)

INDICATIONS & DOSAGES
➤ **Postanesthesia respiratory stimulation**
Adults: 0.5 to 1 mg/kg as a single I.V. injection (not to exceed 1.5 mg/kg) or as multiple injections every 5 minutes, total not to exceed 2 mg/kg. Or, 250 mg in 250 ml of normal saline solution or D_5W infused at initial rate of 5 mg/minute I.V. until satisfactory response is achieved. Maintain at 1 to 3 mg/minute. Don't exceed total dose for infusion of 4 mg/kg.
➤ **Drug-induced CNS depression**
Adults: For injection, priming dose of 2 mg/kg I.V., repeated in 5 minutes and again every 1 to 2 hours until patient awakens (and if relapse occurs). Maximum daily dose is 3 g.

For infusion, priming dose of 2 mg/kg I.V., repeated in 5 minutes and again in 1 to 2 hours, if needed. If response occurs, give I.V. infusion (1 mg/ml) at 1 to 3 mg/minute until patient awakens. Don't infuse for longer than 2 hours or give more than 3 g/day. May resume I.V. infusion after rest period of 30 minutes to 2 hours, if needed.

➤ **Chronic pulmonary disease related to acute hypercapnia**
Adults: 1 to 2 mg/minute by I.V. infusion using 2 mg/ml solution. Maximum, 3 mg/minute for up to 2 hours.

ADMINISTRATION
I.V.
• Drug is compatible with D_5W, $D_{10}W$, and normal saline solution.
• Give slowly; rapid infusion may cause hemolysis.
• Watch for irritation and infiltration; it can cause tissue damage and necrosis.
• **Incompatibilities:** Aminophylline, ascorbic acid, cefoperazone, cefotaxime, cefuroxime sodium, dexamethasone sodium phosphate, diazepam, digoxin, dobutamine, folic acid, furosemide, hydrocortisone sodium phosphate, hydrocortisone sodium succinate, ketamine, methylprednisolone sodium succinate, minocycline, sodium bicarbonate, thiopental, ticarcillin disodium.

ACTION
Not clearly defined. Directly stimulates the central respiratory centers in the medulla and may indirectly act on carotid, aortic, or other peripheral chemoreceptors.

Route	Onset	Peak	Duration
I.V.	20–40 sec	1–2 min	5–12 min

Half-life: $2\frac{1}{2}$ to 4 hours.

ADVERSE REACTIONS
CNS: *headache, dizziness, seizures,* apprehension, disorientation, hyperactivity, bilateral Babinski's signs, paresthesia.
CV: *chest pain and tightness, variations in heart rate, hypertension,* **arrhythmias,** T-wave depression on ECG, flushing.
EENT: *laryngospasm,* sneezing.
GI: nausea, vomiting, diarrhea.

GU: urine retention, bladder stimulation with incontinence, albuminuria.
Musculoskeletal: muscle spasms.
Respiratory: *bronchospasm,* cough, dyspnea, rebound hypoventilation, hiccups.
Skin: pruritus, diaphoresis.

INTERACTIONS
Drug-drug. *General anesthetics:* May cause self-limiting arrhythmias. Avoid using doxapram within 10 minutes of an anesthetic that sensitizes the myocardium to catecholamines.
MAO inhibitors, sympathomimetics: May increase adverse CV effects. Use together cautiously.

EFFECTS ON LAB TEST RESULTS
• May increase BUN level. May decrease hemoglobin level and hematocrit.
• May decrease erythrocyte, RBC, and WBC counts.

CONTRAINDICATIONS & CAUTIONS
• Contraindicated in patients with seizure disorders; head injury; CV disorders; frank, uncompensated heart failure; severe hypertension; stroke; respiratory failure or incompetence secondary to neuromuscular disorders, muscle paresis, flail chest, obstructed airway, pulmonary embolism, pneumothorax, restrictive respiratory disease, acute bronchial asthma, or extreme dyspnea; or hypoxia unrelated to hypercapnia.
• Use cautiously in patients with bronchial asthma, severe tachycardia or arrhythmias, cerebral edema, increased intracranial pressure, hyperthyroidism, pheochromocytoma, or metabolic disorders.

NURSING CONSIDERATIONS
• Drug is used only in surgical or emergency department situations.
• Separate end of anesthetic treatment and start of this drug by at least 10 minutes.
• *Alert:* Establish an adequate airway before giving drug. Prevent patient from aspirating vomitus by placing him on his side.
• Monitor blood pressure, heart rate, deep tendon reflexes, and arterial blood gases

before giving drug and every 30 minutes afterward.

• Monitor patient for evidence of overdose, such as hypertension, tachycardia, arrhythmias, skeletal muscle hyperactivity, and dyspnea. Hold drug and notify prescriber if patient needs mechanical ventilation or shows signs of increased arterial carbon dioxide or oxygen tension.

• *Look alike–sound alike:* Don't confuse doxapram with doxorubicin, doxepin, or doxazosin.

PATIENT TEACHING
• Inform family and patient about need for drug.
• Answer patient's questions and address his concerns.

---

doxepin hydrochloride
DOKS-eh-pin

Sinequan

Pharmacologic class: tricyclic antidepressant (TCA)
Pregnancy risk category C

AVAILABLE FORMS
Capsules: 10 mg, 25 mg, 50 mg, 75 mg, 100 mg, 150 mg
Oral concentrate: 10 mg/ml

INDICATIONS & DOSAGES
➤ **Depression; anxiety**
Adults: Initially, 75 mg P.O. daily. Usual dosage range is 75 to 150 mg daily to maximum of 300 mg daily in divided doses. Or, entire maintenance dose may be given once daily with maximum dose of 150 mg.

ADMINISTRATION
P.O.
• Dilute oral concentrate with 4 ounces (120 ml) of water, milk, or juice (orange, grapefruit, tomato, prune, or pineapple, but not grape); don't mix preparation with carbonated beverages.
• Give at bedtime, if possible, because it may cause drowsiness and dizziness.

ACTION
Unknown. Increases amount of norepinephrine, serotonin, or both in the CNS by blocking their reuptake by the presynaptic neurons.

Route	Onset	Peak	Duration
P.O.	Unknown	2 hr	Unknown

Half-life: 6 to 8 hours.

ADVERSE REACTIONS
CNS: *drowsiness, dizziness, seizures,* confusion, numbness, hallucinations, paresthesia, ataxia, weakness, headache, extrapyramidal reactions.
CV: *orthostatic hypotension, tachycardia,* ECG changes.
EENT: *blurred vision,* tinnitus.
GI: *dry mouth, constipation,* nausea, vomiting, anorexia.
GU: urine retention.
Metabolic: *hypoglycemia,* hyperglycemia.
Skin: *diaphoresis,* rash, urticaria, photosensitivity reactions.
Other: hypersensitivity reactions.

INTERACTIONS
Drug-drug. *Barbiturates, CNS depressants:* May enhance CNS depression. Avoid using together.
Cimetidine, **fluoxetine, fluvoxamine, paroxetine, sertraline:** May increase doxepin level. Monitor drug levels and patient for signs of toxicity.
Clonidine: May cause life-threatening hypertension. Avoid using together.
Epinephrine, norepinephrine: May increase hypertensive effect. Use together cautiously.
MAO inhibitors: May cause severe excitation, hyperpyrexia, or seizures, usually with high dosage. Avoid using within 14 days of MAO inhibitor therapy.
Quinolones: May increase the risk of life-threatening arrhythmias. Avoid using together.
Drug-herb. *Evening primrose oil:* May cause additive or synergistic effect, resulting in lower seizure threshold and increasing the risk of seizure. Discourage use together.

St. John's wort, SAM-e, yohimbe: May cause serotonin syndrome. Discourage use together.

Drug-lifestyle. *Alcohol use:* May enhance CNS depression. Discourage use together.

Sun exposure: May increase risk of photosensitivity reactions. Advise patient to avoid excessive sunlight exposure.

EFFECTS ON LAB TEST RESULTS
● May increase or decrease glucose level.
● May increase liver function test values.

CONTRAINDICATIONS & CAUTIONS
● Contraindicated in patients hypersensitive to drug and in those with glaucoma or tendency toward urine retention; also contraindicated in those who have received an MAO inhibitor within past 14 days and during acute recovery phase of an MI.

NURSING CONSIDERATIONS
● Don't withdraw drug abruptly.
● Monitor patient for nausea, headache, and malaise after abrupt withdrawal of long-term therapy; these symptoms don't indicate addiction.
● *Alert:* Because hypertensive episodes may occur during surgery in patients receiving drug, stop it gradually several days before surgery.
● If signs or symptoms of psychosis occur or increase, expect prescriber to reduce dosage. Record mood changes. Monitor patient for suicidal tendencies and allow only a minimum supply of drug.
● *Alert:* Drug may increase risk of suicidal thinking and behavior in children, adolescents, and young adults ages 18 to 24 during the first 2 months of treatment, especially in those with major depressive disorder or other psychiatric disorder.
● Drug has strong anticholinergic effects and is one of the most sedating TCAs. Adverse anticholinergic effects can occur rapidly.
● Recommend use of sugarless hard candy or gum to relieve dry mouth.
● *Look alike–sound alike:* Don't confuse doxepin with doxazosin, digoxin, doxapram, or Doxidan; don't confuse Sinequan with saquinavir.

PATIENT TEACHING
● Tell patient to dilute oral concentrate with 4 ounces (120 ml) of water, milk, or juice (orange, grapefruit, tomato, prune, or pineapple, but not grape); preparation shouldn't be mixed with carbonated beverages.
● Tell patient to take full dose at bedtime whenever he can, but warn him of possible morning dizziness on standing up quickly.
● Advise patient to consult prescriber before taking other prescription or OTC drugs.
● Warn patient to avoid hazardous activities that require alertness and good psychomotor coordination until effects of drug are known. Drowsiness and dizziness usually subside after a few weeks.
● Tell patient to avoid alcohol during drug therapy.
● Tell patient that maximal effect may not be evident for 2 to 3 weeks.
● Warn patient not to stop drug suddenly.
● To prevent sensitivity to the sun, advise patient to use sunblock, wear protective clothing, and avoid prolonged exposure to strong sunlight.

---

duloxetine hydrochloride
do-LOCKS-ah-teen

Cymbalta

Pharmacologic class: SSNRI
Pregnancy risk category C

AVAILABLE FORMS
Capsules (delayed-release): 20 mg, 30 mg, 60 mg

INDICATIONS & DOSAGES
➤ **Major depressive disorder**
Adults: Initially, 20 mg P.O. b.i.d.; then, 60 mg P.O. once daily or divided in two equal doses. Maximum, 60 mg daily.
✱*NEW INDICATION:* **Generalized anxiety disorder**
Adults: 60 mg P.O. daily. Or, 30 mg P.O. daily for 1 week; then increase to 60 mg P.O. daily.
➤ **Neuropathic pain related to diabetic peripheral neuropathy**
Adults: 60 mg P.O. once daily.

Adjust-a-dose: In patients with impaired renal function, reduce starting dose and increase gradually.

ADMINISTRATION
P.O.
● Give drug whole; don't crush or open capsule.

ACTION
May inhibit serotonin and norepinephrine reuptake in the CNS.

Route	Onset	Peak	Duration
P.O.	Unknown	6 hr	Unknown

Half-life: 12 hours.

ADVERSE REACTIONS
CNS: *dizziness, fatigue, headache, insomnia, somnolence,* **suicidal thoughts,** fever, hypoesthesia, initial insomnia, irritability, lethargy, nervousness, nightmares, restlessness, sleep disorder, anxiety, asthenia, tremor.
CV: hot flushes, hypertension, increased heart rate.
EENT: blurred vision, nasopharyngitis, pharyngolaryngeal pain.
GI: *constipation, diarrhea, dry mouth, nausea,* dyspepsia, gastritis, vomiting.
GU: abnormal orgasm, abnormally increased frequency of urinating, delayed or dysfunctional ejaculation, dysuria, erectile dysfunction, urinary hesitation.
Metabolic: *decreased appetite,* **hypoglycemia,** increased appetite, weight gain or loss.
Musculoskeletal: muscle cramps, myalgia.
Respiratory: cough.
Skin: increased sweating, night sweats, pruritus, rash.
Other: decreased libido, rigors.

INTERACTIONS
Drug-drug. *Antiarrhythmics of type 1C (flecainide, propafenone), phenothiazines:* May increase levels of these drugs. Use together cautiously.
CNS drugs: May increase adverse effects. Use together cautiously.

CYP1A2 inhibitors (cimetidine, fluvoxamine, certain quinolones): May increase duloxetine level. Avoid using together.
CYP2D6 inhibitors (fluoxetine, paroxetine, quinidine): May increase duloxetine level. Use together cautiously.
Drugs that reduce gastric acidity: May cause premature breakdown of duloxetine's protective coating and early release of the drug. Monitor patient for effects.
MAO inhibitors: May cause hyperthermia, rigidity, myoclonus, autonomic instability, rapid fluctuations of vital signs, agitation, delirium, and coma. Avoid use within 2 weeks after MAO inhibitor therapy; wait at least 5 days after stopping duloxetine before starting MAO inhibitor.
Thioridazine: May prolong the QT interval and increase risk of serious ventricular arrhythmias and sudden death. Avoid using together.
Tricyclic antidepressants (amitriptyline, nortriptyline, imipramine): May increase levels of these drugs. Reduce tricyclic antidepressant dose, and monitor drug levels closely.
Triptans: May cause serotonin syndrome (restlessness, hallucinations, loss of coordination, fast heartbeat, rapid changes in blood pressure, increased body temperature, hyperreflexia, nausea, vomiting, and diarrhea). Use cautiously and with increased monitoring, especially when starting or increasing dosages.
Drug-lifestyle. *Alcohol use:* May increase risk of liver damage. Discourage use together.

EFFECTS ON LAB TEST RESULTS
● May increase alkaline phosphatase, ALT, AST, bilirubin, and CK levels.

CONTRAINDICATIONS & CAUTIONS
● Contraindicated in patients hypersensitive to drug or its ingredients, patients taking MAO inhibitors, patients with uncontrolled angle-closure glaucoma, and patients with a creatinine clearance less than 30 ml/minute. Drug isn't recommended for patients with hepatic dysfunction or end-stage renal disease.
● Use cautiously in patients with a history of mania or seizures, patients who drink substantial amounts of alcohol, patients

---

with hypertension, patients with controlled angle-closure glaucoma, and those with conditions that slow gastric emptying.

NURSING CONSIDERATIONS
• Monitor patient for worsening of depression or suicidal behavior, especially when therapy starts or dosage changes.
• *Alert:* Drug may increase risk of suicidal thinking and behavior in children, adolescents, and young adults ages 18 to 24 during the first 2 months of treatment, especially in those with major depressive disorder or other psychiatric disorder.
• Treatment of overdose is symptomatic. Don't induce emesis; gastric lavage or activated charcoal may be performed soon after ingestion or if patient is still symptomatic. Because drug undergoes extensive distribution, forced diuresis, dialysis, hemoperfusion, and exchange transfusion aren't useful. Contact a poison control center for information.
• If taken with tricyclic antidepressants, duloxetine metabolism will be prolonged, and patient will need extended monitoring.
• Periodically reassess patient to determine the need for continued therapy.
• Decrease dosage gradually, and watch for symptoms that may arise when drug is stopped, such as dizziness, nausea, headache, paresthesia, vomiting, irritability, and nightmares.
• If intolerable symptoms arise when decreasing or stopping drug, restart at previous dose and decrease even more gradually.
• Monitor blood pressure periodically during treatment.
• Use during the third trimester of pregnancy may cause neonatal complications including respiratory distress, cyanosis, apnea, seizures, vomiting, hypoglycemia, and hyperreflexia, which may require prolonged hospitalization, respiratory support, and tube feeding. Consider potential benefit of drug to the mother versus risks to the fetus.
• Older patients may be more sensitive to drug effects than younger adults.
• *Alert:* Combining triptans with an SSRI or an SSNRI may cause serotonin syndrome. Signs and symptoms may include restlessness, hallucinations, loss of coordination, fast heartbeat, rapid changes in blood pressure, increased body temperature, overactive reflexes, nausea, vomiting, and diarrhea. Serotonin syndrome may be more likely to occur when starting or increasing the dose of triptan, SSRI, or SSNRI.

PATIENT TEACHING
• *Alert:* Warn families or caregivers to report signs of worsening depression (such as agitation, irritability, insomnia, hostility, impulsivity) and signs of suicidal behavior to prescriber immediately.
• Tell patient to consult his prescriber or pharmacist if he plans to take other prescription or OTC drugs or an herbal or other dietary supplement.
• Instruct patient to swallow capsules whole and not to chew, crush, or open them because they have an enteric coating.
• Urge patient to avoid activities that are hazardous or require mental alertness until he knows how the drug affects him.
• Warn against drinking alcohol during therapy.
• If patient takes drug for depression, explain that it may take 1 to 4 weeks to notice an effect.

---

escitalopram oxalate
ess-si-TAL-oh-pram

Lexapro

Pharmacologic class: SSRI
Pregnancy risk category C

AVAILABLE FORMS
Oral solution: 5 mg/5 ml
Tablets: 5 mg, 10 mg, 20 mg

INDICATIONS & DOSAGES
➤ **Treatment and maintenance therapy for patients with major depressive disorder; general anxiety disorder**
Adults: Initially, 10 mg P.O. once daily, increasing to 20 mg if needed after at least 1 week.
Adjust-a-dose: For elderly patients and those with hepatic impairment, 10 mg P.O. daily, initially and as maintenance dosages.

ADMINISTRATION
P.O.
● Give drug without regard for food.

ACTION
Action may be linked to increase of serotonergic activity in the CNS from inhibition of neuronal reuptake of serotonin.
Drug is closely related to citalopram,
which may be the active component.

Route	Onset	Peak	Duration
P.O.	Unknown	5 hr	Unknown

Half-life: 27 to 32 hours.

ADVERSE REACTIONS
CNS: *suicidal behavior,* fever, insomnia,
dizziness, somnolence, paresthesia, light-
headedness, migraine, tremor, vertigo,
abnormal dreams, irritability, impaired
concentration, fatigue, lethargy.
CV: palpitations, hypertension, flushing,
chest pain.
EENT: rhinitis, sinusitis, blurred vision,
tinnitus, earache.
GI: *nausea,* diarrhea, constipation, indigestion, abdominal pain, vomiting, increased or decreased appetite, dry mouth,
flatulence, heartburn, cramps, gastro-
esophageal reflux.
GU: ejaculation disorder, impotence,
anorgasmia, menstrual cramps, UTI,
urinary frequency.
Metabolic: weight gain or loss.
Musculoskeletal: arthralgia, myalgia,
muscle cramps, pain in arms or legs.
Respiratory: bronchitis, cough.
Skin: rash, increased sweating.
Other: decreased libido, yawning, flulike
symptoms.

INTERACTIONS
Drug-drug. *Aspirin, NSAIDs, other drugs
known to affect coagulation:* May increase the risk of bleeding. Use together
cautiously.
Carbamazepine: May increase escitalopram clearance. Monitor patient for expected antidepressant effect and adjust
dose as needed.
Cimetidine: May increase escitalopram
level. Monitor patient for increased adverse reactions to escitalopram.

Citalopram: May cause additive effects.
Using together is contraindicated.
CNS drugs: May cause additive effects.
Use together cautiously.
*Desipramine, other drugs metabolized by
CYP2D6:* May increase levels of these
drugs. Use together cautiously.
Lithium: May enhance serotonergic effect
of escitalopram. Use together cautiously,
and monitor lithium level.
MAO inhibitors: May cause fatal serotonin
syndrome. Avoid using within 14 days of
MAO inhibitor therapy.
Triptans: May increase serotonergic ef-
fects, leading to weakness, hyperreflexia,
incoordination, rapid changes in blood
pressure, nausea, and diarrhea. Use
together cautiously, especially at the start
of therapy or at dosage increases.
Tramadol: May cause serotonin syndrome.
Monitor patient closely.
Drug-lifestyle. *Alcohol use:* May increase
CNS effects. Discourage use together.

EFFECTS ON LAB TEST RESULTS
None reported.

CONTRAINDICATIONS & CAUTIONS
● Contraindicated in patients taking pimozide, MAO inhibitors, or within 14 days
of MAO inhibitor therapy and in those
hypersensitive to escitalopram, citalopram,
or any of its inactive ingredients.
● Use cautiously in patients with a history of mania, seizure disorders, suicidal
thoughts, or renal or hepatic impairment.
● Use cautiously in patients with diseases
that produce altered metabolism or hemodynamic responses.
● Use with caution in elderly patients
because they may have greater sensitivity
to drug.
● Use in third trimester of pregnancy may
cause complications at birth. Consider the
risk versus benefit of treatment during this
time.
● Drug appears in breast milk. Patient
should either stop breast-feeding or stop
taking drug.

NURSING CONSIDERATIONS
● Closely monitor patients at high risk of
suicide.

Reactions may be *common,* uncommon, ***life-threatening,*** or COMMON AND LIFE-THREATENING.
Interaction may have a *rapid onset* or ***delayed onset***.

• *Alert:* Drug may increase risk of suicidal thinking and behavior in children, adolescents, and young adults ages 18 to 24 during the first 2 months of treatment, especially in those with major depressive disorder or other psychiatric disorder.

• *Look alike–sound alike:* Don't confuse escitalopram with estazolam.

• Evaluate patient for history of drug abuse and observe for signs of misuse or abuse.

• Periodically reassess patient to determine need for maintenance treatment and appropriate dosing.

• *Alert:* Combining triptans with an SSRI or an SSNRI may cause serotonin syndrome. Signs and symptoms may include restlessness, hallucinations, loss of coordination, fast heart beat, rapid changes in blood pressure, increased body temperature, overactive reflexes, nausea, vomiting, and diarrhea. Serotonin syndrome may be more likely to occur when starting or increasing the dose of triptan, SSRI, or SSNRI.

PATIENT TEACHING
• Inform patient that symptoms should improve gradually over several weeks, rather than immediately.

• Tell patient that although improvement may occur within 1 to 4 weeks, he should continue drug as prescribed.

• *Alert:* Caution patient and patient's family to report signs of worsening depression (such as agitation, irritability, insomnia, hostility, impulsivity) and signs of suicidal behavior to prescriber immediately.

• Tell patient to use caution while driving or operating hazardous machinery because of drug's potential to impair judgment, thinking, and motor skills.

• Advise patient to consult health care provider before taking other prescription or OTC drugs.

• Tell patient that drug may be taken in the morning or evening without regard to meals.

• Encourage patient to avoid alcohol while taking drug.

• Tell woman to notify health care provider if she's pregnant or breast-feeding.

esterified estrogens
ESS-tehr-eh-fide ESS-troe-jenz

Menest, Neo-Estrone

Pharmacologic class: estrogen
Pregnancy risk category X

AVAILABLE FORMS
Tablets: 0.3 mg, 0.625 mg, 1.25 mg, 2.5 mg
Tablets (film-coated): 0.3 mg, 0.625 mg, 1.25 mg, 2.5 mg

INDICATIONS & DOSAGES
➤ **Inoperable prostate cancer**
Men: 1.25 to 2.5 mg P.O. t.i.d.
➤ **Palliative treatment for metastatic breast cancer**
Men and postmenopausal women: 10 mg P.O. t.i.d. for 3 or more months.
➤ **Hypogonadism**
Women: 2.5 to 7.5 mg daily in divided doses in cycles of 20 days on, 10 days off.
➤ **Castration, primary ovarian failure**
Women: 1.25 mg daily in cycles of 3 weeks on, 1 week off. Adjust for symptoms. Can be given continuously.
➤ **Vasomotor menopausal symptoms**
Women: 1.25 mg P.O. daily in cycles of 3 weeks on, 1 week off. Dosage may be increased to 2.5 to 3.75 mg P.O. daily, if needed.
➤ **Atrophic vaginitis, atrophic urethritis**
Women: 0.3 to 1.25 mg or more P.O. daily in cycles of 3 weeks on, 1 week off.

ADMINISTRATION
P.O.
• Use lowest effective dose needed for specific indication.

ACTION
Increases synthesis of DNA, RNA, and protein in responsive tissues; reduces release of follicle-stimulating and luteinizing hormones from pituitary gland.

Route	Onset	Peak	Duration
P.O.	Unknown	Unknown	Unknown

Half-life: Unknown.

ADVERSE REACTIONS

CNS: headache, dizziness, chorea, depression, ***stroke, seizures.***
CV: thrombophlebitis, ***thromboembolism,*** hypertension, *edema,* ***pulmonary embolism, MI.***
EENT: worsening myopia or astigmatism, intolerance of contact lenses.
GI: *nausea,* vomiting, abdominal cramps, bloating, anorexia, increased appetite, ***pancreatitis,*** increased risk of gallbladder disease.
GU: breakthrough bleeding, altered menstrual flow, dysmenorrhea, amenorrhea, ***increased risk of endometrial cancer,*** cervical erosion, altered cervical secretions, enlargement of uterine fibromas, vaginal candidiasis, testicular atrophy, impotence.
Hepatic: cholestatic jaundice, ***hepatic adenoma.***
Metabolic: hypercalcemia, weight changes.
Skin: melasma, rash, hirsutism or hair loss, erythema nodosum, dermatitis.
Other: *breast tenderness, enlargement, or secretion, gynecomastia,* ***increased risk of breast cancer.***

INTERACTIONS

Drug-drug. *Carbamazepine, fosphenytoin, phenobarbital, phenytoin, rifampin:* May decrease effectiveness of estrogen therapy. Monitor patient closely.
Corticosteroids: May enhance effects. Monitor patient closely.
Cyclosporine: May increase risk of toxicity. Use together with caution, and monitor cyclosporine level frequently.
Dantrolene, hepatotoxic drugs: May increase risk of hepatotoxicity. Monitor liver function closely.
Oral anticoagulants: May decrease anticoagulant effects. Adjust dosage if needed. Monitor PT and INR.
Tamoxifen: May interfere with tamoxifen effectiveness. Avoid using together.
Drug-herb. *St. John's wort:* May decrease effects of drug. Discourage use together.

Drug-food. *Caffeine:* May increase caffeine level. Urge caution.
Grapefruit, grapefruit juice: May increase risk of adverse effects. Discourage use together.
Drug-lifestyle. *Smoking:* May increase risk of CV effects. If smoking continues, may need another form of therapy.

EFFECTS ON LAB TEST RESULTS

● May increase calcium, thyroid-binding globulin, serum triglyceride, serum phospholipid, and clotting factor VII, VIII, IX, and X levels.
● May increase norepinephrine-induced platelet aggregation and PT.
● May reduce metyrapone test results and cause impaired glucose tolerance.

CONTRAINDICATIONS & CAUTIONS

● Contraindicated in pregnant women, in patients hypersensitive to drug, and in patients with breast cancer (except metastatic disease), estrogen-dependent neoplasia, active thrombophlebitis, thromboembolic disorders, undiagnosed abnormal genital bleeding, or history of thromboembolic disease.
● Use cautiously in patients with history of hypertension, mental depression, cardiac or renal dysfunction, liver impairment, bone disease, migraine, seizures, or diabetes.

NURSING CONSIDERATIONS

● When used for vasomotor symptoms in menstruating women, cyclic administration is started on day 5 of bleeding.
● Make sure patient has thorough physical examination before starting estrogen therapy. Patients receiving long-term therapy should have annual examinations. Periodically monitor body weight, blood pressure, lipid levels, and hepatic function.
● Notify pathologist about patient's estrogen therapy when sending specimens to laboratory for evaluation.
● Because of risk of thromboembolism, stop therapy at least 1 month before procedures that cause prolonged immobilization or increased risk of thromboembolism, such as knee or hip surgery.

Reactions may be *common,* uncommon, ***life-threatening,*** or COMMON AND LIFE-THREATENING.
Interaction may have a *rapid onset* or ***delayed onset***.

• Glucose tolerance may be impaired. Monitor glucose level closely in patients with diabetes.

PATIENT TEACHING
• Tell patient to read package insert describing estrogen's adverse effects; also, give patient verbal explanation.
• Emphasize importance of regular physical examinations. Postmenopausal women who use estrogen replacement for longer than 5 years to treat menopausal symptoms may be at increased risk for endometrial cancer. This risk is reduced by using cyclic rather than continuous therapy and the lowest possible estrogen dosage. Adding progestins to the regimen decreases risk of endometrial hyperplasia, but it's unknown whether progestins affect risk of endometrial cancer.
• *Alert:* Warn patient to immediately report abdominal pain; pain, numbness, or stiffness in legs or buttocks; pressure or pain in chest or shortness of breath; severe headaches; visual disturbances, such as blind spots, flashing lights, or blurriness; vaginal bleeding or discharge; breast lumps; swelling of hands or feet; yellow skin or sclera; dark urine; or light-colored stools.
• Tell diabetic patient to report elevated glucose level so that antidiabetic dosage can be adjusted.
• Explain to woman receiving cyclic therapy for postmenopausal symptoms that she may experience withdrawal bleeding during week off drug. Tell her to report unusual vaginal bleeding.
• Teach woman to perform routine breast self-examination.
• Advise woman of childbearing age to consult prescriber before taking drug and to advise prescriber immediately if she becomes pregnant.
• Teach patient methods to decrease risk of blood clots.
• Encourage patient to stop smoking or reduce number of cigarettes smoked because of the risk of CV complications.

estradiol (oestradiol)
ess-tra-DYE-ole

Alora, Climara, Esclim, Estrace, Estrace Vaginal Cream, Estraderm, Estring Vaginal Ring, FemPatch, Femtrace, Femring, Gynodiol, Menostar, Vivelle, Vivelle-Dot

estradiol cypionate
Depo-Estradiol

estradiol gel
Divigel, Elestrin, EstroGel

estradiol hemihydrate
Estrasorb, Vagifem

estradiol valerate (oestradiol valerate)
Delestrogen

Pharmacologic class: estrogen
Pregnancy risk category X

AVAILABLE FORMS
estradiol
Tablets: 0.45 mg, 0.9 mg, 1.8 mg
Tablets (micronized): 0.5 mg, 1 mg, 1.5 mg, 2 mg
Transdermal: 0.014 mg/24 hours, 0.025 mg/24 hours, 0.0375 mg/24 hours, 0.05 mg/24 hours, 0.06 mg/24 hours, 0.075 mg/24 hours, 0.1 mg/24 hours
Vaginal cream (in nonliquefying base): 0.1 mg/g
Vaginal ring: 0.0075 mg/24 hours; 0.05 mg/24 hours; 0.1 mg/24 hours
estradiol cypionate
Injection (in oil): 5 mg/ml
estradiol gel
Transdermal gel: 0.06% (1.25 g/metered dose), 0.1% (in 0.25-, 0.5-, and 1-g single-dose packets)
estradiol hemihydrate
Topical emulsion: 0.25%
Vaginal tablets: 25 mcg
estradiol valerate
Injection (in oil): 10 mg/ml, 20 mg/ml, 40 mg/ml

INDICATIONS & DOSAGES

➤ **Vasomotor menopausal symptoms, female hypogonadism, female castration, primary ovarian failure**
Women: 0.5 to 2 mg P.O. estradiol daily in cycles of 21 days on and 7 days off or cycles of 5 days on and 2 days off. Or, for vasomotor symptoms, 1 to 5 mg cypionate I.M. once every 3 to 4 weeks; for female hypogonadism, 1.5 to 2 mg cypionate I.M. once every month.
Transdermal patch
Women: 0.025 mg/24 hours Esclim, 0.05 mg/24 hours Estraderm, 0.0375 mg/24 hours or 0.05 mg/24 hours twice weekly Vivelle, 0.05 mg/24 hours Climara, or 0.025 mg/24 hours FemPatch once weekly. Apply to clean, dry area of the trunk. Adjust dose, if necessary, after the first 2 or 3 weeks of therapy; then every 3 to 6 months as needed. Rotate application sites weekly with an interval of at least 1 week between particular sites used. Adjust dosage as needed.
➤ **Postmenopausal urogenital symptoms**
Women: One ring inserted into the upper third of the vagina. Ring is kept in place for 3 months.
➤ **Atrophic vaginitis, kraurosis vulvae**
Women: 0.05 mg/24 hours Estraderm applied twice weekly in a cyclic regimen. Or, 0.05 mg/24 hours Climara applied weekly in a cyclic regimen. Or, 2 to 4 g vaginal applications of cream daily for 1 to 2 weeks. When vaginal mucosa is restored, maintenance dose is 1 g one to three times weekly in a cyclic regimen. If using Vagifem for atrophic vaginitis, give 1 tablet vaginally once daily for 2 weeks. Maintenance dose is 1 tablet inserted vaginally twice weekly. Or, 10 to 20 mg valerate I.M. every 4 weeks as needed. Or, 1 to 5 mg estradiol cypionate I.M. once every 3 to 4 weeks.
➤ **Moderate to severe vasomotor symptoms, as well as vulval and vaginal atrophy associated with menopause**
Women: 1.25 g EstroGel applied once daily to skin in a thin layer from wrist to shoulder of one upper extremity.

➤ **Palliative treatment of advanced, inoperable breast cancer**
Men and postmenopausal women: 10 mg P.O. estradiol t.i.d. for 3 months.
➤ **Palliative treatment of advanced, inoperable prostate cancer**
Men: 30 mg valerate I.M. every 1 to 2 weeks, or 1 to 2 mg P.O. estradiol t.i.d.
➤ **To prevent postmenopausal osteoporosis**
Women: Place a 6.5-cm^2 (0.025 mg/24 hours) Climara patch once weekly on clean, dry skin of lower abdomen or upper quadrant of buttock. Or, place a 3.25-cm^2 (0.014 mg/24 hours) Menostar patch once weekly to clean, dry area of the lower abdomen. For each system, press firmly in place for about 10 seconds; ensure complete contact, especially around edges. Or, 0.025-mg/24 hours Vivelle, Vivelle-Dot, or Alora system applied to a clean, dry area of the trunk twice weekly. Or, 0.5 mg P.O. daily for 21 days, followed by 7 days without drug.
➤ **Moderate to severe vasomotor symptoms from menopause**
Women: Apply contents of two 1.74-g foil pouches (total 3.48 g) of Estrasorb daily. Or, Divigel 0.1% at dose of 0.25, 0.5, or 1 g/day. Start with Divigel 0.25 g daily and adjust dose based on individual patient response.

ADMINISTRATION
P.O.
● Give drug without regard for food. If stomach upset occurs, give with food.
● Don't give drug with grapefruit juice.
● Store at controlled room temperature.
I.M.
● To give I.M. injection, make sure drug is well dispersed by rolling vial between palms. Inject deep into large muscle. Rotate injection sites to prevent muscle atrophy. Never give drug I.V.
Transdermal
● Open each pouch of Estrasorb individually and use contents of one pouch for each leg. Rub emulsion into thigh and calf for 3 minutes until thoroughly absorbed; rub emulsion remaining on hands onto the buttocks. Allow areas to dry before covering with clothing. Wash hands with soap and water to remove excess drug.

Reactions may be *common*, uncommon, *life-threatening*, or COMMON AND LIFE-THREATENING.
Interaction may have a *rapid onset* or *delayed onset*.

• Apply Divigel once daily on skin of either right or left upper thigh. Application surface area should be about 5 by 7 inches (about the size of two palm prints). Apply entire contents of a unit dose packet each day. To avoid potential skin irritation, apply Divigel to right or left upper thigh on alternating days. Don't apply Divigel on face, breasts, or irritated skin, or in or around the vagina. After application, allow gel to dry before dressing. Don't wash application site within 1 hour after applying Divigel. Avoid contact of gel with eyes. Wash hands after application.

• Apply transdermal patch to clean, dry, hairless, intact skin on abdomen or buttock. Don't apply to breasts, waistline, or other areas where clothing can loosen patch. When applying, ensure thorough contact between patch and skin, especially around edges, and hold in place for about 10 seconds. Apply patch immediately after opening and removing protective cover. Rotate application sites.

Vaginal
• Using the applicator, insert Vagifem as far into vagina as it can comfortably go, without using force.

ACTION
Increases synthesis of DNA, RNA, and protein in responsive tissues; reduces release of follicle-stimulating and luteinizing hormones from the pituitary gland.

Route	Onset	Peak	Duration
P.O., I.M., vaginal	Unknown	Unknown	Unknown
Transdermal (Esclim)	Unknown	27–30 hr	Unknown
Transdermal (Estrasorb)	Immediate	Unknown	Unknown
Transdermal gel (EstroGel)	Immediate	1 hr	24–36 hr

Half-life: Unknown.

ADVERSE REACTIONS
CNS: *stroke, headache,* dizziness, chorea, depression, *seizures,* insomnia (Vagifem).

CV: thrombophlebitis, ***thromboembolism,*** hypertension, *edema, pulmonary embolism (PE), MI.*
EENT: worsening myopia or astigmatism, intolerance of contact lenses, sinusitis (Vagifem).
GI: *nausea,* vomiting, abdominal cramps, bloating, increased appetite, ***pancreatitis,*** anorexia, gallbladder disease, dyspepsia (Vagifem).
GU: breakthrough bleeding, altered menstrual flow, dysmenorrhea, amenorrhea, ***increased risk of endometrial cancer,*** cervical erosion, abnormal Pap smear, altered cervical secretions, enlargement of uterine fibromas, vaginal candidiasis in women, testicular atrophy, impotence in men, genital pruritus, hematuria, vaginal discomfort, vaginitis (Vagifem).
Hepatic: cholestatic jaundice, ***hepatic adenoma.***
Metabolic: weight changes, hypothyroidism.
Respiratory: *upper respiratory tract infection,* allergy, bronchitis (Vagifem).
Skin: melasma, urticaria, erythema nodosum, dermatitis, hair loss, pruritus.
Other: *gynecomastia; **increased risk of breast cancer;** hot flashes; pain (Vagifem); breast tenderness, enlargement, or secretion;* flulike syndrome.

INTERACTIONS
Drug-drug. *Carbamazepine, fosphenytoin, phenobarbital, phenytoin, rifampin:* May decrease effectiveness of estrogen therapy. Monitor patient closely.
Corticosteroids: May enhance effects of corticosteroids. Monitor patient closely.
Cyclosporine: May increase risk of toxicity. Use together with caution, and monitor cyclosporine level frequently.
Dantrolene, other hepatotoxic drugs: May increase risk of hepatotoxicity. Monitor liver function closely.
Oral anticoagulants: May decrease anticoagulant effect. Dosage adjustments may be needed. Monitor PT and INR.
Tamoxifen: May interfere with tamoxifen effectiveness. Avoid using together.
Drug-herb. *Black cohosh:* May increase drug's adverse effects. Discourage use together.

Saw palmetto: May negate drug's effects. Discourage use together.

St. John's wort: May decrease effects of drug. Discourage use together.

Drug-food. *Caffeine:* May increase caffeine level. Advise patient to avoid or minimize use of caffeine.

Grapefruit juice: May elevate drug level. Tell patient to take drug with liquid other than grapefruit juice.

Drug-lifestyle. *Smoking:* May increase risk of adverse CV effects. If smoking continues, may need another therapy.

Sunscreen use: May increase absorption of Estrasorb. Tell patient to separate application times.

EFFECTS ON LAB TEST RESULTS

● May increase clotting factor VII, VIII, IX, and X; total T_4; thyroid-binding globulin; and triglyceride levels.

● May increase norepinephrine-induced platelet aggregation and PT.

● May decrease metyrapone test results.

CONTRAINDICATIONS & CAUTIONS

● Contraindicated in pregnant patients and patients with thrombophlebitis or thromboembolic disorders, estrogen-dependent neoplasia, breast or reproductive organ cancer (except for palliative treatment), undiagnosed abnormal genital bleeding, or history of thrombophlebitis or thromboembolic disorders linked to previous estrogen use (except for palliative treatment of breast and prostate cancer).

● Contraindicated in patients with liver dysfunction or disease.

● Use cautiously in patients with cerebrovascular or coronary artery disease, asthma, bone disease, migraine, seizures, or cardiac or renal dysfunction.

● Use cautiously in women who have a strong family history (grandmother, mother, sister) of breast cancer, breast nodules, fibrocystic breasts, or abnormal mammogram findings.

● *Alert:* Postmenopausal women ages 50 to 79 who are taking estrogen and progestin have an increased risk of MI, stroke, invasive breast cancer, PE, and thrombosis. Postmenopausal women age 65 or older also have an increased risk of dementia.

NURSING CONSIDERATIONS

● Ensure that patient has physical examination before starting therapy. Patients receiving long-term therapy should have yearly examinations. Monitor lipid levels, blood pressure, body weight, and hepatic function.

● Ask patient about allergies, especially to foods and plants. Estradiol is available as an aqueous solution or as a solution in peanut oil; estradiol cypionate, as a solution in cottonseed oil; estradiol valerate, as a solution in castor oil or sesame oil.

● *Alert:* EstroGel contains alcohol. Avoid fire, flame, or smoking until area dries in 2 to 5 minutes.

● In women also taking oral estrogen, treatment with the Estraderm transdermal patch can begin 1 week after withdrawal of oral therapy, or sooner if menopausal symptoms appear before the end of the week.

● Transdermal systems may be used continually rather than cyclically. Other alternative regimens are 1 to 5 mg cypionate I.M. every 3 to 4 weeks and 10 to 20 mg (valerate) I.M. every 4 weeks, as needed.

● Instruct patients using Vagifem who have severely atrophic vaginal mucosa to be careful when inserting the applicator. After gynecologic surgery, tell patient to use any vaginal applicator cautiously and only if clearly indicated.

● The prescriber should assess the patient's need to continue Vagifem therapy. Make attempts to stop or taper at 3- to 6-month intervals.

● Because of risk of thromboembolism, stop therapy at least 1 month before high-risk procedures or those that cause prolonged immobilization, such as knee or hip surgery.

● Glucose tolerance may be impaired. Monitor glucose level closely in patients with diabetes.

● Notify pathologist about estrogen therapy when sending specimens to laboratory for evaluation.

● Estrace may contain tartrazine.

PATIENT TEACHING

• Tell patient to read package insert describing estrogen's adverse effects and give verbal explanation.

• Emphasize importance of regular physical examinations. Postmenopausal women who use estrogen replacement for longer than 5 years may be at increased risk for endometrial cancer. Risk is reduced by using cyclic rather than continuous therapy and the lowest possible dosages of estrogen. Adding progestins to the regimen decreases risk of endometrial hyperplasia; however, it isn't known whether progestins affect risk of endometrial cancer. No increased risk of breast cancer has been reported.

• Teach woman how to use cream. She should wash vaginal area with soap and water before applying and insert cream high into the vagina (about two-thirds the length of the applicator). She should take drug at bedtime, or lie flat for 30 minutes after instillation to minimize drug loss.

• Tell patient using Estrasorb emulsion not to apply it with sunscreen.

• Tell patient to use transdermal system correctly, to rotate sites, to avoid breasts and waistline, and to reapply patch if it falls off.

• Teach patient using transdermal gel (EstroGel) to apply in a thin layer on one arm and allow to dry before smoking, getting near flames, dressing, or touching the arm. Recommend bathing before application to maintain full dosage.

• Tell patient to insert Vagifem by the applicator as far into vagina as it can comfortably go, without using force.

• *Alert:* Warn patient to immediately report abdominal pain, pressure or pain in chest, shortness of breath, severe headaches, visual disturbances, vaginal bleeding or discharge, breast lumps, swelling of hands or feet, yellow skin or sclera, dark urine, light-colored stools, and pain, numbness, or stiffness in legs or buttocks.

• Explain to patient receiving cyclic therapy for postmenopausal symptoms that withdrawal bleeding may occur during week off drug. Tell her to report unusual vaginal bleeding.

• Tell diabetic patient to report elevated glucose level so that antidiabetic dosage can be adjusted.

• Teach woman how to perform routine breast self-examination.

• Teach patient methods to decrease risk of blood clots.

• Advise woman not to become pregnant during estrogen therapy.

• Advise woman of childbearing age to consult prescriber before taking drug and to advise prescriber immediately if she becomes pregnant.

• Encourage patient to stop or reduce smoking because of the risk of CV complications.

---

estrogens, conjugated (estrogenic substances, conjugated; oestrogens, conjugated)
ESS-troe-jenz

C.E.S†, Cenestin, Enjuvia, Premarin, Premarin Intravenous

Pharmacologic class: estrogen
Pregnancy risk category X

AVAILABLE FORMS
Injection: 25 mg/5 ml
Tablets: 0.3 mg, 0.45 mg, 0.625 mg, 0.9 mg, 1.25 mg
Vaginal cream: 0.625 mg/g

INDICATIONS & DOSAGES
➤ **Abnormal uterine bleeding (hormonal imbalance)**
Adults: 25 mg I.V. or I.M. Repeat dose in 6 to 12 hours, if necessary.
➤ **Vulvar or vaginal atrophy**
Adults: 0.5 to 2 g cream intravaginally once daily in cycles of 3 weeks on, 1 week off.
➤ **Castration and primary ovarian failure**
Adults: Initially, 1.25 mg Premarin P.O. daily in cycles of 3 weeks on, 1 week off. Adjust dose as needed.
➤ **Female hypogonadism**
Adults: 0.3 to 0.625 mg Premarin P.O. daily, given cyclically 3 weeks on, 1 week off.

➤ **Moderate to severe vasomotor symptoms with or without moderate to severe symptoms of vulvar and vaginal atrophy associated with menopause**
Adults: Initially, 0.3 mg Premarin or Enjuvia P.O. daily, or cyclically 25 days on, 5 days off. Adjust dosage based on patient response.

➤ **Moderate to severe vasomotor symptoms from menopause**
Adults: 0.45 mg Cenestin P.O. daily. Adjust dose based on patient response.

➤ **Moderate to severe symptoms of vulvar and vaginal atrophy from menopause**
Adults: 0.3 mg Cenestin P.O. daily.

➤ **To prevent osteoporosis**
Adults: 0.3 mg Premarin P.O. daily, or cyclically, 25 days on, 5 days off. Adjust dose based on response of bone mineral density testing.

➤ **Palliative treatment of inoperable prostatic cancer**
Adults: 1.25 to 2.5 mg Premarin P.O. t.i.d.

➤ **Palliative treatment of breast cancer**
Adults: 10 mg Premarin P.O. t.i.d. for at least 3 months.

ADMINISTRATION
P.O.
● Give drug at same time each day.
I.V.
● Refrigerate before reconstituting.
● Reconstitute only with diluent provided. Agitate gently after adding diluent.
● Drug is compatible with normal saline, dextrose, or invert sugar solutions.
● Use reconstituted solution within a few hours, if possible. Reconstituted solution is stable under refrigeration for 60 days. Don't use if solution darkens or precipitates.
● Give direct injection slowly to avoid flushing reaction.
● **Incompatibilities:** Acidic solutions, ascorbic acid, protein hydrolysate.
I.M.
● Reconstitute only with diluent provided. Agitate gently after adding diluent.
● Inject deep into large muscle. Rotate injection sites to prevent muscle atrophy.

Vaginal
● Wash the vaginal area with soap and water, insert about two-thirds the length of the applicator into the vagina, and release drug. Give drug at bedtime or when the patient will lie flat for 30 minutes after use to minimize drug loss.

ACTION
Increases synthesis of DNA, RNA, and protein in responsive tissues. Also reduces release of follicle-stimulating and luteinizing hormones from the pituitary gland.

Route	Onset	Peak	Duration
P.O., I.V., I.M., vaginal	Unknown	Unknown	Unknown

Half-life: Unknown.

ADVERSE REACTIONS
CNS: headache, dizziness, chorea, depression, *stroke, seizures.*
CV: flushing with rapid I.V. administration, thrombophlebitis, *thromboembolism,* hypertension, *edema, pulmonary embolism, MI.*
EENT: worsening myopia or astigmatism, intolerance of contact lenses.
GI: *nausea,* vomiting, abdominal cramps, bloating, anorexia, increased appetite, *pancreatitis,* gallbladder disease.
GU: breakthrough bleeding, altered menstrual flow, dysmenorrhea, amenorrhea, *increased risk of endometrial cancer,* cervical erosion, altered cervical secretions, enlargement of uterine fibromas, vaginal candidiasis, testicular atrophy, impotence.
Hepatic: cholestatic jaundice, *hepatic adenoma.*
Metabolic: weight changes.
Skin: melasma, chloasma, urticaria, hirsutism or hair loss, erythema nodosum, dermatitis.
Other: *breast tenderness, enlargement, or secretion, gynecomastia,* **increased risk of breast cancer.**

INTERACTIONS
Drug-drug. *Carbamazepine, fosphenytoin, phenobarbital, phenytoin, rifampin:* May decrease effectiveness of estrogen therapy. Monitor patient closely.

Reactions may be *common,* uncommon, *life-threatening,* or COMMON AND LIFE-THREATENING.
Interaction may have a *rapid onset* or *delayed onset.*

Corticosteroids: May enhance corticosteroid effects. Monitor patient closely.
Cyclosporine: May increase risk of toxicity. Use together with caution, and monitor cyclosporine level frequently.
Dantrolene, other hepatotoxic drugs: May increase risk of hepatotoxicity. Monitor liver function closely.
Oral anticoagulants: May decrease anticoagulant effects. May need to adjust dosage. Monitor PT and INR.
Tamoxifen: May interfere with tamoxifen effectiveness. Avoid using together.
Drug-herb. *Black cohosh:* May increase adverse effects of drug. Discourage use together.
Red clover: May interfere with hormonal therapies. Discourage use together.
Saw palmetto: May have antiestrogenic effects. Discourage use together.
St. John's wort: May decrease effects of drug. Discourage use together.
Drug-food. *Caffeine:* May increase caffeine level. Advise caution.
Grapefruit juice: May increase concentration of estrogen. Avoid using together.
Drug-lifestyle. *Smoking:* May increase risk of adverse CV effects. If smoking continues, recommend nonhormonal contraception.

EFFECTS ON LAB TEST RESULTS
• May increase clotting factor VII, VIII, IX, and X; total T_4; phospholipid; thyroid-binding globulin; and triglyceride levels.
• May increase norepinephrine-induced platelet aggregation and PT.
• May cause a false-positive metyrapone test result.

CONTRAINDICATIONS & CAUTIONS
• Contraindicated in pregnant patients and in patients with thrombophlebitis, thromboembolic disorders, estrogen-dependent neoplasia, breast or reproductive cancer (except for palliative treatment), or undiagnosed abnormal genital bleeding.
• Use cautiously in patients with cerebrovascular or coronary artery disease, asthma, bone disease, migraine, seizures, or cardiac, hepatic, or renal dysfunction.

• Use cautiously in women who have a strong family history (mother, grandmother, sister) of breast or genital tract cancer, breast nodules, fibrocystic breasts, or abnormal mammogram findings.

NURSING CONSIDERATIONS
• Make sure patient has thorough physical exam before starting therapy, and patients receiving long-term therapy should have yearly exams. Periodically monitor lipid levels, blood pressure, body weight, and hepatic function.
• Rapid treatment of dysfunctional uterine bleeding or reduction of surgical bleeding usually requires delivery by I.V. or I.M. route.
• *Alert:* Don't use to prevent CV disease. In postmenopausal women receiving therapy for more than 5 years, drugs may increase risks of MI, stroke, invasive breast cancer, pulmonary emboli, and deep vein thrombosis. Use the lowest effective doses for the shortest time, considering the benefits and risks.
• *Alert:* In postmenopausal women receiving therapy for more than 5 years, drug may increase risk of endometrial cancer. Cyclic therapy and the lowest possible dose reduces risk. Adding progestins decreases risk of endometrial hyperplasia, but it's unknown whether they affect risk of endometrial cancer.
• When used solely for the treatment of vulval and vaginal atrophy, consider topical products.
• Notify pathologist about estrogen therapy when sending specimens to laboratory for evaluation.
• Because of thromboembolism risk, stop therapy at least 1 month before procedures that prolong immobilization or raise the risk of thromboembolism, such as knee or hip surgery.
• Glucose tolerance may be impaired. Monitor glucose level closely in patients with diabetes.
• *Look alike–sound alike:* Don't confuse Premarin with Primaxin.

PATIENT TEACHING
• Tell patient to read package insert describing estrogen's adverse effects and to explain them back to you.

• Emphasize importance of regular physical exams.

• Teach woman how to use vaginal cream. Tell patient to wash the vaginal area with soap and water, insert about two-thirds the length of the applicator into the vagina, and release drug. Tell her to use drug at bedtime or to lie flat for 30 minutes after use to minimize drug loss.

• Explain to patient that cyclic therapy for postmenopausal symptoms may cause withdrawal bleeding during week off drug. Tell her to report unusual vaginal bleeding.

• *Alert:* Warn patient to immediately report abdominal pain; pain, numbness, or stiffness in legs or buttocks; pressure or pain in chest; shortness of breath; severe headaches; visual disturbances, such as blind spots, flashing lights, or blurriness; vaginal bleeding or discharge; breast lumps; swelling of hands or feet; yellow skin or sclera; dark urine; and light-colored stools.

• Tell diabetic patient to report elevated glucose level so that antidiabetic dosage can be adjusted.

• Teach woman how to perform routine breast self-examination.

• Advise woman not to become pregnant during estrogen therapy.

• Advise woman of childbearing age to consult prescriber before taking drug and to advise prescriber immediately if she becomes pregnant.

• Encourage patient to stop smoking or reduce number of cigarettes smoked because of the risk of CV complications.

---

estropipate
ess-troe-PIH-pate

Ogen, Ortho-Est

Pharmacologic class: estrogen
Pregnancy risk category X

AVAILABLE FORMS
Tablets: 0.75 mg, 1.5 mg, 3 mg, 6 mg
Vaginal cream: 1.5 mg/g

INDICATIONS & DOSAGES
➤ **Vulval and vaginal atrophy**
Women: 0.75 to 6 mg P.O. daily, 3 weeks on and 1 week off; or 2 to 4 g vaginal cream daily. Drug usually given on a cyclic, short-term basis but can be given continuously.
➤ **Primary ovarian failure, female castration, female hypogonadism**
Women: 1.5 to 9 mg P.O. daily for first 3 weeks; then a rest period of 8 to 10 days. If bleeding doesn't occur by end of rest period, cycle is repeated. Can be given continuously.
➤ **Vasomotor menopausal symptoms**
Women: 0.75 to 6 mg P.O. daily in cyclic method, 3 weeks on and 1 week off. Can be given continuously.
➤ **To prevent osteoporosis**
Women: 0.75 mg P.O. daily for 25 consecutive days of a 31-day cycle, followed by 6 days without drug. Repeat regimen as indicated.

ADMINISTRATION
P.O.
• Give drug with meals to minimize GI upset.
Vaginal
• Wash vaginal area with soap and water and then insert vaginal cream high into vagina (about two-thirds the length of applicator). Use drug at bedtime or when patient is able to lie flat for 30 minutes after application to minimize drug loss.

ACTION
Increases synthesis of DNA, RNA, and proteins in responsive tissues; reduces follicle-stimulating and luteinizing hormones.

Route	Onset	Peak	Duration
P.O., vaginal	Unknown	Unknown	Unknown

Half-life: Unknown.

ADVERSE REACTIONS
CNS: depression, headache, dizziness, migraine, *seizures, stroke.*
CV: *edema,* thrombophlebitis, *pulmonary embolism (PE), MI, thromboembolism.*

GI: nausea, vomiting, gallbladder disease, abdominal cramps, bloating.
GU: increased size of uterine fibromas, *endometrial cancer,* vaginal candidiasis, cystitis-like syndrome, dysmenorrhea, amenorrhea, breakthrough bleeding, condition resembling premenstrual syndrome.
Hepatic: cholestatic jaundice, *hepatic adenoma.*
Metabolic: weight changes.
Skin: hemorrhagic eruption, erythema nodosum, *erythema multiforme,* hirsutism or hair loss, melasma.
Other: breast engorgement or enlargement, *breast cancer,* breast tenderness.

INTERACTIONS

Drug-drug. *Carbamazepine, fosphenytoin, phenobarbital, phenytoin, rifampin:* May decrease estrogen effect. Monitor patient closely.
Corticosteroids: May enhance corticosteroid effect. Monitor patient closely.
Cyclosporine: May increase risk of toxicity. Use together with caution; frequently monitor cyclosporine level.
Dantrolene, other hepatotoxic drugs: May increase risk of hepatotoxicity. Monitor liver function closely.
Oral anticoagulants: May decrease anticoagulant effect. Dosage adjustments may be needed. Monitor PT and INR.
Tamoxifen: May interfere with tamoxifen effect. Avoid using together.
Drug-herb. *Black cohosh:* May increase adverse effects of estrogen. Discourage use together.
Red clover: May interfere with hormonal therapies. Discourage use together.
Saw palmetto: May have antiestrogenic effect. Discourage use together.
St. John's wort: May decrease estrogen effect. Discourage use together.
Drug-food. *Caffeine:* May increase caffeine level. Advise caution.
Drug-lifestyle. *Smoking:* May increase risk of adverse CV effects. If smoking continues, may need alternative therapy.

EFFECTS ON LAB TEST RESULTS
• May increase clotting factor VII, VIII, IX, and X; total T_4; phospholipid; thyroid-binding globulin; and triglyceride levels.

• May increase norepinephrine-induced platelet aggregation and PT.
• May reduce metyrapone test results.

CONTRAINDICATIONS & CAUTIONS
• Contraindicated in pregnant patients and those with active thrombophlebitis; thromboembolic disorders; estrogen-dependent neoplasia; undiagnosed genital bleeding; and breast, reproductive organ, or genital cancer.
• Use cautiously in patients with cerebrovascular or coronary artery disease; asthma; mental depression; bone disease; migraine; seizures; or cardiac, hepatic, or renal dysfunction.
• Use cautiously in women who have a family history (mother, grandmother, sister) of breast or genital tract cancer, breast nodules, fibrocystic breasts, or abnormal mammogram findings.

NURSING CONSIDERATIONS
• Make sure patient has thorough physical examination before starting estrogen therapy. Patients receiving long-term therapy should have examinations yearly. Periodically monitor lipid levels, blood pressure, body weight, and hepatic function.
• *Alert:* Estrogens and progestins shouldn't be used to prevent CV disease. The Women's Health Initiative study reported increased risks of MI, stroke, invasive breast cancer, PE, and deep vein thrombosis in postmenopausal women during 5 years of combination therapy. Because of these risks, estrogens and progestins should be prescribed at the lowest effective doses and for the shortest duration consistent with treatment goals and risks for the individual woman.
• When used to treat hypogonadism, duration of therapy needed to produce withdrawal bleeding depends on patient's endometrial response to drug. If satisfactory withdrawal bleeding doesn't occur, an oral progestin is added to the regimen. Explain to patient that, despite return of withdrawal bleeding, pregnancy can't occur because she doesn't ovulate.

• Estropipate-estrone equivalents are:

0.75 mg estropipate = 0.625 mg estrone

1.5 mg estropipate = 1.25 mg estrone

3 mg estropipate = 2.5 mg estrone

6 mg estropipate = 5 mg estrone

• Because of risk of thromboembolism, stop therapy at least 1 month before procedures that prolong immobilization or raise the risk of thromboembolism, such as knee or hip surgery.
• Glucose tolerance may be impaired. Monitor glucose level closely in patients with diabetes.

PATIENT TEACHING
• Tell patient to read package insert describing estrogen's adverse effects; also, explain effects verbally.
• Teach woman how to use vaginal cream. Patient should wash the vaginal area with soap and water and then insert vaginal cream high into the vagina (about two-thirds the length of the applicator). Tell her to use drug at bedtime or to lie flat for 30 minutes after application to minimize drug loss.
• Tell diabetic patient to report elevated glucose level to prescriber.
• Stress importance of regular physical examinations. Postmenopausal women who use estrogen replacement for longer than 5 years may have increased risk of endometrial cancer. Using cyclic therapy and lowest possible estrogen dosage reduces risk. Adding progestins to regimen decreases risk of endometrial hyperplasia; however, it isn't known whether progestins affect risk of endometrial cancer.
• *Alert:* Warn patient to immediately report abdominal pain; pain, stiffness, or numbness in legs or buttocks; pressure or pain in chest; shortness of breath; severe headaches; visual disturbances, such as blind spots or flashing lights; vaginal bleeding or discharge; breast lumps; swelling of hands or feet; yellow skin or sclera; dark urine; and light-colored stools.

• Teach woman how to perform routine breast self-examination.
• Advise woman not to become pregnant while on estrogen therapy.
• Encourage patient to stop or reduce smoking because of the risk of CV complications.
• Advise woman of childbearing age to consult prescriber before taking drug and to tell prescriber immediately if she becomes pregnant.

SAFETY ALERT!

eszopiclone
ess-ZOP-ah-klone

Lunesta

Pharmacologic class: pyrrolopy-razine derivative
Pregnancy risk category C
Controlled substance schedule IV

AVAILABLE FORMS
Tablets: 1 mg, 2 mg, 3 mg

INDICATIONS & DOSAGES
➤ **Insomnia**
Adults: 2 mg P.O. immediately before bedtime. Increase to 3 mg as needed.
Elderly patients having trouble falling asleep: 1 mg P.O. immediately before bedtime. Increase to 2 mg as needed.
Elderly patients having trouble staying asleep: 2 mg P.O. immediately before bedtime.
Adjust-a-dose: In patients with severe hepatic impairment, start with 1 mg P.O. In patients who also take a potent CYP3A4 inhibitor, start with 1 mg and increase to 2 mg as needed.

ADMINISTRATION
P.O.
• Avoid giving drug after a high-fat meal.
• Give drug immediately before bedtime because drug may cause dizziness or light-headedness.

ACTION
Probably interacts with GABA receptors at binding sites close or connected to benzodiazepine receptors.

Route	Onset	Peak	Duration
P.O.	Rapid	1 hr	Unknown

Half-life: 6 hours.

ADVERSE REACTIONS
CNS: abnormal dreams, anxiety, complex sleep-related behavior, confusion, decreased libido, depression, dizziness, hallucinations, *headache,* nervousness, pain, *somnolence,* neuralgia.
EENT: *unpleasant taste.*
GI: diarrhea, dry mouth, dyspepsia, nausea, vomiting.
GU: UTI.
Respiratory: *respiratory tract infection.*
Skin: pruritus, rash.
Other: *anaphylaxis, angioedema,* accidental injury, viral infection.

INTERACTIONS
Drug-drug. *CNS depressants:* May have additive CNS effects. Adjust dosage of either drug as needed.
CYP3A4 inhibitors (clarithromycin, itraconazole, ketoconazole, nefazodone, nelfinavir, ritonavir, troleandomycin): May decrease eszopiclone elimination, increasing the risk of toxicity. Use together cautiously.
Olanzapine: May impair cognitive function or memory. Use together cautiously.
Rifampicin: May decrease eszopiclone activity. Don't use together.
Drug-food. *High-fat meals:* May decrease drug absorption and effects. Discourage high-fat meals with or just before taking drug.
Drug-lifestyle. *Alcohol use:* May decrease psychomotor ability. Discourage use together.

EFFECTS ON LAB TEST RESULTS
None reported.

CONTRAINDICATIONS & CAUTIONS
• Use cautiously in patients with diseases or conditions that could affect metabolism or hemodynamic responses. Also use cautiously in patients with compromised respiratory function, severe hepatic impairment, or signs and symptoms of depression.

NURSING CONSIDERATIONS
• *Alert:* Anaphylaxis and angioedema may occur as early as the first dose; monitor the patient closely.
• Evaluate patient for physical and psychiatric disorders before treatment.
• Use the lowest effective dose.
• *Alert:* Give drug immediately before patient goes to bed or after patient has gone to bed and has trouble falling asleep.
• Use only for short periods (for example, 7 to 10 days). If patient still has trouble sleeping, check for other psychological disorders.
• Monitor patient for changes in behavior, including those that suggest depression or suicidal thinking.

PATIENT TEACHING
• *Alert:* Warn patient that drug may cause allergic reactions, facial swelling, and complex sleep-related behaviors, such as driving, eating, and making phone calls while asleep. Advise patient to report these adverse effects.
• Urge patient to take drug immediately before going to bed because drug may cause dizziness or light-headedness.
• Caution patient not to take drug unless he can get a full night's sleep.
• Advise patient to avoid taking drug after a high-fat meal.
• Tell patient to avoid activities that require mental alertness until the drug's effects are known.
• Advise patient to avoid alcohol while taking drug.
• Urge patient to immediately report changes in behavior and thinking.
• Warn patient not to stop drug abruptly or change dose without consulting the prescriber.
• Inform patient that tolerance or dependence may develop if drug is taken for a prolonged period.

finasteride
fin-AS-teh-ride

Propecia, Proscar

Pharmacologic class: steroid
derivative
Pregnancy risk category X

AVAILABLE FORMS
Tablets: 1 mg, 5 mg

INDICATIONS & DOSAGES
➤ **Male pattern hair loss (androge-
netic alopecia) in men only**
Men: 1 mg P.O. Propecia daily.
➤ **To improve symptoms of BPH
and reduce risk of acute urine reten-
tion and need for surgery, including
transurethral resection of prostate
and prostatectomy**
Men: 5 mg P.O. Proscar daily.
➤ **With doxazosin, to reduce the
risk of BPH symptom progression
(Proscar)**
Men: 5 mg P.O. daily.

ADMINISTRATION
P.O.
● Give drug without regard for food.

ACTION
Inhibits conversion of testosterone to di-
hydrotestosterone (DHT), the androgen
primarily responsible for the initial development and subsequent enlargement of
the prostate gland. In male pattern baldness, the scalp contains miniaturized hair
follicles and increased DHT level; drug
decreases scalp DHT level in such cases.

Route	Onset	Peak	Duration
P.O.	Unknown	1–2 hr	24 hr

Half-life: Unknown.

ADVERSE REACTIONS
GU: impotence, decreased volume of
ejaculate, decreased libido.

INTERACTIONS
None significant.

EFFECTS ON LAB TEST RESULTS
● May decrease prostate-specific antigen
(PSA) level.

CONTRAINDICATIONS & CAUTIONS
● Contraindicated in patients hypersensitive to drug or to other 5-alpha-reductase
inhibitors, such as dutasteride. Although
drug isn't used in women or children,
manufacturer indicates pregnancy as a
contraindication.
● Use cautiously in patients with liver
dysfunction.

NURSING CONSIDERATIONS
● Before therapy, evaluate patient for
conditions that mimic BPH, including hy-
potonic bladder, prostate cancer, infection,
or stricture.
● Carefully monitor patients who have a
large residual urine volume or severely
diminished urine flow.
● Sustained increase in PSA level could
indicate noncompliance with therapy.
● A minimum of 6 months of therapy may
be needed for treatment of BPH.

PATIENT TEACHING
● Tell patient that drug may be taken with
or without meals.
● Warn woman who is or may become pregnant not to handle crushed tablets because
of risk of adverse effects on male fetus.
● Inform patient that signs of improvement
may require at least 3 months of daily use
when drug is used to treat hair loss or at
least 6 months when taken for BPH.
● Reassure patient that drug may decrease
volume of ejaculate without impairing
normal sexual function.

flumazenil
floo-MAZ-eh-nill

Romazicon

Pharmacologic class: benzodiazepine antagonist
Pregnancy risk category C

AVAILABLE FORMS
Injection: 0.1 mg/ml in 5-ml and 10-ml
multiple-dose vials

INDICATIONS & DOSAGES

➤ **Complete or partial reversal of sedative effects of benzodiazepines after anesthesia or conscious sedation**

Adults: Initially, 0.2 mg I.V. over 15 seconds. If patient doesn't reach desired level of consciousness after 45 seconds, repeat dose. Repeat at 1-minute intervals, if needed, until cumulative dose of 1 mg has been given (first dose plus four more doses). Most patients respond after 0.6 to 1 mg of drug. In case of resedation, dosage may be repeated after 20 minutes, but never give more than 1 mg at any one time or exceed 3 mg/hour.

Children age 1 year and older: 0.01 mg/kg I.V. over 15 seconds. If patient doesn't reach desired level of consciousness after 45 seconds, repeat dose. Repeat at 1-minute intervals, if needed, until cumulative dose of 0.05 mg/kg or 1 mg, whichever is lower, has been given (first dose plus four more doses).

➤ **Suspected benzodiazepine overdose**

Adults: Initially, 0.2 mg I.V. over 30 seconds. If patient doesn't reach desired level of consciousness after 30 seconds, give 0.3 mg over 30 seconds. If patient still doesn't respond adequately, give 0.5 mg over 30 seconds. Repeat 0.5-mg doses, as needed, at 1-minute intervals until cumulative dose of 3 mg has been given. Most patients with benzodiazepine overdose respond to cumulative doses between 1 and 3 mg; rarely, patients who respond partially after 3 mg may need additional doses, up to 5 mg total. If patient doesn't respond in 5 minutes after receiving 5 mg, sedation is unlikely to be caused by benzodiazepines. In case of resedation, dosage may be repeated after 20 minutes, but never give more than 1 mg at any one time or exceed 3 mg/hour.

ADMINISTRATION

I.V.
- Store drug in vial until use.
- Make sure airway is secure and patent.
- Compatible solutions include D₅W, lactated Ringer's injection, and normal saline solution.

- To minimize pain at injection site, inject drug over 15 to 30 seconds into large vein through free-flowing solution.
- Monitor patient for signs of extravasation.
- Drug is stable in a syringe for 24 hours.
- **Incompatibilities:** None reported.

ACTION

Competitively inhibits the actions of benzodiazepines on the GABA-benzodiazepine receptor complex.

Route	Onset	Peak	Duration
I.V.	1–2 min	6–10 min	Variable

Half-life: 54 minutes.

ADVERSE REACTIONS

CNS: *dizziness, abnormal or blurred vision, headache, seizures,* agitation, emotional lability, tremor, insomnia.
CV: *arrhythmias,* cutaneous vasodilation, palpitations.
GI: *nausea, vomiting.*
Respiratory: dyspnea, hyperventilation.
Skin: *diaphoresis.*
Other: *pain at injection site.*

INTERACTIONS

Drug-drug. *Antidepressants, drugs that may cause seizures or arrhythmias:* May increase risk of seizures or arrhythmias. Don't use flumazenil when overdose involves more than one drug, especially when seizures (from any cause) are likely.

EFFECTS ON LAB TEST RESULTS

None reported.

CONTRAINDICATIONS & CAUTIONS

- Contraindicated in patients hypersensitive to flumazenil or benzodiazepines, in those with evidence of serious tricyclic antidepressant overdose, and in those who have received benzodiazepines to treat a potentially life-threatening condition, such as status epilepticus.
- Use cautiously in patients with head injury, psychiatric disorders, or alcohol dependence.
- Use cautiously in patients at high risk for developing seizures and in those who have recently received multiple doses of

a parenteral benzodiazepine, who display signs of seizure activity, or who may be at risk for benzodiazepine dependence, such as intensive care unit patients.

NURSING CONSIDERATIONS
• Monitor patient closely for resedation that may occur after reversal of benzodiazepine effects; drug's duration of action is the shortest of all benzodiazepines. Length of monitoring period depends on specific drug being reversed. Monitor patient closely after doses of long-acting benzodiazepines, such as diazepam, or after high doses of short-acting benzodiazepines, such as 10 mg of midazolam. In most cases, severe resedation is unlikely in patients who fail to show signs of resedation 2 hours after a 1-mg dose.

PATIENT TEACHING
• Warn patient not to perform hazardous activities within 24 hours of procedure because of resedation risk.
• Tell patient to avoid alcohol, CNS depressants, and OTC drugs for 24 hours.
• Give family necessary instructions or provide patient with written instructions. Patient won't recall information given after the procedure; drug doesn't reverse amnesic effects of benzodiazepines.

---

fluoxetine hydrochloride
floo-OX-e-teen

Prozac, Prozac Weekly, Sarafem

Pharmacologic class: SSRI
Pregnancy risk category C

AVAILABLE FORMS
Capsules (delayed-release): 90 mg
Capsules (pulvules): 10 mg, 20 mg, 40 mg
Oral solution: 20 mg/5 ml
Tablets: 10 mg, 20 mg

INDICATIONS & DOSAGES
➤ **Depression, obsessive-compulsive disorder (OCD)**
Adults: Initially, 20 mg P.O. in the morning; increase dosage based on patient response. Maximum daily dose is 80 mg.

Children ages 7 to 17 (OCD): 10 mg P.O. daily. After 2 weeks, increase to 20 mg daily. Dosage is 20 to 60 mg daily.
Children ages 8 to 18 (depression): 10 mg P.O. once daily for 1 week; then increase to 20 mg daily.
➤ **Depression in elderly patients**
Adults age 65 and older: Initially, 20 mg P.O. daily in the morning. Increase dose based on response. Doses may be given b.i.d., morning and noon. Maximum daily dose is 80 mg. Consider using a lower dosage or less-frequent doses in these patients, especially those with systemic illness and those who are receiving drugs for other illnesses.
➤ **Maintenance therapy for depression in stabilized patients (not for newly diagnosed depression)**
Adults: 90 mg Prozac Weekly P.O. once weekly. Start once-weekly doses 7 days after the last daily dose of Prozac 20 mg.
➤ **Short-term and long-term treatment of bulimia nervosa**
Adults: 60 mg P.O. daily in the morning.
➤ **Short-term treatment of panic disorder with or without agoraphobia**
Adults: 10 mg P.O. once daily for 1 week; then increase dose as needed to 20 mg daily. Maximum daily dose is 60 mg.
Adjust-a-dose: For patients with renal or hepatic impairment, reduce dose or increase interval.
➤ **Anorexia nervosa in weight-restored patients ◆**
Adults: 40 mg P.O. daily.
➤ **Depression caused by bipolar disorder ◆**
Adults: 20 to 60 mg P.O. daily.
➤ **Cataplexy ◆**
Adults: 20 mg P.O. once or twice daily with CNS stimulant therapy.
➤ **Alcohol dependence ◆**
Adults: 60 mg P.O. daily.
➤ **Premenstrual dysphoric disorder**
Adults: 20 mg Sarafem P.O. daily continuously (every day of the menstrual cycle) or intermittently (daily dose starting 14 days before the anticipated onset of menstruation through the first full day of menses and repeating with each new cycle). Maximum daily dose is 80 mg P.O.

Adjust-a-dose: For patients with renal or hepatic impairment and those taking several drugs at the same time, reduce dose or increase dosing interval.

ADMINISTRATION
P.O.
- Give drug without regard for food.
- Avoid giving drug in the afternoon, whenever possible, because doing so commonly causes nervousness and insomnia.
- Delayed-release capsules must be swallowed whole; don't crush or open.

ACTION
Thought to be linked to drug's inhibition of CNS neuronal uptake of serotonin.

Route	Onset	Peak	Duration
P.O.	Unknown	6–8 hr	Unknown

Half-life: Fluoxetine, 2 to 3 days; norfluoxetine, 7 to 9 days.

ADVERSE REACTIONS
CNS: *nervousness, somnolence, anxiety, insomnia, headache, drowsiness, tremor, dizziness, asthenia,* **suicidal behavior,** fatigue, fever.
CV: palpitations, hot flashes.
EENT: nasal congestion, pharyngitis, sinusitis.
GI: *nausea, diarrhea, dry mouth, anorexia,* dyspepsia, constipation, abdominal pain, vomiting, flatulence, increased appetite.
GU: sexual dysfunction.
Metabolic: weight loss.
Musculoskeletal: muscle pain.
Respiratory: upper respiratory tract infection, cough, ***respiratory distress.***
Skin: rash, pruritus, diaphoresis.
Other: flulike syndrome.

INTERACTIONS
Drug-drug. *Amphetamines, buspirone, dextromethorphan, dihydroergotamine, lithium salts, meperidine, other SSRIs or SSNRIs (duloxetine, venlafaxine),* **tramadol,** *trazodone, tricyclic antidepressants, tryptophan:* May increase the risk of serotonin syndrome. Avoid combinations of drugs that increase the availability of serotonin in the CNS; monitor patient closely if used together.
Benzodiazepines, lithium, tricyclic antidepressants: May increase CNS effects. Monitor patient closely.
Beta blockers, carbamazepine, flecainide, vinblastine: May increase levels of these drugs. Monitor drug levels and monitor patient for adverse reactions.
Cyproheptadine: May reverse or decrease fluoxetine effect. Monitor patient closely.
Dextromethorphan: May cause unusual side effects such as visual hallucinations. Advise use of cough suppressant that doesn't contain dextromethorphan while taking fluoxetine.
Highly protein-bound drugs: May increase level of fluoxetine or other highly protein-bound drugs. Monitor patient closely.
Insulin, oral antidiabetics: May alter glucose level and antidiabetic requirements. Adjust dosage.
MAO inhibitors (phenelzine, selegiline, tranylcypromine): May cause serotonin syndrome. Avoid using at the same time and for at least 5 weeks after stopping.
Phenytoin: May increase phenytoin level and risk of toxicity. Monitor phenytoin level and adjust dosage.
Triptans: May cause weakness, hyperreflexia, incoordination, rapid changes in blood pressure, nausea, and diarrhea. Monitor patient closely, especially at the start of treatment and when dosage increases.
Thioridazine: May increase thioridazine level, increasing risk of serious ventricular arrhythmias and sudden death. Avoid using at the same time and for at least 5 weeks after stopping.
Warfarin: May increase risk for bleeding. Monitor PT and INR.
Drug-herb. *St. John's wort:* May increase sedative and hypnotic effects; may cause serotonin syndrome. Discourage use together.
Drug-lifestyle. *Alcohol use:* May increase CNS depression. Discourage use together.

EFFECTS ON LAB TEST RESULTS
None reported.

CONTRAINDICATIONS & CAUTIONS
- Contraindicated in patients hypersensitive to drug and in those taking MAO

---

inhibitors within 14 days of starting therapy. MAO inhibitors shouldn't be started within 5 weeks of stopping fluoxetine. Avoid using thioridazine with fluoxetine or within 5 weeks after stopping fluoxetine.
• Use cautiously in patients at high risk for suicide and in those with history of diabetes mellitus, seizures, mania, or hepatic, renal, or CV disease.
• Use in third trimester of pregnancy may be associated with neonatal complications at birth. Consider the risk versus benefit of treatment during this time.

NURSING CONSIDERATIONS
• Use antihistamines or topical corticosteroids to treat rashes or pruritus.
• Watch for weight change during therapy, particularly in underweight or bulimic patients.
• Record mood changes. Watch for suicidal tendencies.
• *Alert:* Drug may increase the risk of suicidal thinking and behavior in children and adolescents with major depressive disorder or other psychiatric disorder.
• *Alert:* Drug may increase the risk of suicidal thinking and behavior in young adults ages 18 to 24 during the first 2 months of treatment.
• Drug has a long half-life; monitor patient for adverse effects for up to 2 weeks after drug is stopped.
• *Alert:* Combining triptans with an SSRI or an SSNRI may cause serotonin syndrome. Signs and symptoms may include restlessness, hallucinations, loss of coordination, fast heartbeat, rapid changes in blood pressure, increased body temperature, overactive reflexes, nausea, vomiting, and diarrhea. Serotonin syndrome may be more likely to occur when starting or increasing the dose of triptan, SSRI, or SSNRI.
• *Look alike–sound alike:* Don't confuse fluoxetine with fluvoxamine or fluvastatin. Don't confuse Prozac with Proscar, Prilosec, or ProSom.

PATIENT TEACHING
• Tell patient to avoid taking drug in the afternoon whenever possible because doing so commonly causes nervousness and insomnia.
• Drug may cause dizziness or drowsiness. Warn patient to avoid driving and other hazardous activities that require alertness and good psychomotor coordination until effects of drug are known.
• Tell patient to consult prescriber before taking other prescription or OTC drugs.
• Advise patient that full therapeutic effect may not be seen for 4 weeks or longer.

---

fluoxymesterone
flew-ox-ee-MESS-teh-rone

Halotestin

Pharmacologic class: androgen
Pregnancy risk category X
Controlled substance schedule III

AVAILABLE FORMS
Tablets: 2 mg, 5 mg, 10 mg

INDICATIONS & DOSAGES
➤ **Hypogonadism from testicular deficiency**
Adults: 5 to 20 mg P.O. daily.
➤ **Delayed puberty in boys**
Adolescents: Highly individualized; usually 2.5 to 10 mg daily for 4 to 6 months.
➤ **Palliation of breast cancer**
Women: 10 to 40 mg P.O. daily in divided doses. Individualize and use lowest effective dose.
➤ **Vasomotor symptoms associated with menopause in combination with estrogen therapy ♦**
Women: 1 to 2 mg P.O. with 0.02 or 0.04 mg of ethinyl estradiol b.i.d. for 21 days, followed by 7 days without drugs. Repeat cycle as necessary.

ADMINISTRATION
P.O.
• Give as a single daily dose or in divided doses.

ACTION
Stimulates target tissues to develop normally in androgen-deficient men. May have some antiestrogen properties, making it useful in treating certain estrogen-dependent breast cancers.

Route	Onset	Peak	Duration
P.O.	Unknown	Unknown	9 hr

Half-life: 9¹/₄ hours.

ADVERSE REACTIONS
CNS: headache, anxiety, depression, paresthesia, sleep apnea.
CV: edema.
GI: nausea.
GU: decreased ejaculatory volume, oligospermia, priapism.
Hematologic: polycythemia, *suppression of clotting factors.*
Hepatic: reversible jaundice, *cholestatic hepatitis.*
Metabolic: hypercalcemia, hypernatremia, *hyperkalemia,* hyperphosphatemia.
Skin: hypersensitivity reactions.
Other: *hypoestrogenic effects in women,* excessive hormonal effects in men, androgenic effects in women, altered libido, male pattern baldness.

INTERACTIONS
Drug-drug. *Hepatotoxic drugs:* May increase risk of hepatotoxicity. Monitor liver function closely.
Insulin, oral antidiabetics: May alter dosage requirements. Monitor glucose levels in diabetic patients.
Oral anticoagulants: May increase sensitivity to oral anticoagulants; may alter dosage requirements. Monitor INR.

EFFECTS ON LAB TEST RESULTS
● May increase calcium, lipid, liver enzyme, phosphate, potassium, and sodium levels. May decrease thyroxine-binding globulin and total T_4 levels.
● May increase RBC count and resin uptake of T_3 and T_4.
● May cause abnormal glucose tolerance test results.

CONTRAINDICATIONS & CAUTIONS
● Contraindicated in patients hypersensitive to drug; in men with breast cancer or known or suspected prostate cancer; in patients with cardiac, hepatic, or renal decompensation; and in pregnant or breast-feeding women.

● Use cautiously in prepubertal boys or patients with benign prostatic hyperplasia or aspirin sensitivity.

NURSING CONSIDERATIONS
● *Alert:* Don't use in women of childbearing age until pregnancy is ruled out.
● Monitor INR in patients taking oral anticoagulants because dosage may need adjustment.
● Unless contraindicated, use with high-calorie, high-protein diet. Give small, frequent meals.
● Watch for evidence of jaundice, and periodically evaluate hepatic function. If liver function test results are abnormal, notify prescriber because therapy should be stopped.
● Edema can be controlled with sodium restriction or diuretics. Monitor weight routinely.
● Monitor boys and men for evidence of excessive hormonal effects. In prepubertal boys, watch for premature epiphyseal closure, acne, priapism, growth of body and facial hair, and phallic enlargement. If postpubertal men, watch for testicular atrophy, oligospermia, decreased ejaculatory volume, impotence, gynecomastia, and epididymitis.
● Evaluate semen routinely every 3 to 4 months, especially in adolescent boys.
● *Alert:* Hypercalcemia symptoms may be difficult to distinguish from those caused by the condition being treated, unless anticipated and thought of as a symptom cluster. Hypercalcemia is particularly likely to occur in immobilized patients and in women with metastatic breast cancer, and may indicate bone metastases.
● *Alert:* Don't give drug to enhance patient's athletic performance or physique.
● Watch for signs and symptoms of hypoglycemia in diabetic patients. Check glucose levels. Dosage of antidiabetic may need adjustment.
● When given for breast cancer, subjective effects may not occur for about 1 month; objective effects on clinical symptoms may take 3 months.
● Hypoestrogenic effects in women include flushing, diaphoresis, vaginal bleeding, nervousness, emotional lability, menstrual

irregularities, and vaginitis, including itching, dryness, and burning.
● Halotestin may contain tartrazine.

PATIENT TEACHING
● If GI upset occurs, tell patient to take drug with food or meals.
● Make sure patient understands importance of using an effective nonhormonal contraceptive during therapy.
● Advise woman to wear cotton underwear and to wash after intercourse to decrease risk of vaginitis.
● Tell woman of childbearing age to report menstrual irregularities and to stop drug until she can be examined.
● Instruct woman to stop drug immediately and notify prescriber if pregnancy is suspected.
● Explain to woman taking drug for palliation of breast cancer that virilization usually occurs. Give emotional support. Tell her to immediately report androgenic effects (acne, swelling, weight gain, increased hair growth, hoarseness, clitoral enlargement, deepening voice, decreased breast size, changes in libido, male pattern baldness, and oily skin or hair).
● Tell patient that stopping drug prevents further androgenic changes but probably won't reverse existing effects.
● Warn patient with diabetes to be alert for signs and symptoms of hypoglycemia and to notify prescriber if these occur.
● Tell patient to report sudden weight gain.

---

fluphenazine decanoate
floo-FEN-a-zeen

Modecate†, Modecate Concentrate†

fluphenazine hydrochloride

Pharmacologic class: phenothiazine
Pregnancy risk category C

AVAILABLE FORMS
fluphenazine decanoate
Depot injection: 25 mg/ml
fluphenazine hydrochloride
Elixir: 2.5 mg/5 ml*
I.M. injection: 2.5 mg/ml

Oral concentrate: 5 mg/ml*
Tablets: 1 mg, 2.5 mg, 5 mg, 10 mg

INDICATIONS & DOSAGES
➤ **Psychotic disorders**
Adults: Initially, 0.5 to 10 mg fluphenazine hydrochloride P.O. daily in divided doses every 6 to 8 hours; may increase cautiously to 20 mg. Maintenance dose is 1 to 5 mg P.O. daily. I.M. doses are one-third to one-half of P.O. doses. Usual I.M. dose is 1.25 mg. Give more than 10 mg daily with caution.
   Or, 12.5 to 25 mg of fluphenazine decanoate I.M. or subcutaneously every 1 to 6 weeks; maintenance dose is 25 to 100 mg, as needed.
Elderly patients: 1 to 2.5 mg fluphenazine hydrochloride P.O. daily.

ADMINISTRATION
P.O.
● Oral liquid forms can cause contact dermatitis. Wear gloves when preparing solutions, and avoid contact with skin and clothing.
● Protect drug from light. Slight yellowing of concentrate is common and doesn't affect potency. Discard markedly discolored solutions.
● Dilute liquid concentrate with water, fruit juice, milk, or semisolid food just before administration.
I.M.
● Parenteral forms can cause contact dermatitis. Wear gloves when preparing solutions, and avoid contact with skin and clothing.
● Protect drug from light. Slight yellowing of injection is common and doesn't affect potency. Discard markedly discolored solutions.
● For long-acting form (decanoate), which is an oil preparation, use a dry needle of at least 21G.
Subcutaneous
● Long-acting form (decanoate) is indicated for subcutaneous administration.
● Use a dry needle of at least 21G.

ACTION
A piperazine phenothiazine that probably blocks postsynaptic dopamine receptors in the brain.

Route	Onset	Peak	Duration
P.O.	< 1 hr	30 min	6–8 hr
I.M. (decanoate)	24–72 hr	Unknown	1–6 wk
I.M. (hydrochloride)	< 1 hr	90–120 min	6–8 hr
Subcut	Unknown	Unknown	Unknown

Half-life: Hydrochloride, 15 hours; decanoate, 7 to 10 days.

ADVERSE REACTIONS
CNS: *extrapyramidal reactions, tardive dyskinesia, pseudoparkinsonism, **seizures, neuroleptic malignant syndrome,*** sedation, EEG changes, drowsiness, dizziness.
CV: orthostatic hypotension, tachycardia, ECG changes.
EENT: *blurred vision,* ocular changes, nasal congestion.
GI: *dry mouth, constipation,* increased appetite.
GU: *urine retention,* dark urine, menstrual irregularities, inhibited ejaculation.
Hematologic: *leukopenia, agranulocytosis, aplastic anemia, thrombocytopenia,* eosinophilia, hemolytic anemia.
Hepatic: cholestatic jaundice.
Metabolic: weight gain.
Skin: *mild photosensitivity reactions,* allergic reactions.
Other: gynecomastia, galactorrhea.

INTERACTIONS
Drug-drug. *Antacids:* May inhibit absorption of oral phenothiazines. Separate antacid and phenothiazine doses by at least 2 hours.
Anticholinergics: May increase anticholinergic effects. Use together cautiously.
Barbiturates, lithium: May decrease phenothiazine effect and increase neurologic adverse effects. Monitor patient.
Centrally acting antihypertensives: May decrease antihypertensive effect. Monitor blood pressure.
CNS depressants: May increase CNS depression. Use together cautiously.
Drug-herb. *St. John's wort:* May increase risk of photosensitivity reactions. Advise patient to avoid excessive sunlight exposure.
Drug-lifestyle. *Alcohol use:* May increase CNS depression, especially that involving psychomotor skills. Strongly discourage alcohol use.
Sun exposure: May increase risk of photosensitivity reactions. Advise patient to avoid excessive sunlight exposure.

EFFECTS ON LAB TEST RESULTS
● May increase liver function test values. May decrease hemoglobin level and hematocrit.
● May increase eosinophil count. May decrease granulocyte, platelet, and WBC counts.
● May cause false-positive results for amylase, 5-hydroxyindoleacetic acid, urinary porphyrin, and urobilinogen tests and for urine pregnancy tests that use human chorionic gonadotropin.

CONTRAINDICATIONS & CAUTIONS
● Contraindicated in patients hypersensitive to drug and in those with coma, CNS depression, bone marrow suppression or other blood dyscrasia, subcortical damage, or liver damage.
● Use cautiously in elderly or debilitated patients and in those with pheochromocytoma, severe CV disease (may cause sudden drop in blood pressure), peptic ulcer, respiratory disorder, hypocalcemia, seizure disorder (may lower seizure threshold), severe reactions to insulin or electroconvulsive therapy, mitral insufficiency, glaucoma, or prostatic hyperplasia.
● Use cautiously in those exposed to extreme heat or cold (including antipyretic therapy) or phosphorus insecticides.
● Use parenteral form cautiously in patients who have asthma or are allergic to sulfites.

NURSING CONSIDERATIONS
● Monitor patient for tardive dyskinesia, which may occur after prolonged use. It may not appear until months or years later and may disappear spontaneously or persist for life, despite ending drug.
● *Alert:* Watch for signs and symptoms of neuroleptic malignant syndrome (extrapyramidal effects, hyperthermia, autonomic disturbance), which is rare but often fatal. It may not be related to length of drug use or type of neuroleptic; more than 60% of affected patients are men.

• Withhold dose and notify prescriber if patient, especially child or pregnant woman, develops signs or symptoms of blood dyscrasia (fever, sore throat, infection, cellulitis, weakness) or extrapyramidal reactions persisting longer than a few hours.
• Don't withdraw drug abruptly unless serious adverse reactions occur.
• Abrupt withdrawal of long-term therapy may cause gastritis, nausea, vomiting, dizziness, tremor, feeling of warmth or cold, diaphoresis, tachycardia, headache, or insomnia.

PATIENT TEACHING

• Warn patient to avoid activities that require alertness and good coordination until effects of drug are known. Drowsiness and dizziness usually subside after first few weeks.
• Warn patient to avoid alcohol while taking drug.
• Tell patient to relieve dry mouth with sugarless gum or hard candy.
• Have patient report signs of urine retention or constipation.
• Advise patient to use sunblock and wear protective clothing to avoid sensitivity to the sun.
• Tell patient that drug may discolor urine.

SAFETY ALERT!

flurazepam hydrochloride
flur-AZ-e-pam

Dalmane

Pharmacologic class: benzodi-azepine
Pregnancy risk category X
Controlled substance schedule IV

AVAILABLE FORMS
Capsules: 15 mg, 30 mg

INDICATIONS & DOSAGES
➤ **Insomnia**
Adults: 15 to 30 mg P.O. at bedtime. May repeat dose once p.r.n.
Elderly patients: 15 mg P.O. at bedtime initially, until response is determined.

ADMINISTRATION
P.O.
• Give drug without regard for food.
• Give drug with a full glass of water.

ACTION
Thought to act on the limbic system, thalamus, and hypothalamus of CNS to produce hypnotic effects.

Route	Onset	Peak	Duration
P.O.	15–45 min	30–60 min	7–8 hr

Half-life: 2 to 4 days.

ADVERSE REACTIONS
CNS: complex sleep-related behavior, daytime sedation, *dizziness, drowsiness, disturbed coordination,* lethargy, confusion, physical or psychological dependence, *headache,* light-headedness, nervousness, hallucinations, staggering, ataxia, disorientation, ***coma.***
GI: nausea, vomiting, heartburn, diarrhea, abdominal pain.
Other: ***anaphylaxis, angioedema.***

INTERACTIONS
Drug-drug. *Cimetidine:* May increase sedation. Monitor patient carefully.
CNS depressants, including opioid analgesics: May cause excessive CNS depression. Use together cautiously.
Digoxin: May increase digoxin level, resulting in toxicity. Monitor patient closely.
Disulfiram, hormonal contraceptives, isoniazid: May decrease metabolism of benzodiazepines, leading to toxicity. Monitor patient closely.
Fluconazole, itraconazole, ketoconazole, miconazole: May increase and prolong drug level, CNS depression, and psychomotor impairment. Avoid using together.
Phenytoin: May increase phenytoin level. Watch for toxicity.
Rifampin: May enhance metabolism of benzodiazepines. Watch for decreased effectiveness of benzodiazepine.
Theophylline: May act as antagonist with flurazepam. Watch for decreased effectiveness of flurazepam.

Reactions may be *common,* uncommon, *life-threatening,* or COMMON AND LIFE-THREATENING.
Interaction may have a *rapid onset* or *delayed onset.*

Drug-herb. *Calendula, hops, kava, lemon balm, passion flower, skullcap, valerian:* May enhance sedative effect of drug. Discourage use together.
Drug-lifestyle. *Alcohol use:* May cause additive CNS effects. Discourage use together.
Smoking: May increase metabolism and clearance and decrease drug half-life. Advise patient to watch for signs of decreased effectiveness.

EFFECTS ON LAB TEST RESULTS
• May increase alkaline phosphatase, ALT, AST, and bilirubin levels.

CONTRAINDICATIONS & CAUTIONS
• Contraindicated in patients hypersensitive to drug and during pregnancy.
• Use cautiously in elderly patients and in those with impaired hepatic or renal function, chronic pulmonary insufficiency, mental depression, suicidal tendencies, or history of drug abuse.

NURSING CONSIDERATIONS
• *Alert:* Anaphylaxis and angioedema may occur as early as the first dose; monitor the patient closely.
• Check hepatic and renal function and CBC before and periodically during long-term therapy.
• Minor changes in EEG patterns (usually low-voltage, fast activity) may occur during and after therapy.
• Assess mental status before starting. Elderly patients are more sensitive to drug's adverse CNS reactions.
• Take precautions to prevent hoarding or self-overdosing by depressed, suicidal, or drug-dependent patients and those with history of drug abuse.
• Patient may become physically and psychologically dependent with long-term use.
• *Look alike–sound alike:* Don't confuse Dalmane with Demulen.

PATIENT TEACHING
• *Alert:* Warn patient that drug may cause allergic reactions, facial swelling, and complex sleep-related behaviors, such as driving, eating, and making phone calls while asleep. Advise patient to report these adverse effects.
• Inform patient that drug is more effective on second, third, and fourth nights of treatment because drug builds up in the body.
• Warn patient not to abruptly stop drug after taking it for 1 month or longer.
• Tell patient to avoid alcohol use while taking drug.
• Caution patient to avoid performing activities that require mental alertness or physical coordination.
• Warn patient that prolonged use of this drug may produce psychological and physical dependence.
• Advise patient to warn prescriber about planned, suspected, or known pregnancy.

fluvoxamine maleate
floo-VOX-a-meen

Pharmacologic class: SSRI
Pregnancy risk category C

AVAILABLE FORMS
Tablets: 25 mg, 50 mg, 100 mg

INDICATIONS & DOSAGES
➤ **Obsessive-compulsive disorder (OCD)**
Adults: Initially, 50 mg P.O. daily at bedtime; increase by 50 mg every 4 to 7 days. Maximum, 300 mg daily. Give total daily amounts above 100 mg in two divided doses.
Children ages 8 to 17: Initially, 25 mg P.O. daily at bedtime; increase by 25 mg every 4 to 7 days. Maximum, 200 mg daily for children ages 8 to 11 and 300 mg daily for children ages 11 to 17. Give total daily amounts over 50 mg in two divided doses.
Adjust-a-dose: In elderly patients and those with hepatic impairment, give lower first dose and adjust dose more slowly.

ADMINISTRATION
P.O.
• Give drug without regard for food.

ACTION
Unknown. Selectively inhibits the presynaptic neuronal uptake of serotonin, which may improve OCD.

Route	Onset	Peak	Duration
P.O.	Unknown	3–8 hr	Unknown

Half-life: 17 hours.

ADVERSE REACTIONS
CNS: *agitation, headache, asthenia, somnolence, insomnia, nervousness, dizziness,* tremor, anxiety, hypertonia, depression, CNS stimulation.
CV: palpitations, vasodilation.
EENT: amblyopia.
GI: *nausea, diarrhea, constipation, dyspepsia, vomiting, dry mouth,* anorexia, flatulence, dysphagia, taste perversion.
GU: abnormal ejaculation, urinary frequency, impotence, anorgasmia, urine retention.
Respiratory: upper respiratory tract infection, dyspnea.
Skin: sweating.
Other: tooth disorder, flulike syndrome, chills, decreased libido, yawning.

INTERACTIONS
Drug-drug. *Benzodiazepines, theophylline, warfarin:* May reduce clearance of these drugs. Use together cautiously (except for diazepam, which shouldn't be used with fluvoxamine). Adjust dosage as needed.
Carbamazepine, clozapine, methadone, metoprolol, propranolol, theophylline, tricyclic antidepressants: May increase levels of these drugs. Use together cautiously, and monitor patient closely for adverse reactions. Dosage adjustments may be needed.
Diltiazem: May cause bradycardia. Monitor heart rate.
Lithium, tryptophan: May enhance effects of fluvoxamine. Use together cautiously.
MAO inhibitors (phenelzine, selegiline, tranylcypromine): May cause serotonin syndrome (CNS irritability, shivering, and altered consciousness). Avoid using within 2 weeks of MAO inhibitor.
Pimozide, thioridazine: May prolong QTc interval. Avoid using together.

Sumatriptan: May cause weakness, hyperreflexia, and incoordination. Monitor patient closely. May cause serotonin syndrome. Avoid using within 2 weeks of MAO inhibitor.
Tramadol: May cause serotonin syndrome. Monitor patient closely.
Drug-lifestyle. *Alcohol use:* May increase CNS effects. Discourage use together.
Smoking: May decrease drug's effectiveness. Urge patient to stop smoking.

EFFECTS ON LAB TEST RESULTS
None reported.

CONTRAINDICATIONS & CAUTIONS
• Contraindicated in patients hypersensitive to drug or to other phenyl piperazine antidepressants, in those receiving pimozide or thioridazine therapy, and within 2 weeks of MAO inhibitor.
• Use cautiously in patients with hepatic dysfunction, other conditions that may affect hemodynamic responses or metabolism, or history of mania or seizures.

NURSING CONSIDERATIONS
• Record mood changes. Monitor patient for suicidal tendencies.
• Don't use for the treatment of major depressive disorders in children younger than age 18 because of an increased risk of suicidal behavior.
• *Alert:* Drug may increase the risk of suicidal thinking and behavior in young adults ages 18 to 24 during the first 2 months of treatment.
• *Alert:* Combining an SSRI with a triptan may cause serotonin syndrome. Signs and symptoms may include restlessness, hallucinations, loss of coordination, fast heartbeat, rapid changes in blood pressure, increased body temperature, hyperreflexia, nausea, vomiting, and diarrhea. Serotonin syndrome is more likely to occur when starting or increasing the dose of a triptan.
• *Look alike–sound alike:* Don't confuse fluvoxamine with fluoxetine.
• Patients shouldn't stop drug without first consulting prescriber; abruptly stopping drug may cause withdrawal syndrome, including headache, muscle ache, and flulike symptoms.

PATIENT TEACHING

• Warn patient to avoid hazardous activities until CNS effects of drug are known.
• Tell woman to notify prescriber about planned, suspected, or known pregnancy.
• Tell patient who develops a rash, hives, or a related allergic reaction to notify prescriber.
• Inform patient that several weeks of therapy may be needed to obtain full therapeutic effect. Once improvement occurs, advise patient not to stop drug until directed by prescriber.
• Suggest that patient keep a diary of changes in mood or behavior. Tell patient to report suicidal thoughts immediately.
• Advise patient to check with prescriber before taking OTC drugs; drug interactions can occur.
• Tell patient drug can be taken with or without food.

---

folic acid (vitamin B$_9$)
FOE-lik

Folvite, Novo-Folacid†

Pharmacologic class: folic acid derivative
Pregnancy risk category A

AVAILABLE FORMS
Injection: 10-ml vials (5 mg/ml with 1.5% benzyl alcohol, 5 mg/ml with 1.5% benzyl alcohol and 0.2% ethylenediaminetetraacetic acid)
Tablets: 0.4 mg, 0.8 mg, 1 mg

INDICATIONS & DOSAGES
➤ **RDA**
Adults and children age 14 and older: Give 400 mcg.
Children ages 9 to 13: Give 300 mcg.
Children ages 4 to 8: Give 200 mcg.
Children ages 1 to 3: Give 150 mcg.
Infants ages 6 months to 1 year: 80 mcg.
Neonates and infants younger than age 6 months: 65 mcg.
Pregnant women: 600 mcg.
Breast-feeding women: 500 mcg.
➤ **Megaloblastic or macrocytic anemia from folic acid or other nutritional deficiency, hepatic disease,**
alcoholism, intestinal obstruction, or excessive hemolysis
Adults and children age 4 and older: 0.4 to 1 mg P.O., I.M., or subcutaneously daily. After anemia caused by folic acid deficiency is corrected, proper diet and RDA supplements are needed to prevent recurrence.
Children younger than age 4: Up to 0.3 mg P.O., I.M., or subcutaneously daily.
Pregnant and breast-feeding women: 0.8 mg P.O., I.M., or subcutaneously daily.
➤ **To prevent fetal neural tube defects during pregnancy**
Adults: 0.4 mg P.O. daily.
➤ **To prevent megaloblastic anemia during pregnancy to prevent fetal damage**
Adults: Up to 1 mg P.O., I.M., or subcutaneously daily throughout pregnancy.
➤ **Test for folic acid deficiency in patients with megaloblastic anemia without masking pernicious anemia**
Adults and children: 0.1 to 0.2 mg P.O. or I.M. for 10 days while maintaining a diet low in folate and vitamin B$_{12}$.
➤ **Tropical sprue**
Adults: 3 to 15 mg P.O. daily.

ADMINISTRATION
P.O.
• Give drug without regard for food.
I.M.
• Don't mix with other drugs in same syringe for I.M. injections.
• Protect drug from light and heat; store at room temperature.
Subcutaneous
• Protect drug from light and heat; store at room temperature.

ACTION
Stimulates normal erythropoiesis and nucleoprotein synthesis.

Route	Onset	Peak	Duration
P.O., I.M., Subcut	Unknown	30–60 min	Unknown

Half-life: Unknown.

ADVERSE REACTIONS
CNS: altered sleep pattern, general malaise, difficulty concentrating,

---

confusion, impaired judgment, irritability, hyperactivity.
GI: anorexia, nausea, flatulence, bitter taste.
Respiratory: *bronchospasm.*
Skin: allergic reactions including rash, pruritus, and erythema.

INTERACTIONS
Drug-drug. *Aminosalicylic acid, chloramphenicol, hormonal contraceptives, methotrexate, sulfasalazine, trimethoprim:* May antagonize folic acid. Watch for decreased folic acid effect. Use together cautiously.
Phenytoin: May increase anticonvulsant metabolism, which decreases anticonvulsant level. Monitor phenytoin level closely.

EFFECTS ON LAB TEST RESULTS
• May decrease serum and RBC folate levels.

CONTRAINDICATIONS & CAUTIONS
• Contraindicated in patients with undiagnosed anemia (it may mask pernicious anemia) and in those with vitamin B_{12} deficiency.

NURSING CONSIDERATIONS
• The U.S. Public Health Service recommends use of folic acid during pregnancy to decrease fetal neural tube defects. Patients with history of fetal neural tube defects in pregnancy should increase folic acid intake for 1 month before and 3 months after conception.
• Patients with small-bowel resections and intestinal malabsorption may need parenteral administration.
• Most CNS and GI adverse reactions occur at higher doses, such as 15 mg daily for 1 month.
• *Look alike–sound alike:* Don't confuse folic acid with folinic acid.

PATIENT TEACHING
• Teach patient about proper nutrition to prevent recurrence of anemia.
• Stress importance of follow-up visits and laboratory studies.

• Teach patient about foods that contain folic acid: liver, oranges, whole wheat, broccoli, and Brussels sprouts.

---

galantamine hydrobromide
gah-LAN-tah-meen

Razadyne, Razadyne ER

Pharmacologic class: cholinesterase inhibitor
Pregnancy risk category B

AVAILABLE FORMS
Capsules (extended-release): 8 mg, 16 mg, 24 mg
Oral solution: 4 mg/ml
Tablets: 4 mg, 8 mg, 12 mg

INDICATIONS & DOSAGES
➤ **Mild to moderate Alzheimer dementia**
Adults: Initially, 4 mg b.i.d., preferably with morning and evening meals. If dose is well tolerated after minimum of 4 weeks of therapy, increase dosage to 8 mg b.i.d. A further increase to 12 mg b.i.d. may be attempted, but only after at least 4 weeks of therapy at the previous dosage. Dosage range is 16 to 24 mg daily in two divided doses.
   Or, 8 mg extended-release capsule P.O. once daily in the morning with food. Increase to 16 mg P.O. once daily after a minimum of 4 weeks. May further increase to 24 mg once daily after a minimum of 4 weeks, based upon patient response and tolerability.
Adjust-a-dose: For patients with Child-Pugh score of 7 to 9, dosage usually shouldn't exceed 16 mg daily. Drug isn't recommended for patients with Child-Pugh score of 10 to 15. For patients with moderate renal impairment, dosage usually shouldn't exceed 16 mg daily. For patients with creatinine clearance less than 9 ml/minute, drug isn't recommended.

ADMINISTRATION
P.O.
• *Alert:* Give Razadyne tablets twice daily; give Razadyne ER capsules once daily. To

---

avoid dosing errors, verify any prescription that suggests a different dosing schedule.
• Give drug with food and antiemetics, and ensure adequate fluid intake to decrease the risk of nausea and vomiting.
• Use proper technique when dispensing the oral solution with the pipette. Dispense measured amount into a beverage and give to patient right away.

ACTION
Thought to enhance cholinergic function by increasing acetylcholine level in brain.

Route	Onset	Peak	Duration
P.O.	Unknown	1 hr	Unknown

Half-life: About 7 hours.

ADVERSE REACTIONS
CNS: depression, dizziness, headache, tremor, insomnia, somnolence, fatigue, syncope.
CV: *bradycardia.*
EENT: rhinitis.
GI: *diarrhea, nausea, vomiting,* anorexia, abdominal pain, dyspepsia, anorexia.
GU: UTI, hematuria.
Hematologic: anemia.
Metabolic: weight loss.

INTERACTIONS
Drug-drug. *Amitriptyline, fluoxetine, fluvoxamine, quinidine:* May decrease galantamine clearance. Monitor patient closely.
Anticholinergics: May antagonize anticholinergic activity. Monitor patient.
Cholinergics (such as bethanechol, succinylcholine): May have synergistic effect. Monitor patient closely. May need to avoid use before procedures using general anesthesia with succinylcholine-type neuromuscular blockers.
Cimetidine, clarithromycin, erythromycin, ketoconazole, paroxetine: May increase galantamine bioavailability. Monitor patient closely.

EFFECTS ON LAB TEST RESULTS
None reported.

CONTRAINDICATIONS & CAUTIONS
• Contraindicated in patients hypersensitive to drug or its components.
• Use cautiously in patients with supraventricular cardiac conduction disorders and in those taking other drugs that significantly slow heart rate.
• Use cautiously during or before procedures involving anesthesia using succinylcholine-type or similar neuromuscular blockers.
• Use cautiously in patients with history of peptic ulcer disease and in those taking NSAIDs. Because of the potential for cholinomimetic effects, use cautiously in patients with bladder outflow obstruction, seizures, asthma, or COPD.

NURSING CONSIDERATIONS
• Drug may cause bradycardia and heart block. Consider all patients at risk for adverse effects on cardiac conduction.
• *Alert:* The original trade name for galantamine, "Reminyl," was changed to "Razadyne" because of name confusion with the antidiabetic Amaryl.
• If drug is stopped for several days or longer, restart at the lowest dose and gradually increase, at 4-week or longer intervals, to the previous dosage level.
• Because of the risk of increased gastric acid secretion, monitor patients closely for symptoms of active or occult GI bleeding, especially those with an increased risk of developing ulcers.

PATIENT TEACHING
• Advise caregiver to give drug with morning and evening meals (for the conventional form), or only in the morning (for the extended-release form).
• Inform patient that nausea and vomiting are common adverse effects.
• Teach caregiver the proper technique when measuring the oral solution with the pipette. Tell her to place measured amount in a nonalcoholic beverage and have patient drink right away.
• Urge patient or caregiver to report slow heartbeat immediately.
• Advise patient and caregiver that although drug may improve cognitive function, it doesn't alter the underlying disease process.

goserelin acetate
GOE-se-rel-in

Zoladex

Pharmacologic class: gonadotropin-releasing hormone analogue
Pregnancy risk category X (endometriosis and endometrial lining); D (breast cancer)

AVAILABLE FORMS
Implants: 3.6 mg, 10.8 mg

INDICATIONS & DOSAGES
➤ **Endometriosis, including pain relief and lesion reduction**
Women: 3.6 mg subcutaneously every 28 days into the anterior abdominal wall below the navel. Maximum length of therapy is 6 months.
➤ **Endometrial thinning before endometrial ablation**
Women: 3.6 mg subcutaneously into the anterior abdominal wall below the navel. Give one or two implants, 4 weeks apart.
➤ **Palliative treatment of advanced breast cancer in premenopausal and perimenopausal women**
Women: 3.6 mg subcutaneously every 28 days into the anterior abdominal wall below the navel.
➤ **Palliative treatment of advanced prostate cancer**
Men: 3.6 mg subcutaneously every 28 days or 10.8 mg subcutaneously every 12 weeks into the anterior abdominal wall below the navel.

ADMINISTRATION
Subcutaneous
• Implant comes in a preloaded syringe. If package is damaged, don't use the syringe. Make sure drug is visible in the translucent chamber of the syringe.
• Give drug into the anterior abdominal wall below the navel using aseptic technique.
• After cleaning area with an alcohol swab and injecting a local anesthetic, stretch patient's skin with one hand while grasping barrel of syringe with the other.
• Insert needle into the subcutaneous fat; then change direction of needle so that it parallels the abdominal wall. Push needle in until hub touches patient's skin; withdraw about 1 cm (this creates a gap for drug to be injected) before depressing plunger completely.
• To avoid need for a new syringe and injection site, don't aspirate after inserting needle. If needle penetrates a blood vessel, blood will appear in the syringe chamber. Withdraw needle, and inject elsewhere with a new syringe.
• Never give by I.V. injection.

ACTION
A luteinizing hormone–releasing hormone (LH-RH) analogue that acts on the pituitary gland to decrease the release of follicle-stimulating hormone and LH, dramatically lowering sex hormone levels (estrogen in women and testosterone in men).

Route	Onset	Peak	Duration
Subcut	Rapid	30–60 min	Throughout therapy

Half-life: About 4½ hours.

ADVERSE REACTIONS
CNS: lethargy, pain, dizziness, *insomnia, anxiety, depression, headache, chills, emotional lability, **stroke**, asthenia.*
CV: edema, ***heart failure, arrhythmias,** peripheral edema,* hypertension, ***MI**, peripheral vascular disorder, chest pain, hot flashes.*
GI: nausea, vomiting, diarrhea, constipation, ulcer, anorexia, abdominal pain.
GU: *sexual dysfunction, impotence, lower urinary tract symptoms,* renal insufficiency, urinary obstruction, *vaginitis,* UTI, *amenorrhea.*
Hematologic: anemia.
Metabolic: hypercalcemia, hyperglycemia, weight increase, gout.
Musculoskeletal: back pain, osteoporosis.
Respiratory: COPD, upper respiratory tract infection.
Skin: rash, *diaphoresis, acne, seborrhea,* hirsutism.

Other: *changes in breast size, changes in libido, infection,* breast swelling, pain, and tenderness.

INTERACTIONS
None significant.

EFFECTS ON LAB TEST RESULTS
• May increase calcium and glucose levels. May decrease hemoglobin level.

CONTRAINDICATIONS & CAUTIONS
• Contraindicated in patients hypersensitive to LH-RH, LH-RH agonist analogues, or goserelin acetate.
• Contraindicated in pregnant or breast-feeding women and in patients with obstructive uropathy or vertebral metastases.
• The 10.8-mg implant is contraindicated in women because of insufficient data supporting reliable suppression of estradiol.
• Because drug may cause bone density loss in women, use cautiously in patients with risk factors for osteoporosis, such as family history of osteoporosis, chronic alcohol or tobacco abuse, or use of drugs such as corticosteroids or anticonvulsants that affect bone density.

NURSING CONSIDERATIONS
• Before giving to women, rule out pregnancy.
• When drug is used for prostate cancer, LH-RH analogues such as goserelin may initially worsen symptoms because drug first increases testosterone level. Some patients may temporarily have increased bone pain. Rarely, disease may get worse (spinal cord compression or ureteral obstruction), although the relationship to therapy is uncertain.
• When drug is used for endometrial thinning, if one implant is given, surgery should be performed 4 weeks later; if two implants are given, surgery should be performed 2 to 4 weeks after patient receives second implant.

PATIENT TEACHING
• Advise patient to return every 28 days for a new implant. A delay of a couple of days is permissible.
• Tell patient that pain may worsen for first 30 days of treatment.

• Tell woman to use a nonhormonal form of contraception during treatment. Caution patient about significant risks to fetus.
• Urge woman to call prescriber if menstruation persists or if breakthrough bleeding occurs. Menstruation should stop during treatment.
• Inform woman that a delayed return of menstruation may occur after therapy ends. Persistent lack of menstruation is rare.

haloperidol
ha-loe-PER-i-dole

Haldol, Novo-Peridol†

haloperidol decanoate
Haldol Decanoate, Haloperidol LA†

haloperidol lactate
Haldol, Haldol Concentrate

Pharmacologic class: phenyl-butylpiperadine derivative
Pregnancy risk category C

AVAILABLE FORMS
haloperidol
Tablets: 0.5 mg, 1 mg, 2 mg, 5 mg, 10 mg, 20 mg
haloperidol decanoate
Injection: 50 mg/ml, 100 mg/ml
haloperidol lactate
Injection: 5 mg/ml
Oral concentrate: 2 mg/ml

INDICATIONS & DOSAGES
➤ **Psychotic disorders**
Adults and children older than age 12:
Dosage varies for each patient. Initially, 0.5 to 5 mg P.O. b.i.d. or t.i.d. Or, 2 to 5 mg I.M. lactate every 4 to 8 hours, although hourly administration may be needed until control is obtained. Maximum, 100 mg P.O. daily.
Children ages 3 to 12 who weigh 15 to 40 kg (33 to 88 lb): Initially, 0.5 mg P.O. daily divided b.i.d. or t.i.d. May increase dose by 0.5 mg at 5- to 7-day intervals, depending on therapeutic response and patient tolerance. Maintenance dose, 0.05 mg/kg to 0.15 mg/kg P.O. daily given

in two or three divided doses. Severely disturbed children may need higher doses.

➤ **Chronic psychosis requiring prolonged therapy**
Adults: 50 to 100 mg I.M. decanoate every 4 weeks.

➤ **Nonpsychotic behavior disorders**
Children ages 3 to 12: 0.05 to 0.075 mg/kg P.O. daily, in two or three divided doses. Maximum, 6 mg daily.

➤ **Tourette syndrome**
Adults: 0.5 to 5 mg P.O. b.i.d., t.i.d., or as needed.
Children ages 3 to 12: 0.05 to 0.075 mg/kg P.O. daily, in two or three divided doses.
Elderly patients: 0.5 to 2 mg P.O. b.i.d. or t.i.d.; increase gradually, as needed.
Adjust-a-dose: For debilitated patients, initially, 0.5 to 2 mg P.O. b.i.d. or t.i.d.; increase gradually, as needed.

➤ **Delirium ◆**
Adults: 1 to 2 mg I.V. lactate every 2 to 4 hours. Severely agitated patients may require higher doses.
Elderly patients: 0.25 to 0.5 mg I.V. every 4 hours.

ADMINISTRATION
P.O.
● Protect drug from light. Slight yellowing of concentrate is common and doesn't affect potency. Discard very discolored solutions.
● Dilute oral dose with water or a beverage, such as orange juice, apple juice, tomato juice, or cola, immediately before administration.
I.V.
● Only the lactate form can be given I.V.
● Monitor patient receiving single doses higher than 50 mg or total daily doses greater than 500 mg closely for prolonged QTc interval and torsades de pointes.
● Store at controlled room temperature, and protect from light.
● **Incompatibilities:** Allopurinol, amphotericin B cholesteryl sulfate complex, benztropine, cefepime, diphenhydramine, fluconazole, foscarnet, heparin, hydromorphone, hydroxyzine, ketorolac, morphine, nitroprusside sodium, piperacillin and tazobactam sodium, sargramostim.

I.M.
● Protect drug from light. Slight yellowing of injection is common and doesn't affect potency. Discard very discolored solutions.
● When switching from tablets to decanoate injection, give 10 to 15 times the oral dose once a month (maximum 100 mg).
● *Alert:* Don't give decanoate form I.V.

ACTION
A butyrophenone that probably exerts antipsychotic effects by blocking postsynaptic dopamine receptors in the brain.

Route	Onset	Peak	Duration
P.O.	Unknown	3–6 hr	Unknown
I.V.	Unknown	Unknown	Unknown
I.M. (decanoate)	Unknown	3–9 days	Unknown
I.M. (lactate)	Unknown	10–20 min	Unknown

Half-life: P.O., 24 hours; I.M., 21 hours.

ADVERSE REACTIONS
CNS: *severe extrapyramidal reactions, tardive dyskinesia,* **neuroleptic malignant syndrome, seizures,** sedation, drowsiness, lethargy, headache, insomnia, confusion, vertigo.
CV: tachycardia, hypotension, hypertension, ECG changes, *torsades de pointes,* with I.V. use.
EENT: blurred vision.
GI: dry mouth, anorexia, constipation, diarrhea, nausea, vomiting, dyspepsia.
GU: urine retention, menstrual irregularities, priapism.
Hematologic: *leukopenia,* leukocytosis.
Hepatic: jaundice.
Skin: rash, other skin reactions, diaphoresis.
Other: gynecomastia.

INTERACTIONS
Drug-drug. *Anticholinergics:* May increase anticholinergic effects and glaucoma. Use together cautiously.
Azole antifungals, buspirone, macrolides: May increase haloperidol level. Monitor patient for increased adverse reactions; haloperidol dose may need to be adjusted.
Carbamazepine: May decrease haloperidol level. Monitor patient.

CNS depressants: May increase CNS depression. Use together cautiously.
Lithium: May cause lethargy and confusion after high doses. Monitor patient.
Methyldopa: May cause dementia. Monitor patient closely.
Rifampin: May decrease haloperidol level. Monitor patient for clinical effect.
Drug-lifestyle. *Alcohol use:* May increase CNS depression. Discourage use together.

EFFECTS ON LAB TEST RESULTS
● May increase liver function test values. May increase or decrease WBC count.

CONTRAINDICATIONS & CAUTIONS
● Contraindicated in patients hypersensitive to drug and in those with parkinsonism, coma, or CNS depression.
● Use cautiously in elderly and debilitated patients; in patients with history of seizures or EEG abnormalities, severe CV disorders, allergies, glaucoma, or urine retention; and in those taking anticonvulsants, anticoagulants, antiparkinsonians, or lithium.

NURSING CONSIDERATIONS
● Monitor patient for tardive dyskinesia, which may occur after prolonged use. It may not appear until months or years later and may disappear spontaneously or persist for life, despite ending drug.
● *Alert:* Watch for signs and symptoms of neuroleptic malignant syndrome (extrapyramidal effects, hyperthermia, autonomic disturbance), which is rare but commonly fatal.
● Don't withdraw drug abruptly unless required by severe adverse reactions.
● *Alert:* Haldol may contain tartrazine.
● *Look alike–sound alike:* Don't confuse Haldol with Halcion or Halog.

PATIENT TEACHING
● Although drug is the least sedating of the antipsychotics, warn patient to avoid activities that require alertness and good coordination until effects of drug are known. Drowsiness and dizziness usually subside after a few weeks.
● Warn patient to avoid alcohol during therapy.

● Tell patient to relieve dry mouth with sugarless gum or hard candy.

---

hydroxyzine hydrochloride
hye-DROX-i-zeen

Anx, Vistaril

hydroxyzine pamoate
Vistaril

Pharmacologic class: piperazine derivative
Pregnancy risk category NR

AVAILABLE FORMS
hydroxyzine hydrochloride
Capsules: 10 mg†, 25 mg†, 50 mg†
Injection: 25 mg/ml, 50 mg/ml
Syrup: 10 mg/5 ml
Tablets: 10 mg, 25 mg, 50 mg, 100 mg
hydroxyzine pamoate
Capsules: 25 mg, 50 mg, 100 mg
Oral suspension: 25 mg/5 ml

INDICATIONS & DOSAGES
➤ **Anxiety**
Adults: 50 to 100 mg P.O. q.i.d.
Children age 6 and older: 50 to 100 mg P.O. daily in divided doses.
Children younger than age 6: 50 mg P.O. daily in divided doses.
➤ **Preoperative and postoperative adjunctive therapy for sedation**
Adults: 25 to 100 mg I.M. or 50 to 100 mg P.O.
Children: 1.1 mg/kg I.M. or 0.6 mg/kg P.O.
➤ **Pruritus from allergies**
Adults: 25 mg P.O. t.i.d. or q.i.d.
Children age 6 and older: 50 to 100 mg P.O. daily in divided doses.
Children younger than age 6: 50 mg P.O. daily in divided doses.
➤ **Psychiatric and emotional emergencies, including acute alcoholism**
Adults: 50 to 100 mg I.M. every 4 to 6 hours, p.r.n.
➤ **Nausea and vomiting (excluding nausea and vomiting of pregnancy)**
Adults: 25 to 100 mg I.M.
Children: 1.1 mg/kg I.M.

➤ **Antepartum and postpartum adjunctive therapy**
Adults: 25 to 100 mg I.M.

ADMINISTRATION
P.O.
● Give drug without regard for meals.
● Shake suspension well before giving.
I.M.
● Parenteral form (hydroxyzine hydrochloride) is for I.M. use only, preferably by Z-track injection. Never give drug I.V. or subcutaneously.
● Aspirate I.M. injection carefully to prevent inadvertent I.V. injection. Inject deeply into a large muscle.

ACTION
Suppresses activity in certain essential regions of the subcortical area of the CNS.

Route	Onset	Peak	Duration
P.O.	15–30 min	2 hr	4–6 hr
I.M.	Unknown	Unknown	4–6 hr

Half-life: 3 hours.

ADVERSE REACTIONS
CNS: *drowsiness,* involuntary motor activity.
GI: *dry mouth,* constipation.
Skin: pain at I.M. injection site.
Other: hypersensitivity reactions.

INTERACTIONS
Drug-drug. *Anticholinergics:* May cause additive anticholinergic effects. Use together cautiously.
CNS depressants: May increase CNS depression. Use together cautiously; dosage adjustments may be needed.
Epinephrine: May inhibit and reverse vasopressor effect of epinephrine. Avoid using together.
Drug-lifestyle. *Alcohol use:* May increase CNS depression. Discourage use together.

EFFECTS ON LAB TEST RESULTS
● May cause false increase in urinary 17-hydroxycorticosteroid level. May cause false-negative skin allergen tests by reducing or inhibiting the cutaneous response to histamine.

CONTRAINDICATIONS & CAUTIONS
● Contraindicated in patients hypersensitive to drug, patients in early pregnancy, and breast-feeding women.

NURSING CONSIDERATIONS
● If patient takes other CNS drugs, watch for oversedation.
● Elderly patients may be more sensitive to adverse anticholinergic effects; monitor these patients for dizziness, excessive sedation, confusion, hypotension, and syncope.
● *Look alike–sound alike:* Don't confuse hydroxyzine with hydroxyurea or hydralazine.

PATIENT TEACHING
● Warn patient to avoid hazardous activities that require alertness and good coordination until effects of drug are known.
● Tell patient to avoid use of alcohol while taking drug.
● Advise patient to use sugarless hard candy or gum to relieve dry mouth.
● Warn woman of childbearing age to avoid use during pregnancy and breast-feeding.

---

imipramine hydrochloride
im-IP-ra-meen

Novo-pramine†, Tofranil

imipramine pamoate
Tofranil-PM

Pharmacologic class: tricyclic antidepressant (TCA)
Pregnancy risk category D

AVAILABLE FORMS
imipramine hydrochloride
Tablets: 10 mg, 25 mg, 50 mg
imipramine pamoate
Capsules: 75 mg, 100 mg, 125 mg, 150 mg

INDICATIONS & DOSAGES
➤ **Depression**
Adults: 75 to 100 mg P.O. daily in divided doses, increased by 25 to 50 mg. Maximum daily dose is 200 mg for outpatients

---

and 300 mg for hospitalized patients. Give entire dose at bedtime.
Adolescents and elderly patients: Initially, 30 to 40 mg daily; maximum shouldn't exceed 100 mg daily.

➤ **Childhood enuresis**
Children age 5 and older: 25 mg P.O. 1 hour before bedtime. If patient doesn't improve within 1 week, increase dose to 50 mg if child is younger than age 12; increase dose to 75 mg for children age 12 and older. In either case, maximum daily dose is 2.5 mg/kg.

ADMINISTRATION
P.O.
● Give drug without regard for food.
● Give full dose at bedtime if possible.

ACTION
Unknown. Increases norepinephrine, serotonin, or both in the CNS by blocking their reuptake by the presynaptic neurons.

Route	Onset	Peak	Duration
P.O.	Unknown	1–2 hr	Unknown

Half-life: 11 to 25 hours.

ADVERSE REACTIONS
CNS: *drowsiness, dizziness, **seizures, stroke,** excitation, tremor, confusion, hallucinations, anxiety, ataxia, paresthesia, nervousness, EEG changes, extrapyramidal reactions.*
CV: *orthostatic hypotension, tachycardia, ECG changes, **MI, arrhythmias, heart block,** hypertension, **precipitation of heart failure.***
EENT: *blurred vision,* tinnitus, mydriasis.
GI: *dry mouth, constipation,* nausea, vomiting, anorexia, paralytic ileus, abdominal cramps.
GU: *urine retention.*
Metabolic: *hypoglycemia,* hyperglycemia.
Skin: rash, urticaria, photosensitivity reactions, pruritus, diaphoresis.
Other: hypersensitivity reactions.

INTERACTIONS
Drug-drug. *Barbiturates, CNS depressants:* May enhance CNS depression. Avoid using together.

*Cimetidine, **fluoxetine, fluvoxamine, paroxetine, sertraline:*** May increase imipramine level. Monitor drug levels and patient for signs of toxicity.
Clonidine: May cause life-threatening hypertension. Avoid using together.
Epinephrine, norepinephrine: May increase hypertensive effect. Use together cautiously.
MAO inhibitors: May cause hyperpyretic crisis, severe seizures, and death. Avoid using within 14 days of MAO inhibitor therapy.
Quinolones: May increase the risk of life-threatening arrhythmias. Avoid using together.
Drug-herb. *Evening primrose oil:* May cause additive or synergistic effect, lowering the seizure threshold and increasing the risk of seizure. Discourage use together.
St. John's wort, SAM-e, yohimbe: May cause serotonin syndrome. Discourage use together.
Drug-lifestyle. *Alcohol use:* May enhance CNS depression. Discourage use together.
Smoking: May lower level of drug. Monitor patient for lack of effect.
Sun exposure: May increase risk of photosensitivity reactions. Advise patient to avoid excessive sunlight exposure.

EFFECTS ON LAB TEST RESULTS
● May increase or decrease glucose level.
● May increase liver function test values.

CONTRAINDICATIONS & CAUTIONS
● Contraindicated in patients hypersensitive to drug and in those receiving MAO inhibitors; also contraindicated during acute recovery phase of MI.
● Use with extreme caution in patients at risk for suicide; in patients with history of urine retention, angle-closure glaucoma, or seizure disorders; in patients with increased intraocular pressure, CV disease, impaired hepatic function, hyperthyroidism, or impaired renal function; and in patients receiving thyroid drugs. Injectable form contains sulfites, which may cause allergic reactions in hypersensitive patients.

NURSING CONSIDERATIONS

- Monitor patient for nausea, headache, and malaise after abrupt withdrawal of long-term therapy; these symptoms don't indicate addiction.
- Don't withdraw drug abruptly.
- Because of hypertensive episodes during surgery in patients receiving TCAs, stop drug gradually several days before surgery.
- If signs or symptoms of psychosis occur or increase, expect prescriber to reduce dosage. Record mood changes. Monitor patient for suicidal tendencies, and allow only a minimum supply of drug.
- *Alert:* Drug may increase the risk of suicidal thinking and behavior in children and adolescents with major depressive disorder or other psychiatric disorder.
- *Alert:* Drug may increase the risk of suicidal thinking and behavior in young adults ages 18 to 24 during the first 2 months of treatment.
- To prevent relapse in children receiving drug for enuresis, withdraw drug gradually.
- Recommend sugarless hard candy or gum to relieve dry mouth. Saliva substitutes may be useful.
- *Alert:* Tofranil and Tofranil-PM may contain tartrazine.
- *Look alike–sound alike:* Don't confuse imipramine with desipramine.

PATIENT TEACHING

- Tell patient to take full dose at bedtime whenever possible, but warn him of possible morning dizziness upon standing up quickly.
- If child is an early-night bed-wetter, tell parents it may be more effective to divide dose and give the first dose earlier in day.
- Tell patient to avoid alcohol while taking this drug.
- Advise patient to consult prescriber before taking other prescription or OTC drugs.
- Warn patient to avoid hazardous activities that require alertness and good coordination until effects of the drug are known. Drowsiness and dizziness usually subside after a few weeks.
- Warn patient not to stop drug suddenly.
- To prevent oversensitivity to the sun, advise patient to use sunblock, wear protective clothing, and avoid prolonged exposure to strong sunlight.

---

lamotrigine
la-MO-tri-geen

Lamictal

Pharmacologic class: phenyltriazine
Pregnancy risk category C

AVAILABLE FORMS
Tablets: 25 mg, 100 mg, 150 mg, 200 mg
Tablets (chewable dispersible): 2 mg, 5 mg, 25 mg

INDICATIONS & DOSAGES
➤ **Adjunct treatment of partial seizures or primary generalized tonic-clonic seizures caused by epilepsy or generalized seizures of Lennox-Gastaut syndrome**
Adults and children older than age 12 taking other enzyme-inducing anticonvulsants with valproic acid: 25 mg P.O. every other day for 2 weeks; then 25 mg P.O. daily for 2 weeks. Continue to increase, as needed, by 25 to 50 mg daily every 1 to 2 weeks until an effective maintenance dosage of 100 to 400 mg daily given in one or two divided doses is reached. When added to valproic acid alone, the usual daily maintenance dose is 100 to 200 mg.
Adults and children older than age 12 taking other enzyme-inducing anticonvulsants but not valproic acid: 50 mg P.O. daily for 2 weeks; then 100 mg P.O. daily in two divided doses for 2 weeks. Increase, as needed, by 100 mg daily every 1 to 2 weeks. Usual maintenance dosage is 300 to 500 mg P.O. daily in two divided doses.
Children ages 2 to 12 weighing 6.7 to 40 kg (15 to 88 lb) taking other enzyme-inducing anticonvulsants with valproic acid: 0.15 mg/kg P.O. daily in one or two divided doses (rounded down to nearest whole tablet) for 2 weeks, followed by 0.3 mg/kg daily in one or two divided doses for another 2 weeks. Thereafter, usual maintenance dosage is 1 to 5 mg/kg daily (maximum, 200 mg daily in one to two divided doses).

Children ages 2 to 12 weighing 6.7 to 40 kg (15 to 88 lb) taking other enzyme-inducing anticonvulsants but not valproic acid: 0.6 mg/kg P.O. daily in two divided doses (rounded down to nearest whole tablet) for 2 weeks; then 1.2 mg/kg daily in two divided doses for another 2 weeks. Usual maintenance dosage is 5 to 15 mg/kg P.O. daily (maximum 400 mg daily in two divided doses).

➤ **To convert patients from therapy with a hepatic enzyme-inducing anticonvulsant alone to lamotrigine therapy**
Adults and children age 16 and older: Add lamotrigine 50 mg P.O. once daily to current drug regimen for 2 weeks, followed by 100 mg P.O. daily in two divided doses for 2 weeks. Then increase daily dosage by 100 mg every 1 to 2 weeks until maintenance dose of 500 mg daily in two divided doses is reached. The concomitant hepatic enzyme-inducing anticonvulsant can then be gradually reduced by 20% decrements weekly for 4 weeks.
Adjust-a-dose: For patients with severe renal impairment, use lower maintenance dosage.

➤ **To convert patients with partial seizures from adjunctive therapy with valproate to therapy with lamotrigine alone**
Adults and children age 16 and older: Add lamotrigine until 200 mg daily is achieved; then gradually decrease valproate to 500 mg daily by decrements of no more than 500 mg daily per week. Maintain these dosages for 1 week, then increase lamotrigine to 300 mg daily while decreasing valproate to 250 mg daily. Maintain these dosages for 1 week, then stop valproate completely while increasing lamotrigine by 100 mg daily every week until a dose of 500 mg daily is reached.

➤ **Bipolar disorder**
Adults: Initially, 25 mg P.O. once daily for 2 weeks; then 50 mg P.O. once daily for 2 weeks. Dosage may then be doubled at weekly intervals, to maintenance dosage of 200 mg daily.
Adults taking carbamazepine or other hepatic enzyme-inducing drugs without valproic acid: Initially, 50 mg P.O. once

daily for 2 weeks; then 100 mg daily in two divided doses for 2 weeks. Dosage is then increased by 100 mg weekly to maintenance dosage of 400 mg daily, given in two divided doses.
Adults taking valproic acid: Initially, 25 mg P.O. every other day for 2 weeks; then 25 mg P.O. once daily for 2 weeks. Dosage may then be doubled at weekly intervals to maintenance dosage of 100 mg daily.

ADMINISTRATION
P.O.
● Chewable dispersible tablets may be swallowed whole, chewed, or dispersed in water or diluted fruit juice.
● If tablets are chewed, give a small amount of water or diluted fruit juice to aid in swallowing.

ACTION
Unknown. May inhibit release of glutamate and aspartate (excitatory neurotransmitters) in the brain via an action at voltage-sensitive sodium channels.

Route	Onset	Peak	Duration
P.O.	Unknown	1–5 hr	Unknown

Half-life: 14½ to 70¼ hours, depending on dosage schedule and use of other anticonvulsants.

ADVERSE REACTIONS
CNS: *ataxia, dizziness, headache, somnolence, seizures,* aggravated reaction, anxiety, concentration disturbance, decreased memory, depression, dysarthria, emotional lability, fever, incoordination, insomnia, irritability, malaise, mind racing, speech disorder, sleep disorder, tremor, vertigo.
CV: palpitations.
EENT: *blurred vision, diplopia, rhinitis,* nystagmus, pharyngitis, vision abnormality.
GI: *nausea, vomiting,* abdominal pain, anorexia, constipation, diarrhea, dry mouth, dyspepsia.
GU: amenorrhea, dysmenorrhea, vaginitis.
Musculoskeletal: muscle spasm, neck pain.
Respiratory: cough, dyspnea.

Skin: *rash, **Stevens-Johnson syndrome,
toxic epidermal necrolysis,** acne, alopecia,
hot flashes, pruritus.
Other: chills, flulike syndrome, infection,
tooth disorder.

INTERACTIONS

Drug-drug. *Acetaminophen:* May decrease therapeutic effects of lamotrigine.
Monitor patient.
Carbamazepine: May decrease effects of
lamotrigine while increasing toxicity of
carbamazepine. Adjust doses and monitor
patient.
*Ethosuximide, oxcarbazepine, phenobar-
bital, phenytoin, primidone:* May decrease
lamotrigine level. Monitor patient closely.
*Folate inhibitors, such as co-trimoxazole
and methotrexate:* May have additive effect
because lamotrigine inhibits dihydrofolate
reductase, an enzyme involved in folic acid
synthesis. Monitor patient.
*Hormonal contraceptives containing estro-
gen, rifampin:* May decrease lamotrigine
levels. Adjust dosage. By the end of the
"pill-free" week, lamotrigine levels may
double.
Valproic acid: May decrease clearance of
lamotrigine, which increases lamotrigine
level; also decreases valproic acid level.
Monitor patient for toxicity.
Drug-lifestyle. *Sun exposure:* May cause
photosensitivity reactions. Advise patient
to avoid excessive sun exposure.

EFFECTS ON LAB TEST RESULTS
None reported.

CONTRAINDICATIONS & CAUTIONS
• Contraindicated in patients hypersensitive to drug or its components.
• Use cautiously in patients with renal,
hepatic, or cardiac impairment.

NURSING CONSIDERATIONS
• Don't stop drug abruptly because this
may increase seizure frequency. Instead,
taper drug over at least 2 weeks.
• **Alert:** Stop drug at first sign of rash,
unless rash is clearly not drug related.
• Reduce lamotrigine dose if drug is
added to a multidrug regimen that includes
valproic acid.

• Evaluate patients for changes in seizure
activity. Check adjunct anticonvulsant
level.
• ***Look alike–sound alike:*** Don't confuse
lamotrigine with lamivudine or Lamictal
with Lamisil, Ludiomil, labetalol, or
Lomotil.

PATIENT TEACHING
• Inform patient that drug may cause rash.
Combination therapy of valproic acid and
lamotrigine may cause a serious rash. Tell
patient to report rash or signs or symptoms
of hypersensitivity promptly to prescriber
because they may warrant stopping drug.
• Warn patient not to engage in hazardous activity until drug's CNS effects are
known.
• Warn patient that the drug may trigger
sensitivity to the sun and to take precautions until tolerance is determined.
• Warn patient not to stop drug abruptly.
• **Alert:** Advise woman of childbearing age
to discuss drug therapy with prescriber
if she's considering pregnancy. Babies
exposed to drug during the first trimester
have a greater risk of cleft lip or palate.
• Advise woman of childbearing age that
breast-feeding isn't recommended during
therapy.

SAFETY ALERT!

leuprolide acetate
loo-PROE-lide

Eligard, Lupron, Lupron Depot,
Lupron Depot-Ped, Lupron
Depot–3 Month, Lupron Depot–
4 Month, Lupron for Pediatric Use,
Viadur

Pharmacologic class: gonadotropin-
releasing hormone analogue
Pregnancy risk category X

AVAILABLE FORMS
Depot injection: 3.75 mg, 7.5 mg,
11.25 mg, 15 mg, 22.5 mg, 30 mg,
45 mg
Injection: 5 mg/ml in 2.8-ml multiple-dose
vials
Implant: 72 mg

INDICATIONS & DOSAGES
➤ **Advanced prostate cancer**
Adults: 1 mg subcutaneously daily. Or,
7.5 mg I.M. depot injection monthly.
Or, 7.5 mg subcutaneous Eligard once
monthly. Or, 22.5 mg I.M. depot injection
every 3 months. Or, 22.5 mg subcutaneous Eligard every 3 months. Or, 30 mg
I.M. depot injection every 4 months. Or,
30 mg subcutaneous Eligard every
4 months. Or, 45 mg subcutaneous Eligard every 6 months. Or, 72-mg Viadur
implant inserted subcutaneously every
12 months.
➤ **Endometriosis**
Adults: 3.75 mg I.M. depot injection as
single injection once monthly for up to
6 months. Or, 11.25 mg I.M. every
3 months for up to 6 months.
➤ **Central precocious puberty**
Children: Initially, 0.3 mg/kg (minimum
7.5 mg) I.M. depot injection as single
injection every 4 weeks. May increase in
increments of 3.75 mg every 4 weeks, if
needed. Stop drug before girl reaches age
11 or boy reaches age 12.
➤ **Anemia related to uterine fi-
broids (with iron therapy)**
Adults: 3.75 mg I.M. depot injection once
monthly for up to 3 consecutive months.
Or, 11.25 mg I.M. depot injection for
1 dose.

ADMINISTRATION
• Products have specific mixing and administration instructions. Read manufacturer's directions closely.
I.M.
• Never give by I.V. injection.
• Give depot injections under medical
supervision.
• Use supplied diluent to reconstitute
drug (extra diluent is provided; discard
remainder).
• Inject into vial; shake well. Suspension
will appear milky. Use immediately.
• Draw 1 ml into a syringe with a 22G
needle.
• When preparing Lupron Depot–3 Month
22.5 mg, use a 23G or larger needle.
Withdraw 1.5 ml from ampule for the
3-month form.

• When using prefilled dual-chamber
syringes, prepare for injection according to
manufacturer's instructions.
• Gently shake syringe to form a uniform
milky suspension. If particles adhere to
stopper, tap syringe against your finger.
• Remove needle guard and advance
plunger to expel air from syringe. Inject
entire contents I.M. as with a normal
injection.
Subcutaneous
• For the two-syringe mixing system,
connect the syringes and inject the liquid
contents according to manufacturer's
instructions.
• Mix product by pushing contents back
and forth between syringes for about
45 seconds; shaking the syringes won't
mix the contents enough.
• Attach the needle provided in the kit and
inject subcutaneously.
• Suspension settles very quickly. Remix
if settling occurs. Must be given within
30 minutes.
• Never give by I.V. injection.

ACTION
Stimulates and then inhibits release of
follicle-stimulating hormone and luteinizing hormone, which suppresses testosterone and estrogen levels.

Route	Onset	Peak	Duration
I.M., Subcut	Variable	1–2 mo	60–90 days
Implant	Unknown	4 hr	12 mo

Half-life: Unknown.

ADVERSE REACTIONS
CNS: *dizziness, depression, headache,
pain,* insomnia, paresthesia, *asthenia.*
CV: *arrhythmias,* angina, *MI, peripheral edema, ECG changes,* hypotension,
hypertension, murmur, *hot flashes.*
GI: *nausea, vomiting,* anorexia, constipation.
GU: *impotence, vaginitis,* urinary frequency, hematuria, UTI, *amenorrhea.*
Hematologic: anemia.
Metabolic: *weight gain or loss.*
Musculoskeletal: transient bone pain during first week of treatment, joint disorder,
myalgia, neuromuscular disorder, bone
loss.

Respiratory: dyspnea, sinus congestion, *pulmonary fibrosis.*
Skin: reactions at injection site, dermatitis, acne.
Other: gynecomastia, androgen-like effects.

INTERACTIONS
None significant.

EFFECTS ON LAB TEST RESULTS
● May increase albumin, alkaline phosphatase, bilirubin, BUN, calcium, creatinine, glucose, LDH, phosphorus, and uric acid levels. May decrease hemoglobin level.
● May alter results of pituitary-gonadal system tests during therapy and for 12 weeks after.

CONTRAINDICATIONS & CAUTIONS
● Contraindicated in patients hypersensitive to drug or other gonadotropin-releasing hormone analogues, in women with undiagnosed vaginal bleeding, and in pregnant or breast-feeding women.
● The 30- and 45-mg depot injections and the Viadur implant are contraindicated in women and children.
● Use cautiously in patients hypersensitive to benzyl alcohol.

NURSING CONSIDERATIONS
● A fractional dose of drug formulated to give every 3, 4, or 6 months isn't equivalent to same dose of once-a-month formulation.
● After starting treatment for central precocious puberty, monitor patient response every 1 to 2 months with a gonadotropin-releasing hormone stimulation test and sex corticosteroid level determinations. Measure bone age for advancement every 6 to 12 months.
● *Alert:* During first few weeks of treatment for prostate cancer, signs and symptoms of disease may temporarily worsen or additional signs and symptoms may occur (tumor flare).

PATIENT TEACHING
● Before starting child on treatment for central precocious puberty, make sure parents understand importance of continuous therapy.
● Carefully instruct patient who will give himself subcutaneous injection about the proper technique and advise him to use only the syringes provided by manufacturer.
● Advise patient that, if another syringe must be substituted, a low-dose insulin syringe (U-100, 0.5 ml) may be an appropriate choice but that needle gauge should be no smaller than 22G (except when using Lupron Depot–3 Month 22.5 mg).
● Instruct patient to store leuprolide acetate powder (depot) and diluent at room temperature, to refrigerate unopened vials of leuprolide acetate injection, and to protect leuprolide acetate injection from heat and light.
● Inform patient with history of undesirable effects from other endocrine therapies that leuprolide is easier to tolerate.
● Reassure patient that adverse effects disappear after about 1 week. Explain that symptoms of prostate cancer or central precocious puberty may worsen at first.
● Advise patient to keep implant insertion site clean and dry for 24 hours after procedure and to avoid heavy physical activity until site has healed. Local insertion site reactions such as bruising, burning, itching, and pain may resolve within 2 weeks.
● Advise woman of childbearing age to use a nonhormonal form of contraception during treatment.

✴ NEW DRUG

lisdexamfetamine dimesylate
lis-DEX-am-FET-a-meen

Vyvanse

Pharmacologic class: amphetamine
Pregnancy risk category C
Controlled substance schedule II

AVAILABLE FORMS
Capsules: 30 mg, 50 mg, 70 mg

INDICATIONS & DOSAGES
➤ **Attention deficit hyperactivity disorder (ADHD)**
Children ages 6 to 12: Initially, 30 mg P.O. once daily in the morning. Increase by

20 mg at weekly intervals to a maximum of 70 mg daily.

ADMINISTRATION
P.O.
● Capsules may be swallowed whole or the contents dissolved in a glass of water and taken immediately.
● Give drug in the morning to prevent insomnia.

ACTION
May increase the release of norepinephrine and dopamine into extraneural spaces by blocking their reuptake into the presynaptic neuron.

Route	Onset	Peak	Duration
P.O.	Rapid	1 hr	Unknown

Half-life: Less than 1 hour.

ADVERSE REACTIONS
CNS: *headache, insomnia, irritability,* aggressive or hostile behavior, delusional thinking, dizziness, fever, hallucinations, labile affect, somnolence, tic.
CV: *ventricular hypertrophy.*
EENT: abnormal vision, blurred vision.
GI: *abdominal pain, decreased appetite,* dry mouth, nausea, vomiting.
Metabolic: slow growth, weight loss.
Skin: rash.

INTERACTIONS
Drug-drug. *Adrenergic blockers:* May inhibit adrenergic blocking effects. Avoid using together.
Antihistamines: May inhibit sedative effects of antihistamines. Monitor patient.
Antihypertensives, veratrum alkaloids: May inhibit antihypertensive effects of these drugs. Avoid using together.
Chlorpromazine, haloperidol: May decrease effectiveness of amphetamines. Monitor patient closely.
Ethosuximide: May delay absorption of this drug. Monitor patient closely.
Lithium: May inhibit anorectic and CNS stimulant effects of amphetamine. Monitor patient closely.
MAO inhibitors: May cause severe hypertension or hypertensive crisis. Avoid using within 14 days of MAO inhibitor therapy.

Meperidine: May increase the analgesic effect of meperidine. Use together cautiously.
Norepinephrine: May increase adrenergic effects of norepinephrine. Monitor patient closely.
Phenobarbital, phenytoin: May delay intestinal absorption of these drugs and enhance their anticonvulsant effects. Monitor patient closely.
Propoxyphene: May cause fatal seizures if overdose of propoxyphene taken. Don't use together.
Tricyclic antidepressants: May cause adverse CV effects. Avoid using together.
Urine acidifiers (ammonium chloride, sodium acid phosphate), methenamine: May decrease serum level due to increased renal excretion of amphetamine. Monitor patient for decreased drug effects.
Drug-food. *Caffeine:* May increase CNS stimulation. Discourage use together.

EFFECTS ON LAB TEST RESULTS
● May increase corticosteroid level.
● May interfere with urinary steroid test.

CONTRAINDICATIONS & CAUTIONS
● Contraindicated in patients hypersensitive to sympathomimetic amines or in those with idiosyncratic reactions to them, in agitated patients, and in those with a history of drug abuse.
● Contraindicated in patients with advanced arteriosclerosis, hyperthyroidism, symptomatic CV disease, structural cardiac abnormalities, moderate to severe hypertension, or glaucoma.
● Contraindicated within 14 days of MAO inhibitor therapy.
● Use cautiously in patients with a history of arrhythmias, MI, stroke, or seizures.
● Use cautiously in patients with pre-existing psychosis, bipolar disorder, or aggressive behavior; or Tourette syndrome.

NURSING CONSIDERATIONS
● Diagnosis of ADHD must be based on complete history and evaluation of the child with consultation of psychological, educational, and social resources.

• Give the lowest effective dose in the morning. Afternoon doses may cause insomnia.
• Monitor patient for signs of drug dependence or abuse.
• Abruptly stopping the drug can cause severe fatigue and depression.
• Monitor patient closely for adverse CV effects, new or worsening behavior (aggression, mania), vision problems, or seizures.
• Monitor blood pressure and pulse routinely.
• Effectiveness of this drug when taken longer than 4 weeks isn't known. Periodically interrupt therapy to determine whether continuation is necessary.
• Growth may be suppressed with long-term stimulant use. Monitor the child for growth and weight gain. Stop treatment if growth is suppressed or if weight gain is lower than expected.
• The drug may trigger Tourette syndrome. Monitor patient, especially at the start of therapy.

PATIENT TEACHING
• Tell patient or caregiver that drug should be taken in the morning to prevent insomnia.
• Advise patient to swallow capsule whole. If he's unable to do so, the contents may be dissolved in a glass of water and taken immediately. Once dissolved, don't store for later use.
• Tell patient or caregiver that abruptly stopping drug can cause severe fatigue, depression, or general withdrawal reaction.
• Caution patient to avoid activities that require alertness or good psychomotor coordination until CNS effects of drug are known.
• Warn patient with seizure disorder that drug may decrease seizure threshold. Urge him to notify his prescriber if a seizure occurs.
• Instruct patient or caregiver to report palpitations or visual disturbances.
• Tell patient or caregiver to report worsening aggression, hallucinations, delusions, or mania.
• Advise patient to avoid caffeine consumption while taking drug.

lithium carbonate
LITH-ee-um

Carbolith†, Duralith†, Eskalith, Lithane†, Lithobid

lithium citrate
Cibalith-S*

Pharmacologic class: alkali metal
Pregnancy risk category D

AVAILABLE FORMS
lithium carbonate
Capsules: 150 mg, 300 mg, 600 mg
Tablets: 300 mg (300 mg equals 8.12 mEq lithium)
Tablets (controlled-release): 300 mg, 450 mg
lithium citrate
Syrup (sugarless): 8 mEq lithium/5 ml; 5 ml lithium citrate liquid contains 8 mEq lithium, equal to 300 mg lithium carbonate

INDICATIONS & DOSAGES
➤ **To prevent or control mania**
Adults: 300 to 600 mg P.O. up to q.i.d. Or, 900-mg controlled-release tablets P.O. every 12 hours. Increase dosage based on blood levels to achieve optimum dosage. Recommended therapeutic lithium levels are 1 to 1.5 mEq/L for acute mania and 0.6 to 1.2 mEq/L for maintenance therapy.

ADMINISTRATION
P.O.
• Give drug after meals with plenty of water to minimize GI upset.
• Don't crush controlled-release tablets.

ACTION
Probably alters chemical transmitters in the CNS, possibly by interfering with ionic pump mechanisms in brain cells, and may compete with or replace sodium ions.

Route	Onset	Peak	Duration
P.O.	Unknown	30 min–3 hr	Unknown

Half-life: 18 hours (adolescents) to 36 hours (elderly).

ADVERSE REACTIONS

CNS: *fatigue, lethargy,* ***coma, epileptiform seizures,*** tremors, drowsiness, headache, confusion, restlessness, dizziness, psychomotor retardation, blackouts, EEG changes, worsened organic mental syndrome, impaired speech, ataxia, incoordination.

CV: ***arrhythmias, bradycardia,*** reversible ECG changes, hypotension.

EENT: tinnitus, blurred vision.

GI: *vomiting, anorexia, diarrhea, thirst,* nausea, metallic taste, dry mouth, abdominal pain, flatulence, indigestion.

GU: *polyuria,* **renal toxicity with long-term use,** glycosuria, decreased creatinine clearance, albuminuria.

Hematologic: *leukocytosis with leukocyte count of 14,000 to 18,000/mm³.*

Metabolic: transient hyperglycemia, goiter, hypothyroidism, hyponatremia.

Musculoskeletal: *muscle weakness.*

Skin: pruritus, rash, diminished or absent sensation, drying and thinning of hair, psoriasis, acne, alopecia.

Other: ankle and wrist edema.

INTERACTIONS

Drug-drug. *ACE inhibitors:* May increase lithium level. Monitor lithium level; adjust lithium dosage, as needed.

Aminophylline, sodium bicarbonate, urine alkalinizers: May increase lithium excretion. Avoid excessive salt, and monitor lithium levels.

Calcium channel blockers (verapamil): May decrease lithium levels and may increase risk of neurotoxicity. Use together cautiously.

Carbamazepine, fluoxetine, methyldopa, NSAIDs, probenecid: May increase effect of lithium. Monitor patient for lithium toxicity.

Neuromuscular blockers: May cause prolonged paralysis or weakness. Monitor patient closely.

Thiazide diuretics: May increase reabsorption of lithium by kidneys, with possible toxic effect. Use with caution, and monitor lithium and electrolyte levels (especially sodium).

Drug-food. *Caffeine:* May decrease lithium level and drug effect. Advise patient who ingests large amounts of caffeine to tell prescriber before stopping caffeine. Adjust lithium dosage, as needed.

EFFECTS ON LAB TEST RESULTS

● May increase glucose and creatinine levels. May decrease sodium, T_3, T_4, and protein-bound iodine levels.

● May increase ^{131}I uptake and WBC and neutrophil counts.

CONTRAINDICATIONS & CAUTIONS

● Contraindicated if therapy can't be closely monitored.

● Avoid using in pregnant patient unless benefits outweigh risks.

● Use with caution in patients receiving neuromuscular blockers and diuretics; in elderly or debilitated patients; and in patients with thyroid disease, seizure disorder, infection, renal or CV disease, severe debilitation or dehydration, or sodium depletion.

NURSING CONSIDERATIONS

● *Alert:* Drug has a narrow therapeutic margin of safety. Determining drug level is crucial to safe use of drug. Don't use drug in patients who can't have regular tests. Monitor level 8 to 12 hours after first dose, the morning before second dose is given, two or three times weekly for the first month, and then weekly to monthly during maintenance therapy.

● When drug level is less than 1.5 mEq/L, adverse reactions are usually mild.

● Monitor baseline ECG, thyroid studies, renal studies, and electrolyte levels.

● Check fluid intake and output, especially when surgery is scheduled.

● Weigh patient daily; check for edema or sudden weight gain.

● Adjust fluid and salt ingestion to compensate if excessive loss occurs from protracted diaphoresis or diarrhea. Under normal conditions, patient fluid intake should be $2^1/_2$ to 3 L daily, and he should follow a balanced diet with adequate salt intake.

● Check urine specific gravity and report level below 1.005, which may indicate diabetes insipidus.

● Drug alters glucose tolerance in diabetics. Monitor glucose level closely.

• Perform outpatient follow-up of thyroid and renal functions every 6 to 12 months. Palpate thyroid to check for enlargement.
• *Look alike–sound alike:* Don't confuse Lithobid with Levbid.

PATIENT TEACHING
• Tell patient to take drug with plenty of water and after meals to minimize GI upset.
• Explain the importance of having regular blood tests to determine drug levels; even slightly high values can be dangerous.
• Warn patient and caregivers to expect transient nausea, large amounts of urine, thirst, and discomfort during first few days of therapy and to watch for evidence of toxicity (diarrhea, vomiting, tremor, drowsiness, muscle weakness, incoordination).
• Instruct patient to withhold one dose and call prescriber if signs and symptoms of toxicity appear, but not to stop drug abruptly.
• Warn patient to avoid hazardous activities that require alertness and good psychomotor coordination until CNS effects of drug are known.
• Tell patient not to switch brands or take other prescription or OTC drugs without prescriber's guidance.
• Tell patient to wear or carry medical identification at all times.

SAFETY ALERT!

lorazepam
lor-AZ-e-pam

Ativan, Lorazepam Intensol, Novo-Lorazem†

Pharmacologic class: benzo-diazepine
Pregnancy risk category D
Controlled substance schedule IV

AVAILABLE FORMS
Injection: 2 mg/ml, 4 mg/ml
Oral solution (concentrated): 2 mg/ml
Tablets: 0.5 mg, 1 mg, 2 mg

INDICATIONS & DOSAGES
➤ **Anxiety**
Adults: 2 to 6 mg P.O. daily in divided doses. Maximum, 10 mg daily.
Elderly patients: 1 to 2 mg P.O. daily in divided doses. Maximum, 10 mg daily.
➤ **Insomnia from anxiety**
Adults: 2 to 4 mg P.O. at bedtime.
➤ **Preoperative sedation**
Adults: 2 mg I.V. total or 0.044 mg/kg I.V., whichever is smaller. Larger doses up to 0.05 mg/kg I.V., to total of 4 mg, may be needed. Or, 0.05 mg/kg I.M. 2 hours before procedure. Total dose shouldn't exceed 4 mg.
➤ **Status epilepticus**
Adults: 4 mg I.V. If seizures continue or recur after 10 to 15 minutes, then an additional 4-mg dose may be given. Drug may be given I.M. if I.V. access isn't available.
Children ♦: 0.05 to 0.1 mg/kg I.V.
➤ **Nausea and vomiting caused by emetogenic cancer chemotherapy ♦**
Adults: 2.5 mg P.O. the evening before and just after starting chemotherapy. Or, 1.5 mg/m^2 (usually max dose of 3 mg) I.V. (over 5 minutes) 45 minutes before starting chemotherapy.

ADMINISTRATION
P.O.
• Mix oral solution with liquid or semisolid food, such as water, juices, carbonated beverages, applesauce, or pudding.
I.V.
• Keep emergency resuscitation equipment and oxygen available.
• Dilute with an equal volume of sterile water for injection, normal saline solution for injection, or D_5W. Give slowly at no more than 2 mg/minute.
• Monitor respirations every 5 to 15 minutes and before each I.V. dose.
• Contains benzyl alcohol. Avoid use in neonates.
• Refrigerate intact vials and protect from light.
• **Incompatibilities:** Aldesleukin, aztreonam, buprenorphine, caffeine citrate, floxacillin, foscarnet, idarubicin, imipenem-cilastatin sodium, omeprazole,

ondansetron hydrochloride, sargramostim, sufentanil citrate, thiopental.

I.M.
• For status epilepticus, drug may be given I.M. if I.V. access isn't available.
• For I.M. use, inject deeply into a muscle. Don't dilute.
• Refrigerate parenteral form to prolong shelf life.

ACTION
May potentiate the effects of GABA, depress the CNS, and suppress the spread of seizure activity.

Route	Onset	Peak	Duration
P.O.	1 hr	2 hr	12–24 hr
I.V.	5 min	60–90 min	6–8 hr
I.M.	15–30 min	60–90 min	6–8 hr

Half-life: 10 to 20 hours.

ADVERSE REACTIONS
CNS: *drowsiness, sedation,* amnesia, insomnia, agitation, dizziness, weakness, unsteadiness, disorientation, depression, headache.
CV: hypotension.
EENT: visual disturbances, nasal congestion.
GI: abdominal discomfort, nausea, change in appetite.

INTERACTIONS
Drug-drug. *CNS depressants:* May increase CNS depression. Use together cautiously.
Digoxin: May increase digoxin level and risk of toxicity. Monitor patient and digoxin level closely.
Drug-herb. *Kava:* May increase sedation. Discourage use together.
Drug-lifestyle. *Alcohol use:* May cause additive CNS effects. Discourage use together.
Smoking: May decrease drug's effectiveness. Monitor patient closely.

EFFECTS ON LAB TEST RESULTS
• May increase liver function test values.

CONTRAINDICATIONS & CAUTIONS
• Contraindicated in patients hypersensitive to drug, other benzodiazepines, or the vehicle used in parenteral dosage form; in patients with acute angle-closure glaucoma; and in pregnant women, especially in the first trimester.
• Use cautiously in patients with pulmonary, renal, or hepatic impairment.
• Use cautiously in elderly, acutely ill, or debilitated patients.

NURSING CONSIDERATIONS
• Monitor hepatic, renal, and hematopoietic function periodically in patients receiving repeated or prolonged therapy.
• *Alert:* Use of this drug may lead to abuse and addiction. Don't stop drug abruptly after long-term use because withdrawal symptoms may occur.
• *Look alike–sound alike:* Don't confuse lorazepam with alprazolam.

PATIENT TEACHING
• When used before surgery, drug causes substantial preoperative amnesia. Patient teaching requires extra care to ensure adequate recall. Provide written materials or inform a family member, if possible.
• Warn patient to avoid hazardous activities that require alertness or good coordination until effects of drug are known.
• Tell patient to avoid use of alcohol while taking drug.
• Notify patient that smoking may decrease drug's effectiveness.
• Warn patient not to stop drug abruptly because withdrawal symptoms may occur.
• Advise woman to avoid becoming pregnant while taking drug.

---

loxapine succinate
LOX-a-peen

Loxitane

Pharmacologic class: dibenzapine derivative
Pregnancy risk category NR

AVAILABLE FORMS
Capsules: 5 mg, 10 mg, 25 mg, 50 mg

INDICATIONS & DOSAGES
➤ **Psychotic disorders**
Adults: 10 mg P.O. b.i.d. to q.i.d., rapidly increasing to 60 to 100 mg P.O. daily for most patients; dosage varies.
Elderly patients: Initially, 5 mg P.O. b.i.d. Adjust dosage as needed and as tolerated.

ADMINISTRATION
P.O.
● Give drug without regard for food.

ACTION
Unknown. Probably exerts antipsychotic effects by blocking postsynaptic dopamine receptors in the brain.

Route	Onset	Peak	Duration
P.O.	30 min	90 min–3 hr	12 hr

Half-life: 8 hours.

ADVERSE REACTIONS
CNS: *extrapyramidal reactions, sedation, tardive dyskinesia,* **neuroleptic malignant syndrome, seizures,** drowsiness, numbness, confusion, syncope, pseudoparkinsonism, EEG changes, dizziness.
CV: orthostatic hypotension, tachycardia, ECG changes, hypertension.
EENT: *blurred vision,* nasal congestion.
GI: *dry mouth, constipation,* nausea, vomiting, paralytic ileus.
GU: *urine retention,* menstrual irregularities.
Hematologic: *leukopenia, agranulocytosis, thrombocytopenia.*
Hepatic: jaundice.
Metabolic: weight gain.
Skin: allergic reactions, rash, pruritus.
Other: gynecomastia, galactorrhea.

INTERACTIONS
Drug-drug. *Anticholinergics:* May increase anticholinergic effect. Use together cautiously.
CNS depressants: May increase CNS depression. Use together cautiously.
Epinephrine: May inhibit vasopressor effect of epinephrine. Avoid using together.
Drug-lifestyle. *Alcohol use:* May increase CNS depression. Discourage use together.

EFFECTS ON LAB TEST RESULTS
● May increase liver function test values. May decrease WBC, granulocyte, and platelet counts.
● May cause false-positive results for urinary porphyrin, urobilinogen, amylase, and 5-hydroxyindoleacetic acid tests and for urine pregnancy tests that use human chorionic gonadotropin.

CONTRAINDICATIONS & CAUTIONS
● Contraindicated in patients hypersensitive to dibenzapines, in those in a coma, and in those with severe CNS depression or drug-induced depressed states.
● Use cautiously in patients with seizure disorder, CV disorder, glaucoma, or history of urine retention.

NURSING CONSIDERATIONS
● Obtain baseline blood pressure measurements before starting therapy and monitor pressure regularly.
● Monitor patient for tardive dyskinesia, which may occur after prolonged use. It may not appear until months or years later and may disappear spontaneously or persist for life, despite ending drug.
● *Alert:* Watch for evidence of neuroleptic malignant syndrome (extrapyramidal effects, hyperthermia, autonomic disturbance), a rare but deadly disorder.

PATIENT TEACHING
● Warn patient to avoid activities that require alertness and good coordination until effects of drug are known. Drowsiness and dizziness usually subside after first few weeks.
● Advise patient to report bruising, fever, or sore throat immediately.
● Tell patient to avoid alcohol while taking drug.
● Advise patient to get up slowly to avoid dizziness upon standing quickly.
● Tell patient to relieve dry mouth with sugarless gum or hard candy.
● Recommend periodic eye examinations.

---

magnesium sulfate
mag-NEE-zee-um

Pharmacologic class: mineral;
electrolyte
Pregnancy risk category A

AVAILABLE FORMS
Injection: 4%, 8%, 10%, 12.5%, 25%,
50%
Injection solution: 1% in D_5W, 2% in D_5W

INDICATIONS & DOSAGES
➤ **To prevent or control seizures in
preeclampsia or eclampsia**
Women: Initially, 4 g I.V. in 250 ml D_5W or
normal saline and 4 to 5 g deep I.M. into
each buttock; then 4 to 5 g deep I.M. into
alternate buttock every 4 hours, as needed.
Or, 4 g I.V. loading dose; then 1 to 3 g
hourly as I.V. infusion. Total dose shouldn't
exceed 30 or 40 g daily.
➤ **Hypomagnesemia**
Adults: For mild deficiency, 1 g I.M.
every 6 hours for four doses; for severe
deficiency, 5 g in 1,000 ml D_5W or normal
saline solution infused over 3 hours.
➤ **Seizures, hypertension, and encephalopathy with acute nephritis in
children**
Children: 20 to 40 mg/kg I.M. as needed to
control seizures. Dilute the 50% concentration to a 20% solution and give 0.1 to
0.2 ml/kg of the 20% solution.
➤ **To manage paroxysmal atrial
tachycardia**
Adults: 3 to 4 g I.V. over 30 seconds, with
extreme caution.
➤ **To manage life-threatening ventricular arrhythmias, such as sustained ventricular tachycardia or
torsades de pointes ♦**
Adults: 1 to 6 g I.V. over several minutes;
then continuous I.V. infusion of 3 to
20 mg/minute for 5 to 48 hours. Base
dosage and duration of therapy on patient
response and magnesium level.
➤ **To manage preterm labor ♦**
Adults: 4 to 6 g I.V. over 20 minutes,
followed by 2 to 4 g/hour I.V. infusion
for 12 to 24 hours, as tolerated, after
contractions have stopped.

ADMINISTRATION
I.V.
● If necessary, dilute to maximum level of
20%. Infuse no faster than 150 mg/minute
(1.5 ml/minute of a 10% solution or
0.75 ml/minute of a 20% solution). Drug
is compatible with D_5W and normal saline
solution.
● Maximum infusion rate is 150 mg/
minute. Too-rapid infusion produces
uncomfortable feeling of heat.
● Monitor vital signs every 15 minutes
when giving drug I.V.
● **Incompatibilities:** Alkali carbonates
and bicarbonates, amiodarone, amphotericin B, calcium gluconate, cefepime,
ciprofloxacin, clindamycin, cyclosporine,
dobutamine, heavy metals, I.V. fat emulsion 10%, polymyxin B, procaine, salicylates, sodium bicarbonate, soluble
phosphates.
I.M.
● For adults, give undiluted 50% concentration by deep injection.
● For children, dilute to concentration of
20% or less with D_5W or normal saline for
injection.

ACTION
May decrease acetylcholine released
by nerve impulses, but anticonvulsant
mechanism is unknown.

Route	Onset	Peak	Duration
I.V.	1–2 min	Rapid	30 min
I.M.	1 hr	Unknown	3–4 hr

Half-life: Unknown.

ADVERSE REACTIONS
CNS: *depressed reflexes,* drowsiness,
flaccid paralysis, hypothermia.
CV: *flushing, hypotension,* **bradycardia,**
circulatory collapse, depressed cardiac
function.
EENT: diplopia.
Metabolic: hypocalcemia.
Respiratory: *respiratory paralysis.*
Skin: diaphoresis.

INTERACTIONS
Drug-drug. *Anesthetics, CNS depressants:*
May cause additive CNS depression. Use
together cautiously.

Cardiac glycosides: May worsen arrhythmias. Use together cautiously.
Neuromuscular blockers: May cause increased neuromuscular blockade. Use together cautiously.

EFFECTS ON LAB TEST RESULTS
• May increase magnesium level. May decrease calcium level.

CONTRAINDICATIONS & CAUTIONS
• Parenteral administration contraindicated in patients with heart block or myocardial damage.
• Contraindicated in patients with toxemia of pregnancy during 2 hours preceding delivery.
• Use cautiously in patients with impaired renal function.
• Use cautiously in pregnant women during labor.

NURSING CONSIDERATIONS
• If used to treat seizures, take appropriate seizure precautions.
• *Alert:* Watch for respiratory depression and signs and symptoms of heart block.
• Keep I.V. calcium gluconate available to reverse magnesium intoxication, but use cautiously in digitalized patients because of danger of arrhythmias.
• Check magnesium level after repeated doses. Disappearance of knee-jerk and patellar reflexes is sign of impending magnesium toxicity.
• Signs of hypermagnesemia begin to appear at levels of 4 mEq/L.
• Effective anticonvulsant level ranges from 2.5 to 7.5 mEq/L.
• Monitor fluid intake and output. Make sure urine output is 100 ml or more in 4-hour period before each dose.
• Observe neonates for signs of magnesium toxicity, including neuromuscular or respiratory depression, when giving I.V. form of drug to toxemic mothers within 24 hours before delivery.
• *Look alike–sound alike:* Don't confuse magnesium sulfate with manganese sulfate.

PATIENT TEACHING
• Inform patient of short-term need for drug and answer any questions and address concerns.
• Review potential adverse reactions and instruct patient to promptly report any occurrences. Reassure patient that, although adverse reactions can occur, vital signs, reflexes, and drug level will be monitored frequently to ensure safety.

---

memantine hydrochloride
meh-MAN-teen

Namenda

Pharmacologic class: N-methyl-D-aspartate (NMDA) receptor antagonist
Pregnancy risk category B

AVAILABLE FORMS
Oral solution: 2 mg/ml
Tablets: 5 mg, 10 mg

INDICATIONS & DOSAGES
➤ **Moderate to severe Alzheimer dementia**
Adults: Initially, 5 mg P.O. once daily. Increase by 5 mg/day every week until target dose is reached. Maximum, 10 mg P.O. b.i.d. Doses greater than 5 mg should be divided b.i.d.
Adjust-a-dose: Reduce dosage in patients with moderate renal impairment.

ADMINISTRATION
P.O.
• Give drug without regard for food.

ACTION
Antagonizes NMDA receptors, the persistent activation of which seems to increase Alzheimer symptoms.

Route	Onset	Peak	Duration
P.O.	Unknown	3–7 hr	Unknown

Half-life: 60 to 80 hours.

ADVERSE REACTIONS
CNS: *stroke,* aggressiveness, agitation, anxiety, ataxia, confusion, depression, dizziness, fatigue, hallucinations,

---

headache, hypokinesia, insomnia, pain, somnolence, syncope, transient ischemic attack, vertigo.

CV: *heart failure,* edema, hypertension.
EENT: cataracts, conjunctivitis.
GI: anorexia, constipation, diarrhea, nausea, vomiting.
GU: incontinence, urinary frequency, UTI.
Hematologic: anemia.
Metabolic: weight loss.
Musculoskeletal: arthralgia, back pain.
Respiratory: bronchitis, coughing, dyspnea, flulike symptoms, pneumonia, upper respiratory tract infection.
Skin: rash.
Other: abnormal gait, falls, injury.

INTERACTIONS

Drug-drug. *Cimetidine, hydrochlorothiazide, quinidine, ranitidine, triamterene:* May alter levels of both drugs. Monitor patient.
NMDA antagonists (amantadine, dextromethorphan, ketamine): Combined use unknown. Use together cautiously.
Urine alkalinizers (carbonic anhydrase inhibitors, sodium bicarbonate): May decrease memantine clearance. Monitor patient for adverse effects.
Drug-herb. *Herbs that alkalinize urine:* May increase drug level and adverse effects. Use together cautiously.
Drug-food. *Foods that alkalinize urine:* May increase drug level and adverse effects. Use together cautiously.
Drug-lifestyle. *Alcohol use:* May alter drug adherence, decrease its effectiveness, or increase adverse effects. Discourage use together.
Nicotine: May alter levels of drug and nicotine. Discourage use together.

EFFECTS ON LAB TEST RESULTS

● May increase alkaline phosphatase level. May decrease hemoglobin level and hematocrit.

CONTRAINDICATIONS & CAUTIONS

● Contraindicated in patients allergic to drug or its components.
● Contraindicated for mild Alzheimer disease or other types of dementia.
● Drug isn't recommended for patients with severe renal impairment.

● Use cautiously in patients with seizures, hepatic impairment, or moderate renal impairment.
● Use cautiously in patients who may have an increased urine pH (from drugs, diet, renal tubular acidosis, or severe UTI, for example).

NURSING CONSIDERATIONS

● In elderly patients, even those with a normal creatinine level, use of this drug may impair renal function. Estimate creatinine clearance; reduce dosage in patients with moderate renal impairment. Don't give drug to patients with severe renal impairment.
● Monitor patient carefully for adverse reactions as he may not be able to recognize changes or communicate effectively.

PATIENT TEACHING

● Explain that drug doesn't cure Alzheimer disease but may improve the symptoms.
● Tell patient or caregiver to report adverse effects.
● Urge patient to avoid alcohol during treatment.
● To avoid possible interactions, advise patient not to take herbal or OTC products without consulting prescriber.

---

methylphenidate hydrochloride
meth-ill-FEN-i-date

Concerta, Metadate CD, Metadate ER, Methylin, Methylin ER, Ritalin, Ritalin LA, Ritalin-SR

methylphenidate transdermal system
Daytrana

Pharmacologic class: piperidine derivative
Pregnancy risk category NR; C; (for Concerta, Daytrana, Metadate CD, Ritalin LA)
Controlled substance schedule II

AVAILABLE FORMS

Oral solution (Methylin): 5 mg/5 ml, 10 mg/5 ml

Tablets (chewable): 2.5 mg, 5 mg, 10 mg
Tablets (Ritalin, Methylin): 5 mg, 10 mg, 20 mg
Extended-release
Capsules (Metadate CD): 10 mg, 20 mg, 30 mg
Capsules (Ritalin LA): 20 mg, 30 mg, 40 mg
Tablets (Concerta): 18 mg, 27 mg, 36 mg, 54 mg
Tablets (Metadate ER, Methylin ER): 10 mg, 20 mg
Sustained-release
Tablets (Ritalin-SR): 20 mg
Transdermal system
Patch: 10 mg, 15 mg, 20 mg, 30 mg

INDICATIONS & DOSAGES
➤ **Attention deficit hyperactivity disorder (ADHD)**
Children age 6 and older: Initially, 5 mg P.O. b.i.d. immediate-release form before breakfast and lunch, increasing by 5 to 10 mg at weekly intervals, as needed, until an optimum daily dose of 2 mg/kg is reached, not to exceed 60 mg/day. To use Ritalin-SR, Metadate ER, and Methylin ER tablets in place of immediate-release methylphenidate tablets, calculate methylphenidate dosage in 8-hour intervals.
Concerta
Adolescents ages 13 to 17 not currently taking methylphenidate, or for patients taking other stimulants: 18 mg P.O. extended-release Concerta once daily in the morning. Adjust dosage by 18 mg at weekly intervals to a maximum of 72 mg P.O. (not to exceed 2 mg/kg) once daily in the morning.
Children ages 6 to 12 not currently taking methylphenidate or patients taking stimulants other than methylphenidate: 18 mg extended-release P.O. once daily every morning. Adjust dosage by 18 mg at weekly intervals to a maximum of 54 mg daily every morning.
Adolescents and children age 6 and older currently taking methylphenidate: If previous methylphenidate dosage was 5 mg b.i.d. or t.i.d. or 20 mg sustained-release, give 18 mg P.O. every morning. If previous dosage was 10 mg b.i.d. or t.i.d. or 40 mg sustained-release, give 36 mg P.O.

every morning. If previous dosage was 15 mg b.i.d. or t.i.d. or 60 mg sustained-release, give 54 mg P.O. every morning. Maximum conversion daily dose is 54 mg. Once conversion is complete, adjust adolescents ages 13 to 17 to maximum dose of 72 mg once daily (not to exceed 2 mg/kg).
Metadate CD
Children age 6 and older: Initially, 20 mg P.O. daily before breakfast, increasing by 10 to 20 mg at weekly intervals to a maximum of 60 mg daily.
Ritalin LA
Children age 6 and older: 20 mg P.O. once daily. Increase by 10 mg at weekly intervals to a maximum of 60 mg daily. If previous methylphenidate dosage was 10 mg b.i.d. or 20 mg sustained-release, give 20 mg P.O. once daily. If previous methylphenidate dosage was 15 mg b.i.d., give 30 mg P.O. once daily. If previous methylphenidate dosage was 20 mg b.i.d. or 40 mg sustained-release, give 40 mg P.O. once daily. If previous methylphenidate dosage was 30 mg b.i.d. or 60 mg sustained-release, give 60 mg P.O. once daily.
Daytrana
Children ages 6 to 12: Initially, apply one 10-mg patch to clean, dry, nonirritated skin on the hip, alternating sites daily. Apply 2 hours before desired effect and remove 9 hours later. Increase dose weekly as needed to a maximum of 30 mg daily. Base final dose and wear time on patient response.
➤ **Narcolepsy**
Adults: 10 mg P.O. b.i.d. or t.i.d. immediate-release, 30 to 45 minutes before meals. Dosage varies; average is 40 to 60 mg/day. To use Ritalin-SR, Metadate ER, or Methylin ER tablets in place of immediate-release methylphenidate tablets, calculate the dose of methylphenidate in 8-hour intervals.

ADMINISTRATION
P.O.
• Give chewable tablet with at least 8 oz (237 ml) of water.
• Give drug after meals to reduce appetite-suppressant effects; give last daily dose

at least 6 hours before bedtime to prevent insomnia.

● Metadate CD or Ritalin LA may be swallowed whole, or the contents of the capsule may be sprinkled onto a small amount of cool applesauce and taken immediately.

Transdermal

● Avoid placing the patch on the waistline or where tight clothing may rub it off.

ACTION

Releases nerve terminal stores of norepinephrine, promoting nerve impulse transmission. At high doses, effects are mediated by dopamine.

Route	Onset	Peak	Duration
P.O. (Methylin, Ritalin)	Unknown	2 hr	Unknown
P.O. (Methylin ER, Ritalin-SR)	Unknown	5 hr	8 hr
P.O. (Metadate CD)	Unknown	1½ hr; 4½ hr	Unknown
P.O. (Ritalin LA)	Unknown	1–3 hr; 4–7 hr	Unknown
P.O. (Concerta)	Unknown	6–8 hr	Unknown
Transdermal	2 hr	Variable	14 hr

Half-life: Conventional, 3 to 6 hours; extended-release (Metadate ER, Methylin ER, Ritalin SR), 3 to 8 hours, (Concerta, Metadate CD, Ritalin LA) 8 to 12 hours; transdermal, 3 to 4 hours.

ADVERSE REACTIONS

CNS: *nervousness, headache, insomnia, **seizures,** tics,* dizziness, akathisia, dyskinesia, drowsiness, mood swings.
CV: *palpitations, tachycardia, **arrhythmias,*** hypertension.
EENT: pharyngitis, sinusitis.
GI: *nausea, abdominal pain, anorexia, decreased appetite, vomiting.*
Hematologic: *thrombocytopenia, thrombocytopenic purpura, leukopenia,* anemia.
Metabolic: weight loss.
Respiratory: cough, upper respiratory tract infection.
Skin: *exfoliative dermatitis, **erythema multiforme,*** rash, urticaria, application site irritation (redness, swelling, papules).
Other: *viral infection.*

INTERACTIONS

Drug-drug. *Anticonvulsants (such as phenobarbital, phenytoin, primidone), SSRIs, tricyclic antidepressants (imipramine, clomipramine, desipramine), warfarin:* May increase levels of these drugs. Monitor patient for adverse reactions and decrease dose of these drugs as needed. Monitor drug levels (or coagulation times if patient is also taking warfarin).
Centrally acting alpha$_2$ agonists, clonidine: May cause serious adverse events. Avoid using together.
Centrally acting antihypertensives: May decrease antihypertensive effect. Monitor blood pressure.
MAO inhibitors: May cause severe hypertension or hypertensive crisis. Avoid using within 14 days of MAO inhibitor therapy.
Drug-food. *Caffeine:* May increase amphetamine and related amine effects. Discourage use together.

EFFECTS ON LAB TEST RESULTS

● May decrease hemoglobin level and hematocrit.
● May decrease platelet and WBC counts.

CONTRAINDICATIONS & CAUTIONS

● Contraindicated in patients hypersensitive to drug and in those with glaucoma, motor tics, family history or diagnosis of Tourette syndrome, or history of marked anxiety, tension, or agitation. Also contraindicated within 14 days of MAO inhibitor therapy. Avoid use in patients with structural cardiac abnormalities.
● Because it doesn't dissolve, Concerta isn't recommended in patients with a history of peritonitis or with severe GI narrowing (such as small bowel inflammatory disease, short-gut syndrome caused by adhesions or decreased transit time, cystic fibrosis, chronic intestinal pseudoobstruction, or Meckel diverticulum).
● Use cautiously in patients with a history of seizures, EEG abnormalities, or hypertension, and in patients whose underlying medical conditions might be compromised by increases in blood pressure or heart rate, such as those with preexisting hypertension, heart failure, recent MI, or hyperthyroidism.

- Use cautiously in patients who are emotionally unstable or who have a history of drug dependence or alcoholism.

NURSING CONSIDERATIONS
- Chewable tablets contain phenylalanine.
- Don't use drug to prevent fatigue or treat severe depression.
- Drug may trigger Tourette syndrome in children. Monitor patient, especially at start of therapy.
- Observe patient for signs of excessive stimulation. Monitor blood pressure.
- Check CBC, differential, and platelet counts with long-term use, particularly if patient shows signs or symptoms of hematologic toxicity (fever, sore throat, easy bruising).
- Monitor height and weight in children on long-term therapy. Drug may delay growth spurt, but children will attain normal height when drug is stopped.
- Monitor patient for tolerance or psychological dependence.
- *Look alike–sound alike:* Don't confuse Ritalin with Rifadin.

PATIENT TEACHING
- Tell patient or caregiver to give last daily dose at least 6 hours before bedtime to prevent insomnia and after meals to reduce appetite-suppressant effects.
- Warn patient against chewing sustained-release tablets.
- Metadate CD or Ritalin LA may be swallowed whole, or the contents of the capsule may be sprinkled onto a small amount of cool applesauce and taken immediately.
- *Alert:* Warn patient to take chewable tablet with at least 8 oz (237 ml) of water. Not using enough water to swallow tablet may cause the tablet to swell and block the throat, causing choking.
- Caution patient to avoid activities that require alertness or good psychomotor coordination until CNS effects of drug are known.
- Warn patient with seizure disorder that drug may decrease seizure threshold. Urge him to notify prescriber if seizure occurs.
- Advise patient to avoid beverages containing caffeine while taking drug.

- Tell parent to apply patch immediately after opening; don't use if pouch seal is broken. Press firmly in place for about 30 seconds using the palm of your hand, being sure there is good contact with the skin, especially around the edges. Once applied correctly, the child may shower, bathe, or swim as usual.
- Inform parent if patch comes off, a new one may be applied on a different site, but the total wear time for that day should be 9 hours. Upon removal, fold patch in half so the sticky sides adhere to itself, then flush down toilet or dispose of in a lidded container.
- Tell parent, if the applied patch is missing, to ask the child when or how the patch came off.
- Encourage parent to use the application chart provided with patch carton to keep track of application and removal.
- Tell parent to remove patch sooner than 9 hours if the child has decreased evening appetite or has difficulty sleeping.
- Tell parent the effects of the patch lasts for several hours after its removal.
- Warn parent and patient to avoid exposing patch to direct external heat sources, such as heating pads, electric blankets, and heated water beds.
- Tell parent to notify prescriber if the child develops bumps, swelling, or blistering at the application site or is experiencing blurred vision or other serious side effects.

methyltestosterone
meth-ill-tes-TOSS-ter-own

Android, Metandren†, Methitest, Testred, Virilon

Pharmacologic class: androgenic anabolic steroid hormone
Pregnancy risk category X
Controlled substance schedule III

AVAILABLE FORMS
Capsules: 10 mg
Tablets: 10 mg, 25 mg
Tablets (buccal): 10 mg

Reactions may be *common,* uncommon, ***life-threatening***, or COMMON AND LIFE-THREATENING.
Interaction may have a *rapid onset* or ***delayed onset***.

INDICATIONS & DOSAGES
➤ **Breast cancer**
Women 1 to 5 years after menopause: 50 to 200 mg P.O. daily or 25 to 100 mg buccally daily.
➤ **Hypogonadism**
Men: 10 to 50 mg P.O. daily or 5 to 25 mg buccally daily.
➤ **Postpubertal cryptorchidism**
Men: 30 mg P.O. daily or 15 mg buccally daily.

ADMINISTRATION
P.O.
• Give without regard for food.
Buccal
• *Alert:* Buccal tablets are twice as potent as oral tablets.
• Have patient place buccal tablet in upper or lower buccal pouch between cheek and gum; it needs 30 to 60 minutes to dissolve. Patient shouldn't eat, drink, chew, or smoke while buccal tablet is in place nor should he swallow tablet.
• Have patient rinse mouth after tablet dissolves.

ACTION
Stimulates target tissues to develop normally in androgen-deficient men. May have some antiestrogen properties, making it useful in treating certain estrogen-dependent breast cancers.

Route	Onset	Peak	Duration
P.O.	Unknown	2 hr	Unknown
Buccal	Unknown	1 hr	Unknown

Half-life: Unknown.

ADVERSE REACTIONS
CNS: headache, anxiety, depression, paresthesia.
CV: edema.
GI: irritation of oral mucosa with buccal administration, nausea.
GU: oligospermia, decreased ejaculatory volume, priapism.
Hematologic: *suppression of clotting factors,* polycythemia.
Hepatic: reversible jaundice, *cholestatic hepatitis.*

Metabolic: hypernatremia, *hyperkalemia,* hyperphosphatemia, hypercholesterolemia, hypercalcemia.
Musculoskeletal: muscle cramps or spasms.
Skin: hypersensitivity reactions.
Other: androgenic effects in women, altered libido, *hypoestrogenic effects in women,* excessive hormonal effects in men, male pattern baldness.

INTERACTIONS
Drug-drug. *Cyclosporine:* May increase cyclosporine toxicity. Monitor cyclosporine levels.
Hepatotoxic drugs: May increase risk of hepatotoxicity. Monitor liver function closely.
Imipramine: May cause dramatic paranoid response. Monitor patient closely.
Insulin, oral antidiabetics: May decrease glucose level; may alter dosage requirements. Monitor glucose level in diabetic patients.
Oral anticoagulants: May increase sensitivity to oral anticoagulants; may alter dosage requirements. Monitor PT and INR.

EFFECTS ON LAB TEST RESULTS
• May increase sodium, potassium, phosphate, liver enzyme, lipid, and calcium levels. May decrease thyroxine-binding globulin and total T_4 levels.
• May increase RBC count and resin uptake of T_3 and T_4.

CONTRAINDICATIONS & CAUTIONS
• Contraindicated in pregnant or breast-feeding women and in men with breast or prostate cancer.
• Contraindicated in patients with cardiac, hepatic, or renal disease.
• Use cautiously in elderly patients; patients with cardiac, renal, or hepatic disease; and healthy males with delayed puberty.

NURSING CONSIDERATIONS
• Don't give to woman of childbearing age until pregnancy is ruled out.
• In children, obtain X-rays of wrist bones before therapy begins to establish bone maturation level. During treatment, bones

may mature more rapidly than they grow in length. Periodically review X-rays to monitor bone maturation.
• Drug is typically used only for intermittent therapy. Because of potential hepatotoxicity, watch closely for jaundice.
• Promptly report evidence of virilization in women, such as deepening of the voice, increased hair growth, acne, or baldness.
• Watch for hypoestrogenic effects in women (flushing, diaphoresis, vaginal bleeding, nervousness, emotional lability, menstrual irregularities, and vaginitis, including itching, dryness, and burning).
• Watch for excessive hormonal effects in men. If patient is prepubertal, watch for premature epiphyseal closure, acne, priapism, growth of body and facial hair, and phallic enlargement. If he's postpubertal, watch for testicular atrophy, oligospermia, decreased ejaculatory volume, impotence, gynecomastia, and epididymitis.
• Unless contraindicated, use with high-calorie, high-protein diet. Give small, frequent meals.
• Periodically check cholesterol, calcium, and hemoglobin levels, hematocrit, and cardiac and liver function test results.
• Check weight regularly. Control edema with sodium restriction or diuretics.
• *Alert:* In breast cancer, therapeutic response usually occurs within 3 months. If disease appears to progress, stop drug.
• Report signs of hypercalcemia. In metastatic breast cancer, hypercalcemia may indicate progression of bone metastases.
• Evaluate semen every 3 to 4 months, especially in adolescent boys.
• *Alert:* Don't use to enhance athletic performance or physique.
• *Look alike–sound alike:* Testosterone and methyltestosterone aren't interchangeable. Don't confuse methyltestosterone with medroxyprogesterone.

PATIENT TEACHING
• Make sure patient understands importance of using effective contraception during therapy.
• Tell woman of childbearing age to report menstrual irregularities and to stop drug while awaiting examination.

• Instruct patient to stop drug immediately and notify prescriber if pregnancy is suspected.
• Tell patient to place buccal tablet in upper or lower buccal pouch between cheek and gum; tablet needs 30 to 60 minutes to dissolve. Tell patient not to eat, drink, chew, or smoke while buccal tablet is in place and not to swallow tablet.
• Instruct patient to change buccal tablet absorption site with each dose to minimize risk of irritation. Advise patient to rinse mouth after using buccal tablet.
• Tell woman to immediately report evidence of virilization, such as acne, swelling, weight gain, increased hair growth, hoarseness, clitoral enlargement, decreased breast size, deepening of voice, changes in libido, male pattern baldness, and oily skin or hair.
• Teach patient signs and symptoms of low glucose level (hypoglycemia) and method for checking glucose level; drug enhances hypoglycemia. Instruct patient to report signs or symptoms of hypoglycemia immediately.
• Advise woman to wear cotton underwear and to wash after intercourse to decrease risk of vaginitis.

SAFETY ALERT!

midazolam hydrochloride
mid-AY-zoh-lam

Pharmacologic class:
benzodiazepine
Pregnancy risk category D
Controlled substance schedule IV

AVAILABLE FORMS
Injection: 1 mg/ml, 5 mg/ml
Syrup: 2 mg/ml

INDICATIONS & DOSAGES
➤ **Preoperative sedation (to induce sleepiness or drowsiness and relieve apprehension)**
Adults: 0.07 to 0.08 mg/kg I.M. about 1 hour before surgery.

➤ **Conscious sedation before short diagnostic or endoscopic procedures**
Adults younger than age 60: Initially, small dose not to exceed 2.5 mg I.V. given slowly; repeat in 2 minutes p.r.n., in small increments of first dose over at least 2 minutes to achieve desired effect. Total dose of up to 5 mg may be used. Additional doses to maintain desired level of sedation may be given by slow titration in increments of 25% of dose used to first reach the sedative end point.

Patients age 60 or older and debilitated patients: 0.5 to 1.5 mg I.V. over at least 2 minutes. Incremental doses shouldn't exceed 1 mg. A total dose of up to 3.5 mg is usually sufficient.

➤ **To induce sleepiness and amnesia and to relieve apprehension before anesthesia or before and during procedures**
P.O.
Children ages 6 to 16 who are cooperative: 0.25 to 0.5 mg/kg P.O. as a single dose, up to 20 mg.

Infants and children ages 6 months to 5 years or less cooperative, older children: 0.25 to 1 mg/kg P.O. as a single dose, up to 20 mg.

I.V.
Children ages 12 to 16: Initially, no more than 2.5 mg I.V. given slowly; repeat in 2 minutes, if needed, in small increments of first dose over at least 2 minutes to achieve desired effect. Total dose of up to 10 mg may be used. Additional doses to maintain desired level of sedation may be given by slow titration in increments of 25% of dose used to first reach the sedative end point.

Children ages 6 to 12: Give 0.025 to 0.05 mg/kg I.V. over 2 to 3 minutes. Additional doses may be given in small increments after 2 to 3 minutes. Total dose of up to 0.4 mg/kg, not to exceed 10 mg, may be used.

Children ages 6 months to 5 years: 0.05 to 0.1 mg/kg I.V. over 2 to 3 minutes. Additional doses may be given in small increments after 2 to 3 minutes. Total dose of up to 0.6 mg/kg, not to exceed 6 mg, may be used.

I.M.
Children: 0.1 to 0.15 mg/kg I.M. Use up to 0.5 mg/kg in more anxious patients.
Adjust-a-dose: For obese children, base dose on ideal body weight; high-risk or debilitated children and children receiving other sedatives need lower doses.

➤ **To induce general anesthesia**
Adults older than age 55: Give 0.3 mg/kg I.V. over 20 to 30 seconds if patient hasn't received premedication, or 0.2 mg/kg I.V. over 20 to 30 seconds if patient has received a sedative or opioid premedication. Additional increments of 25% of first dose may be needed to complete induction.

Adults younger than age 55: Give 0.3 to 0.35 mg/kg I.V. over 20 to 30 seconds if patient hasn't received premedication, or 0.25 mg/kg I.V. over 20 to 30 seconds if patient has received a sedative or opioid premedication. Additional increments of 25% of first dose may be needed to complete induction.

Adjust-a-dose: For debilitated patients, initially, 0.2 to 0.25 mg/kg. As little as 0.15 mg/kg may be needed.

➤ **As continuous infusion to sedate intubated patients in critical care unit**
Adults: Initially, 0.01 to 0.05 mg/kg may be given I.V. over several minutes, repeated at 10- to 15-minute intervals until adequate sedation is achieved. To maintain sedation, usual initial infusion rate is 0.02 to 0.1 mg/kg/hour. Higher loading dose or infusion rates may be needed in some patients. Use the lowest effective rate.
Children: Initially, 0.05 to 0.2 mg/kg may be given I.V. over 2 to 3 minutes or longer; then continuous infusion at rate of 0.06 to 0.12 mg/kg/hour. Increase or decrease infusion to maintain desired effect.
Neonates more than 32 weeks' gestational age: Initially, 0.06 mg/kg/hour. Adjust rate, as needed, using lowest possible rate.
Neonates less than 32 weeks' gestational age: Initially, 0.03 mg/kg/hour. Adjust rate, as needed, using lowest possible rate.

ADMINISTRATION
P.O.
● Give drug without regard for food, but don't give with grapefruit juice or grapefruit.

I.V.
• Drug may be mixed in the same syringe with morphine sulfate, meperidine, atropine, or scopolamine.
• When mixing infusion, use 5-mg/ml vial and dilute to 0.5 mg/ml with D_5W or normal saline solution.
• Give slowly over at least 2 minutes, and wait at least 2 minutes when titrating doses to produce therapeutic effect.
• **Incompatibilities:** Albumin, amoxicillin sodium, amphotericin B, ampicillin sodium, bumetanide, butorphanol, ceftazidime, cefuroxime, clonidine, dexamethasone sodium phosphate, dimenhydrinate, dobutamine, foscarnet, fosphenytoin, furosemide, heparin sodium, hydrocortisone, imipenem-cilastatin sodium, lactated Ringer injection, methotrexate sodium, nafcillin, omeprazole sodium, pentobarbital sodium, perphenazine, prochlorperazine edisylate, ranitidine hydrochloride, sodium bicarbonate, thiopental, some total parenteral nutrition formulations, trimethoprim-sulfamethoxazole.
I.M.
• Inject deeply into a large muscle.

ACTION
May potentiate the effects of GABA, depress the CNS, and suppress the spread of seizure activity.

Route	Onset	Peak	Duration
P.O.	10–20 min	45–60 min	2–6 hr
I.V.	90 sec–5 min	Rapid	2–6 hr
I.M.	15 min	15–60 min	2–6 hr

Half-life: 2 to 6 hours.

ADVERSE REACTIONS
CNS: *oversedation, drowsiness,* amnesia, headache, involuntary movements, nystagmus, paradoxical behavior or excitement.
CV: variations in blood pressure and pulse rate.
GI: *nausea,* vomiting.
Respiratory: APNEA, *decreased respiratory rate,* hiccups.
Other: *pain at injection site.*

INTERACTIONS
Drug-drug. *CNS depressants:* May cause apnea. Use together cautiously. Adjust dosage of midazolam if used with opiates or other CNS depressants.
Diltiazem: May increase CNS depression and prolonged effects of midazolam. Use lower dose of midazolam.
Erythromycin: May alter metabolism of midazolam. Use together cautiously.
Fluconazole, itraconazole, ketoconazole, miconazole: May increase and prolong midazolam level, CNS depression, and psychomotor impairment. Avoid using together.
Hormonal contraceptives: May prolong half-life of midazolam. Use together cautiously.
Rifampin: May decrease midazolam level. Monitor for midazolam effectiveness.
Theophylline: May antagonize sedative effect of midazolam. Use together cautiously.
Verapamil: May increase midazolam level. Monitor patient closely.
Drug-herb. *St. John's wort:* May decrease drug level. Discourage use together.
Drug-food. *Grapefruit juice:* May increase bioavailability of oral drug. Discourage use together.
Drug-lifestyle. *Alcohol use:* May cause additive CNS effects. Discourage use together.

EFFECTS ON LAB TEST RESULTS
None reported.

CONTRAINDICATIONS & CAUTIONS
• Contraindicated in patients hypersensitive to drug and in those with acute angle-closure glaucoma, shock, coma, or acute alcohol intoxication.
• Use cautiously in patients with uncompensated acute illness and in elderly or debilitated patients.

NURSING CONSIDERATIONS
• *Alert:* Have oxygen and resuscitation equipment available in case of severe respiratory depression. Excessive amounts and rapid infusion have been linked to respiratory arrest. Continuously monitor patient, including children taking syrup form, for life-threatening respiratory depression.
• Monitor blood pressure, heart rate and rhythm, respirations, airway integrity,

---

and arterial oxygen saturation during procedure.

PATIENT TEACHING
• Because drug diminishes patient's recall of events around the time of surgery, provide written information, family member instructions, and follow-up contact.
• Warn patient to avoid hazardous activities that require alertness or good coordination until effects of drug are known.

mirtazapine
mer-TAH-zah-peen

Remeron, Remeron Soltab

Pharmacologic class: tetracyclic antidepressant
Pregnancy risk category C

AVAILABLE FORMS
Orally disintegrating tablets (ODTs): 15 mg, 30 mg, 45 mg
Tablets: 15 mg, 30 mg, 45 mg

INDICATIONS & DOSAGES
➤ **Depression**
Adults: Initially, 15 mg P.O. at bedtime. Maintenance dose is 15 to 45 mg daily. Adjust dosage at intervals of at least 1 week.

ADMINISTRATION
P.O.
• Give drug without regard for food.
• Remove ODT from blister pack and immediately place on patient's tongue.
• ODT may be given with or without water.
• Don't split or crush ODT.

ACTION
Thought to enhance central noradrenergic and serotonergic activity.

Route	Onset	Peak	Duration
P.O.	Unknown	2 hr	Unknown

Half-life: About 20 to 40 hours.

ADVERSE REACTIONS
CNS: *somnolence,* **suicidal behavior,** dizziness, asthenia, abnormal dreams, abnormal thinking, tremors, confusion.
CV: edema, peripheral edema.
GI: *increased appetite, dry mouth, constipation,* nausea.
GU: urinary frequency.
Metabolic: *weight gain.*
Musculoskeletal: back pain, myalgia.
Respiratory: dyspnea.
Other: flulike syndrome.

INTERACTIONS
Drug-drug. *Diazepam, other CNS depressants:* May cause additive CNS effects. Avoid using together.
MAO inhibitors: May sometimes cause fatal reactions. Avoid using within 14 days of MAO inhibitor therapy.
Drug-lifestyle. *Alcohol use:* May cause additive CNS effects. Discourage use together.

EFFECTS ON LAB TEST RESULTS
• May increase ALT, cholesterol and triglyceride levels.

CONTRAINDICATIONS & CAUTIONS
• Contraindicated in patients hypersensitive to drug and within 14 days of MAO inhibitor therapy.
• Use cautiously in patients with CV or cerebrovascular disease, seizure disorders, suicidal thoughts, hepatic or renal impairment, or history of mania or hypomania.
• Use cautiously in patients with conditions that predispose them to hypotension, such as dehydration, hypovolemia, or antihypertensive therapy.
• Give drug cautiously to elderly patients; decreased clearance has occurred in this age group.

NURSING CONSIDERATIONS
• Don't use within 14 days of MAO inhibitor therapy.
• Record mood changes. Watch for suicidal tendencies.
• *Alert:* Drug may increase risk of suicidal thinking and behavior in children and adolescents with major depressive or other psychiatric disorder.

• Although agranulocytosis occurs rarely, stop drug and monitor patient closely if he develops a sore throat, fever, stomatitis, or other signs and symptoms of infection with a low WBC count.

• Lower dosages tend to be more sedating than higher dosages.

PATIENT TEACHING

• Caution patient not to perform hazardous activities if he gets too sleepy.

• Tell patient to report signs and symptoms of infection, such as fever, chills, sore throat, mucous membrane irritation, or flulike syndrome.

• Instruct patient not to use alcohol or other CNS depressants while taking drug.

• Stress importance of following prescriber's orders.

• Instruct patient not to take other drugs without prescriber's approval.

• Tell woman of childbearing age to report suspected pregnancy immediately and to notify prescriber if she is breast-feeding.

• Instruct patient to remove ODTs from blister pack and place immediately on tongue. Tell patient to be sure his hands are clean and dry if he touches the tablet.

• Advise patient not to break or split tablet.

---

modafinil
moe-DAFF-in-ill

Provigil

Pharmacologic class: analeptic
Pregnancy risk category C
Controlled substance schedule IV

AVAILABLE FORMS
Tablets: 100 mg, 200 mg

INDICATIONS & DOSAGES
➤ **To improve wakefulness in patients with excessive daytime sleepiness caused by narcolepsy, obstructive sleep apnea-hypopnea syndrome, and shift-work sleep disorder**
Adults: 200 mg P.O. daily, as single dose in the morning. Patients with shift-work sleep disorder should take dose about 1 hour before the start of their shift.

Adjust-a-dose: In patients with severe hepatic impairment, give 100 mg P.O. daily, as single dose in the morning.

ADMINISTRATION
P.O.
• Give drug without regard for food; however, food may delay effect of drug.

ACTION
Unknown. Similar to action of sympathomimetics, including amphetamines, but drug is structurally distinct from amphetamines and doesn't alter release of dopamine or norepinephrine to produce CNS stimulation.

Route	Onset	Peak	Duration
P.O.	Unknown	2–4 hr	Unknown

Half-life: 15 hours.

ADVERSE REACTIONS
CNS: *headache, nervousness, dizziness, insomnia,* fever, depression, anxiety, cataplexy, paresthesia, dyskinesia, hypertonia, confusion, syncope, amnesia, emotional lability, ataxia, tremor, mania, hallucination, *suicidal ideation.*
CV: *arrhythmias,* hypotension, hypertension, vasodilation, chest pain.
EENT: *rhinitis,* pharyngitis, epistaxis, amblyopia, abnormal vision.
GI: *nausea,* diarrhea, dry mouth, anorexia, vomiting, mouth ulcer, gingivitis, thirst.
GU: abnormal urine, urine retention, abnormal ejaculation, albuminuria.
Hematologic: eosinophilia.
Metabolic: hyperglycemia.
Musculoskeletal: joint disorder, neck pain, neck rigidity.
Respiratory: asthma, dyspnea, lung disorder.
Skin: sweating.
Other: herpes simplex, chills.

INTERACTIONS
Drug-drug. *Carbamazepine, phenobarbital, rifampin, and other inducers of CYP3A4:* May alter modafinil level. Monitor patient closely.
Cyclosporine, theophylline: May reduce levels of these drugs. Use together cautiously.

Diazepam, phenytoin, propranolol, other drugs metabolized by CYP2C19: May inhibit CYP2C19 and lead to higher levels of drugs metabolized by this enzyme. Use together cautiously; adjust dosage as needed.

Hormonal contraceptives: May reduce contraceptive effectiveness. Advise patient to use alternative or additional method of contraception during modafinil therapy and for 1 month after drug is stopped.

Itraconazole, ketoconazole, other inhibitors of CYP3A4: May alter modafinil level. Monitor patient closely.

Methylphenidate: May cause 1-hour delay in modafinil absorption. Separate dosage times.

Phenytoin, warfarin: May inhibit CYP2C9 and increase phenytoin and warfarin levels. Monitor patient closely for toxicity.

Tricyclic antidepressants (such as clomipramine, desipramine): May increase tricyclic antidepressant level. Reduce dosage of these drugs.

EFFECTS ON LAB TEST RESULTS
● May increase glucose, GGT, and AST levels.
● May increase eosinophil count.

CONTRAINDICATIONS & CAUTIONS
● Contraindicated in patients hypersensitive to drug and in those with a history of left ventricular hypertrophy or ischemic ECG changes, chest pain, arrhythmias, or other evidence of mitral valve prolapse linked to CNS stimulant use.
● Use cautiously in patients with recent MI or unstable angina and in those with history of psychosis.
● Use cautiously and give reduced dosage to patients with severe hepatic impairment, with or without cirrhosis.
● Use cautiously in patients taking MAO inhibitors.
● Safety and efficacy in patients with severe renal impairment haven't been determined.

NURSING CONSIDERATIONS
● Monitor hypertensive patients closely.
● Although single daily 400-mg doses have been well tolerated, the larger dose is no more beneficial than the 200-mg dose.

PATIENT TEACHING
● *Alert:* Advise patient to stop drug and notify prescriber if rash, peeling skin, trouble swallowing or breathing, or other symptoms of allergic reaction occur. Rare cases of serious rash including Stevens-Johnson syndrome, toxic epidermal necrolysis, and drug rash with eosinophilia and hypersensitivity have been reported.
● Advise woman to notify prescriber about planned, suspected, or known pregnancy, or if she's breast-feeding.
● Caution patient that use of hormonal contraceptives (including depot or implantable contraceptives) together with modafinil tablets may reduce contraceptive effectiveness. Recommend an alternative method of contraception during modafinil therapy and for 1 month after drug is stopped.
● Instruct patient to confer with prescriber before taking prescription or OTC drugs to avoid drug interactions.
● Tell patient to avoid alcohol while taking drug.
● Warn patient to avoid activities that require alertness or good coordination until CNS effects of drug are known.

naloxone hydrochloride
nal-OX-one

Narcan

Pharmacologic class: opioid antagonist
Pregnancy risk category C

AVAILABLE FORMS
Injection: 0.02 mg/ml, 0.4 mg/ml

INDICATIONS & DOSAGES
➤ **Known or suspected opioid-induced respiratory depression, including that caused by pentazocine and propoxyphene**
Adults: 0.4 to 2 mg I.V., I.M., or subcutaneously. Repeat dose every 2 to 3 minutes, p.r.n. If patient doesn't respond after 10 mg have been given, question diagnosis of opioid-induced toxicity.
Children: 0.01 mg/kg I.V.; then, second dose of 0.1 mg/kg I.V., if needed. If I.V.

route isn't available, drug may be given I.M. or subcutaneously in divided doses.
Neonates: 0.01 mg/kg I.V., I.M., or subcutaneously. Repeat dose every 2 to 3 minutes, p.r.n.

➤ **Postoperative opioid depression**
Adults: 0.1 to 0.2 mg I.V. every 2 to 3 minutes, p.r.n. Repeat dose within 1 to 2 hours, if needed.
Children: 0.005 to 0.01 mg I.V. repeated every 2 to 3 minutes, p.r.n.
Neonates (asphyxia neonatorum):
0.01 mg/kg I.V. into umbilical vein. May be repeated every 2 to 3 minutes.

ADMINISTRATION
I.V.
● Give continuous infusion to control adverse effects of epidural morphine.
● Dilute 2 mg of drug in 500 ml D_5W or normal saline solution to yield a concentration of 0.004 mg/ml.
● Titrate rate to patient's response.
● If 0.02 mg/ml isn't available, adult concentration (0.4 mg) may be diluted by mixing 0.5 ml with 9.5 ml of sterile water for injection to make neonatal concentration (0.02 mg/ml).
● **Incompatibilities:** Alkaline solutions, amphotericin B cholesteryl sulfate, preparations containing bisulfite, sulfite, long-chain or high-molecular-weight anions.
I.M.
● Use mixtures within 24 hours. After 24 hours, discard.
Subcutaneous
● Use mixtures within 24 hours. After 24 hours, discard.

ACTION
May displace opioid analgesics from their receptors (competitive antagonism); drug has no pharmacologic activity of its own.

Route	Onset	Peak	Duration
I.V.	1–2 min	5–15 min	Variable
I.M., Subcut	2–5 min	5–15 min	Variable

Half-life: 30 to 81 minutes in adults; 3 hours in neonates.

ADVERSE REACTIONS
CNS: *seizures,* tremors.
CV: *ventricular fibrillation,* tachycardia, hypertension with higher than recommended doses, hypotension.
GI: nausea, vomiting.
Respiratory: *pulmonary edema.*
Skin: diaphoresis.
Other: withdrawal symptoms in opioid-dependent patients with higher than recommended doses.

INTERACTIONS
None significant.

EFFECTS ON LAB TEST RESULTS
None reported.

CONTRAINDICATIONS & CAUTIONS
● Contraindicated in patients hypersensitive to drug.
● Use cautiously in patients with cardiac irritability or opioid addiction. Abrupt reversal of opioid-induced CNS depression may result in nausea, vomiting, diaphoresis, tachycardia, CNS excitement, and increased blood pressure.

NURSING CONSIDERATIONS
● Duration of action of the opioid may exceed that of naloxone, and patients may relapse into respiratory depression.
● Respiratory rate increases within 1 to 2 minutes.
● *Alert:* Drug is only effective for reversing respiratory depression caused by opioids and not for other drug-induced respiratory depression, including that caused by benzodiazepines.
● Patients who receive drug to reverse opioid-induced respiratory depression may exhibit tachypnea.
● Monitor respiratory depth and rate. Provide oxygen, ventilation, and other resuscitation measures.
● *Look alike–sound alike:* Don't confuse naloxone with naltrexone.

PATIENT TEACHING
● Reassure family that patient will be monitored closely until effects of opioid resolve.

naltrexone
nal-TREX-one

Vivitrol

naltrexone hydrochloride
ReVia

Pharmacologic class: opioid
antagonist
Pregnancy risk category C

AVAILABLE FORMS
naltrexone
Injection: 380 mg/vial dose kit
naltrexone hydrochloride
Tablets: 50 mg

INDICATIONS & DOSAGES
➤ **Adjunct for maintaining opioid-free state in detoxified patients**
Adults: Initially, 25 mg P.O. If no withdrawal signs occur within 1 hour, patient may be started on 50 mg every 24 hours the following day. From 50 to 150 mg may be given daily, depending on schedule prescribed.
➤ **Alcohol dependence**
Adults: 50 mg P.O. once daily or 380 mg I.M. in the gluteal muscle once monthly.

ADMINISTRATION
P.O.
● Keep container tightly closed and protect from light.
I.M.
● Use only the diluent, needles, and other components supplied with the dose kit. Don't substitute.

ACTION
Probably reversibly blocks the effects of I.V. opioids by competitively occupying opiate receptors in the brain.

Route	Onset	Peak	Duration
P.O.	15–30 min	1 hr	24 hr
I.M.	Unknown	2–3 days	>30 days

Half-life: About 4 hours.

ADVERSE REACTIONS
CNS: *insomnia, anxiety, nervousness, headache,* **suicidal ideation,** *depression, dizziness, fatigue, somnolence.*
GI: *nausea, vomiting, abdominal pain, anorexia, constipation, increased thirst.*
GU: delayed ejaculation, decreased potency.
Hepatic: *hepatotoxicity.*
Musculoskeletal: *muscle and joint pain.*
Skin: injection site reaction, rash.
Other: chills.

INTERACTIONS
Drug-drug. *Products that contain opioids:* May decrease effect of opioid. Avoid using together.
Thioridazine: May increase somnolence and lethargy. Monitor patient closely.

EFFECTS ON LAB TEST RESULTS
● May increase AST, ALT, and LDH levels.
● May increase lymphocyte count.

CONTRAINDICATIONS & CAUTIONS
● Contraindicated in patients hypersensitive to drug or dependent on opioids, those receiving opioid analgesics, those who fail the naloxone challenge test or who have a positive urine screen for opioids, those in acute opioid withdrawal, or with acute hepatitis or liver failure.
● Use cautiously in patients with mild hepatic disease or history of recent hepatic disease.

NURSING CONSIDERATIONS
● Don't begin treatment for opioid dependence until patient receives naloxone challenge, a test of opioid dependence. If signs and symptoms of opioid withdrawal persist after naloxone challenge, don't give drug.
● Patient must be completely free from opioids before taking naltrexone or severe withdrawal symptoms may occur. Patients who have been addicted to short-acting opioids, such as heroin and meperidine, must wait at least 7 days after last opioid dose before starting drug. Patients who have been addicted to longer-acting opioids such as methadone should wait at least 10 days.

• In an emergency, patient may be given an opioid analgesic, but dose must be higher than usual to overcome naltrexone's effect. Watch for respiratory depression from the opioid; it may be longer and deeper.

• For patients expected to be noncompliant because of history of opioid dependence, use a flexible maintenance-dose regimen of 100 mg on Monday and Wednesday and 150 mg on Friday.

• Use drug only as part of a comprehensive rehabilitation program.

• *Look alike–sound alike:* Don't confuse naltrexone with naloxone.

PATIENT TEACHING

• Advise patient to carry medical identification and to tell medical personnel that he takes naltrexone.

• Tell patient that drug can block the effects of opioids or opioid-like drugs, including heroin, pain medicine, antidiarrheals, or cough medicine.

• *Alert:* Warn patient if he uses large doses of heroin or any other opioid; serious injury, coma, or death can occur.

• Advise patient who previously used opioids that he may be more sensitive to lower doses of opioids once naltrexone therapy is stopped.

• Tell patient to report adverse effects, especially those related to liver injury, to prescriber immediately.

• Tell caregiver of alcohol-dependent patient to monitor him closely for signs of depression or suicide ideation and to report this immediately to prescriber.

• Give patient the names of nonopioid drugs that he can continue to take for pain, diarrhea, or cough.

---

nefazodone hydrochloride
ne-FAZ-oh-dohn

Pharmacologic class:
phenylpiperazine
Pregnancy risk category C

AVAILABLE FORMS
Tablets: 50 mg, 100 mg, 150 mg, 250 mg

INDICATIONS & DOSAGES
➤ **Depression**
Adults: Initially, 200 mg daily P.O. in two divided doses. Dosage may be increased by 100 to 200 mg daily at intervals of at least 1 week, as needed. Usual dosage range is 300 to 600 mg daily.
Elderly patients: Initially, 100 mg daily P.O. in two divided doses.
Adjust-a-dose: For debilitated patients, initially, 100 mg daily P.O. in two divided doses.

ADMINISTRATION
P.O.
• Give drug without regard for food.

ACTION
Thought to be linked to drug's inhibition of CNS neuronal uptake of serotonin ($5-HT_2$) and norepinephrine; it also occupies serotonin and $alpha_1$-adrenergic receptors in the CNS.

Route	Onset	Peak	Duration
P.O.	Unknown	1 hr	Unknown

Half-life: 2 to 4 hours.

ADVERSE REACTIONS
CNS: *headache, somnolence, dizziness, asthenia, insomnia, light-headedness, confusion,* **suicidal behavior,** memory impairment, paresthesia, vasodilation, abnormal dreams, impaired concentration, ataxia, incoordination, psychomotor retardation, tremor, hypertonia.
CV: orthostatic hypotension, hypotension, peripheral edema.
EENT: blurred vision, abnormal vision, tinnitus, visual field defect, pharyngitis.
GI: *dry mouth, nausea, constipation,* taste perversion, dyspepsia, diarrhea, increased appetite, vomiting.
GU: urinary frequency, UTI, urine retention, vaginitis.
Hepatic: *liver failure.*
Musculoskeletal: neck rigidity, arthralgia.
Respiratory: cough.
Skin: pruritus, rash.
Other: infection, flulike syndrome, chills, breast tenderness, thirst.

Reactions may be *common,* uncommon, *life-threatening,* or COMMON AND LIFE-THREATENING.
Interaction may have a *rapid onset* or *delayed onset.*

INTERACTIONS

Drug-drug. *Alprazolam, triazolam:*
May potentiate effects of these drugs.
Avoid using together; if use together is
unavoidable, greatly reduce doses of
alprazolam and triazolam.
CNS drugs: May alter CNS activity. Avoid
using together.
Cyclosporine: May cause cyclosporine
toxicity. Monitor cyclosporine level.
Digoxin: May increase digoxin level. Use
together cautiously and monitor digoxin
level.
Haloperidol: May increase haloperidol
level. Monitor patient for increased adverse reactions.
HMG-CoA reductase inhibitors: May
increase atorvastatin, lovastatin, and
simvastatin levels. Monitor patient for
increased adverse effects.
*MAO inhibitors, such as phenelzine,
selegiline, tranylcypromine:* May cause
serotonin syndrome. Avoid using within
14 days of MAO inhibitor therapy.
Other highly protein-bound drugs: May
increase risk and severity of adverse
reactions. Monitor patient closely.
Tramadol: May cause serotonin syndrome.
Monitor patient closely.
Drug-herb. *St. John's wort:* May cause
additive effects and serotonin syndrome.
Discourage use together.
Drug-lifestyle. *Alcohol use:* May enhance
CNS depression. Discourage use together.

EFFECTS ON LAB TEST RESULTS

● May decrease hemoglobin level and
hematocrit.
● May increase liver function test values.

CONTRAINDICATIONS & CAUTIONS

● Contraindicated in patients hypersensitive to drug or other phenylpiperazine
antidepressants; also contraindicated
within 14 days of MAO inhibitor therapy.
● Contraindicated in patients with liver
disease or who stopped using drug because
of liver injury.
● Use cautiously in patients with CV or
cerebrovascular disease that could be worsened by hypotension (such as history of
MI, angina, or stroke) and conditions that
would predispose patients to hypotension

(such as dehydration, hypovolemia, and
antihypertensive therapy).
● Use cautiously in patients with a history
of mania.

NURSING CONSIDERATIONS

● **Alert:** Drug may cause hepatic failure.
Don't start drug in patients with active
liver disease or with elevated baseline
transaminase level. Although preexisting hepatic disease doesn't increase the
likelihood of developing hepatic failure,
baseline abnormalities can complicate
patient monitoring. Stop drug if clinical
signs and symptoms of hepatic dysfunction
appear, such as increased AST or ALT
level exceeding three times the upper limit
of normal. Don't restart therapy.
● **Alert:** Do a thorough risk-versus-benefit
assessment before using drug to treat
depression, taking into account the risk of
hepatic failure and emergence of suicidal
thoughts and attempts.
● **Alert:** Drug may increase the risk of
suicidal thinking and behavior in children
and adolescents with major depressive
disorder or other psychiatric disorders.
● **Alert:** Drug may increase the risk of
suicidal thinking and behavior in young
adults ages 18 to 24 during the first
2 months of treatment.

PATIENT TEACHING

● Warn patient not to engage in hazardous
activity until effects of drug are known.
● **Alert:** Instruct men who experience prolonged or inappropriate erections to stop
drug immediately and notify prescriber.
● Instruct woman of childbearing age to
notify prescriber if she becomes pregnant
or is planning pregnancy during therapy or
if she's breast-feeding.
● **Alert:** Teach patient the signs and symptoms of liver problems, including yellowed
skin or eyes, appetite loss, GI complaints,
and malaise. Tell patient to report these
adverse events to prescriber immediately.
● **Alert:** Inform family members to be
particularly vigilant for suicidal tendencies
during therapy.
● Tell patient to notify prescriber if rash,
hives, or related allergic reactions occur.
● Instruct patient to avoid alcohol during
therapy.

• Tell patient to notify prescriber before taking OTC drugs.
• Inform patient that several weeks of therapy may be needed to obtain full antidepressant effect. Once improvement occurs, advise him not to stop drug until directed by prescriber.

---

nortriptyline hydrochloride
nor-TRIP-ti-leen

Aventyl, Pamelor*

Pharmacologic class: tricyclic antidepressant
Pregnancy risk category D

AVAILABLE FORMS
Capsules: 10 mg, 25 mg, 50 mg, 75 mg
Oral solution: 10 mg/5 ml*

INDICATIONS & DOSAGES
➤ **Depression**
Adults: 25 mg P.O. t.i.d. or q.i.d., gradually increased to maximum of 150 mg daily. Give entire dose at bedtime. Monitor level when doses above 100 mg daily are given.
Adolescents and elderly patients: 30 to 50 mg daily given once or in divided doses.

ADMINISTRATION
P.O.
• Give drug without regard for food.
• Whenever possible, give full dose at bedtime.

ACTION
Unknown. Increases the amount of norepinephrine, serotonin, or both in the CNS by blocking reuptake by the presynaptic neurons.

Route	Onset	Peak	Duration
P.O.	Unknown	7–8½ hr	Unknown

Half-life: 18 to 24 hours.

ADVERSE REACTIONS
CNS: *drowsiness, dizziness, **seizures, stroke,*** tremor, weakness, confusion, headache, nervousness, EEG changes, extrapyramidal syndrome, insomnia, nightmares, hallucinations, paresthesia, ataxia, agitation.
CV: *tachycardia, **heart block, MI,*** ECG changes, hypertension, hypotension.
EENT: *blurred vision,* tinnitus, mydriasis.
GI: *constipation,* dry mouth, nausea, vomiting, anorexia, paralytic ileus.
GU: *urine retention.*
Hematologic: ***agranulocytosis, thrombocytopenia,*** bone marrow depression, eosinophilia.
Metabolic: ***hypoglycemia,*** hyperglycemia.
Skin: rash, urticaria, photosensitivity reactions, diaphoresis.
Other: hypersensitivity reactions.

INTERACTIONS
Drug-drug. *Barbiturates, CNS depressants:* May enhance CNS depression. Avoid using together.
*Cimetidine, **fluoxetine, fluvoxamine, paroxetine, sertraline:*** May increase nortriptyline level. Monitor drug levels and patient for signs of toxicity.
Clonidine: May cause life-threatening hypertension. Avoid using together.
Epinephrine, norepinephrine: May increase hypertensive effect. Use together cautiously.
MAO inhibitors: May cause severe excitation, hyperpyrexia, or seizures, usually with high doses. Avoid using within 14 days of MAO inhibitor therapy.
Quinolones: May increase the risk of life-threatening arrhythmias. Avoid using together.
Drug-herb. *Evening primrose oil:* May cause additive or synergistic effect, lowering seizure threshold and increasing the risk of seizure. Discourage use together.
St. John's wort, SAM-e, yohimbe: May cause serotonin syndrome and reduced drug level. Discourage use together.
Drug-lifestyle. *Alcohol use:* May enhance CNS depression. Discourage use together.
Smoking: May decrease drug level. Monitor patient for lack of effect.
Sun exposure: May increase risk of photosensitivity reactions. Advise patient to avoid excessive sunlight exposure.

EFFECTS ON LAB TEST RESULTS
• May increase or decrease glucose level.

Reactions may be *common*, uncommon, ***life-threatening***, or COMMON AND LIFE-THREATENING.
Interaction may have a *rapid onset* or ***delayed onset***.

● May increase eosinophil count and liver function test values. May decrease WBC, RBC, granulocyte, and platelet counts.

CONTRAINDICATIONS & CAUTIONS
● Contraindicated in patients hypersensitive to drug and during acute recovery phase of MI; also contraindicated within 14 days of MAO inhibitor therapy.
● Use with extreme caution in patients with glaucoma, suicidal tendency, history of urine retention or seizures, CV disease, or hyperthyroidism and in those receiving thyroid drugs.

NURSING CONSIDERATIONS
● Monitor patient for nausea, headache, and malaise after abrupt withdrawal of long-term therapy; these symptoms don't indicate addiction.
● Because patients using tricyclic antidepressants may suffer hypertensive episodes during surgery, stop drug gradually several days before surgery.
● If signs or symptoms of psychosis occur or increase, expect to reduce dosage. Record mood changes. Monitor patient for suicidal tendencies and allow him only a minimum supply of drug.
● *Alert:* Drug may increase the risk of suicidal thinking and behavior in children and adolescents with major depressive disorder or other psychiatric disorder.
● *Alert:* Drug may increase the risk of suicidal thinking and behavior in young adults ages 18 to 24 during the first 2 months of treatment.
● *Look alike–sound alike:* Don't confuse nortriptyline with amitriptyline.

PATIENT TEACHING
● Advise patient to take full dose at bedtime whenever possible to reduce risk of dizziness upon standing quickly.
● Warn patient to avoid activities that require alertness and good coordination until effects of drug are known. Drowsiness and dizziness usually subside after a few weeks.
● Recommend use of sugarless hard candy or gum to relieve dry mouth. Saliva substitutes may be needed.
● Tell patient to consult prescriber before taking other prescription or OTC drugs.

● Warn patient not to stop drug suddenly.
● To prevent oversensitivity to the sun, advise patient to use sunblock, wear protective clothing, and avoid prolonged exposure to strong sunlight.

olanzapine
oh-LAN-za-peen

Zyprexa, Zyprexa Zydis

Pharmacologic class: dibenzapine derivative
Pregnancy risk category C

AVAILABLE FORMS
Injection: 10 mg
Tablets: 2.5 mg, 5 mg, 7.5 mg, 10 mg, 15 mg, 20 mg
Tablets (orally disintegrating): 5 mg, 10 mg, 15 mg, 20 mg

INDICATIONS & DOSAGES
➤ **Schizophrenia**
Adults: Initially, 5 to 10 mg P.O. once daily with the goal to be at 10 mg daily within several days of starting therapy. Adjust dose in 5-mg increments at intervals of 1 week or more. Most patients respond to 10 to 15 mg daily. Safety of dosages greater than 20 mg daily hasn't been established.
➤ **Short-term treatment of acute manic episodes linked to bipolar I disorder**
Adults: Initially, 10 to 15 mg P.O. daily. Adjust dosage as needed in 5-mg daily increments at intervals of 24 hours or more. Maximum, 20 mg P.O. daily. Duration of treatment is 3 to 4 weeks.
➤ **Short-term treatment, with lithium or valproate, of acute manic episodes linked to bipolar I disorder**
Adults: 10 mg P.O. once daily. Dosage range is 5 to 20 mg daily. Duration of treatment is 6 weeks.
➤ **Long-term treatment of bipolar I disorder**
Adults: 5 to 20 mg P.O. daily.
➤ **Adjunct to lithium or valproate to treat bipolar mania**
Adults: 10 mg P.O. daily. Usual range 5 to 20 mg daily.

Adjust-a-dose: In elderly or debilitated patients, those predisposed to hypotensive reactions, patients who may metabolize olanzapine more slowly than usual (non-smoking women older than age 65) or may be more pharmacodynamically sensitive to olanzapine, initially, 5 mg P.O. Increase dose cautiously.

➤ **Agitation caused by schizophrenia and bipolar I mania**
Adults: 10 mg I.M. (range 2.5 to 10 mg). Subsequent doses of up to 10 mg may be given 2 hours after the first dose or 4 hours after the second dose, up to 30 mg I.M. daily. If maintenance therapy is required, convert patient to 5 to 20 mg P.O. daily.
Adjust-a-dose: In elderly patients, give 5 mg I.M. In debilitated patients, in those predisposed to hypotension, and in patients sensitive to effects of drug, give 2.5 mg I.M.

ADMINISTRATION
P.O.
● Give drug without regard for food.
● Don't crush or break orally disintegrating tablet (ODT).
● Place immediately on patient's tongue after opening package.
● ODT may be given without water.
I.M.
● Inspect I.M. solution for particulate matter and discoloration before administration.
● To reconstitute I.M. injection, dissolve contents of one vial with 2.1 ml of sterile water for injection to yield a clear yellow 5 mg/ml solution. Store at room temperature and give within 1 hour of reconstitution. Discard any unused solution.

ACTION
May block dopamine and 5-HT$_2$ receptors.

Route	Onset	Peak	Duration
P.O.	Unknown	6 hr	Unknown
I.M.	Rapid	15–45 min	Unknown

Half-life: 21 to 54 hours.

ADVERSE REACTIONS
CNS: *somnolence, insomnia, parkinsonism, dizziness, **neuroleptic malignant syndrome, suicide attempt,*** abnormal gait, asthenia, personality disorder, akathisia, tremor, articulation impairment, tardive dyskinesia, fever, extrapyramidal events (I.M.).
CV: orthostatic hypotension, tachycardia, chest pain, hypertension, ecchymosis, peripheral edema, hypotension (I.M.).
EENT: amblyopia, rhinitis, pharyngitis, conjunctivitis.
GI: *constipation, dry mouth, dyspepsia,* increased appetite, increased salivation, vomiting, thirst.
GU: hematuria, metrorrhagia, urinary incontinence, UTI, amenorrhea, vaginitis.
Hematologic: *leukopenia.*
Metabolic: *hyperglycemia,* weight gain.
Musculoskeletal: joint pain, extremity pain, back pain, neck rigidity, twitching, hypertonia.
Respiratory: increased cough, dyspnea.
Skin: sweating, injection site pain (I.M.).
Other: flulike syndrome, injury.

INTERACTIONS
Drug-drug. *Antihypertensives:* May potentiate hypotensive effects. Monitor blood pressure closely.
Carbamazepine, omeprazole, rifampin: May increase clearance of olanzapine. Monitor patient.
Ciprofloxacin: May increase olanzapine level. Monitor patient for increased adverse effects.
Diazepam: May increase CNS effects. Monitor patient.
Dopamine agonists, levodopa: May cause antagonized activity of these drugs. Monitor patient.
Fluoxetine: May increase olanzapine level. Use together cautiously.
Fluvoxamine: May increase olanzapine level. May need to reduce olanzapine dose.
Drug-herb. *St. John's wort:* May decrease drug level. Discourage use together.
Drug-lifestyle. *Alcohol use:* May increase CNS effects. Discourage use together.
Smoking: May increase drug clearance. Urge patient to quit smoking.

EFFECTS ON LAB TEST RESULTS
● May increase AST, ALT, GGT, CK, triglyceride, and prolactin levels.
● May increase eosinophil count. May decrease WBC count.

Reactions may be *common,* uncommon, *life-threatening,* or COMMON AND LIFE-THREATENING.
Interaction may have a *rapid onset* or *delayed onset.*

CONTRAINDICATIONS & CAUTIONS
• Contraindicated in patients hypersensitive to drug.
• Use cautiously in patients with heart disease, cerebrovascular disease, conditions that predispose patient to hypotension, history of seizures or conditions that might lower the seizure threshold, and hepatic impairment.
• Use cautiously in elderly patients, those with a history of paralytic ileus, and those at risk for aspiration pneumonia, prostatic hyperplasia, or angle-closure glaucoma.

NURSING CONSIDERATIONS
• ODTs contain phenylalanine.
• Monitor patient for abnormal body temperature regulation, especially if he exercises, is exposed to extreme heat, takes anticholinergics, or is dehydrated.
• Obtain baseline and periodic liver function test results.
• Monitor patient for weight gain.
• *Alert:* Watch for evidence of neuroleptic malignant syndrome (hyperpyrexia, muscle rigidity, altered mental status, autonomic instability), which is rare but commonly fatal. Stop drug immediately; monitor and treat patient as needed.
• *Alert:* Drug may cause hyperglycemia. Monitor patients with diabetes regularly. In patients with risk factors for diabetes, obtain fasting blood glucose test results at baseline and periodically.
• *Alert:* Monitor patient for symptoms of metabolic syndrome (significant weight gain and increased body mass index, hypertension, hyperglycemia, hypercholesterolemia, and hypertriglyceridemia).
• Monitor patient for tardive dyskinesia, which may occur after prolonged use. It may not appear until months or years later and may disappear spontaneously or persist for life, despite stopping drug.
• Periodically reevaluate the long-term usefulness of olanzapine.
• Drug may increase risk of stroke and death in elderly patients with dementia. Olanzapine isn't approved to treat patients with dementia-related psychosis.
• A patient who feels dizzy or drowsy after an I.M. injection should remain recumbent until he can be assessed for orthostatic hypotension and bradycardia. He should rest until the feeling passes.
• *Alert:* Drug may increase the risk of suicidal thinking and behavior in young adults ages 18 to 24 during the first 2 months of treatment.
• *Look alike–sound alike:* Don't confuse olanzapine with olsalazine or Zyprexa with Zyrtec.

PATIENT TEACHING
• Warn patient to avoid hazardous tasks until full effects of drug are known.
• Warn patient against exposure to extreme heat; drug may impair body's ability to reduce temperature.
• Inform patient that he may gain weight.
• Advise patient to avoid alcohol.
• Tell patient to rise slowly to avoid dizziness upon standing up quickly.
• Inform patient that ODTs contain phenylalanine.
• Tell patient to peel foil away from ODT, not to push tablet through. Have patient take tablet immediately, allowing tablet to dissolve on tongue and be swallowed with saliva; no additional fluid is needed.
• Tell patient to take drug with or without food.
• Urge woman of childbearing age to notify prescriber if she becomes pregnant or plans or suspects pregnancy. Tell her not to breast-feed during therapy.

SAFETY ALERT!

oxazepam
ox-AZ-e-pam

Serax

Pharmacologic class:
benzodiazepine
Pregnancy risk category D
Controlled substance schedule IV

AVAILABLE FORMS
Capsules: 10 mg, 15 mg, 30 mg
Tablets: 15 mg

INDICATIONS & DOSAGES
➤ **Alcohol withdrawal, severe anxiety**
Adults: 15 to 30 mg P.O. t.i.d. or q.i.d.
➤ **Mild to moderate anxiety**
Adults: 10 to 15 mg P.O. t.i.d. or q.i.d.
Elderly patients: Initially, 10 mg t.i.d.; cautiously increase to 15 mg t.i.d. to q.i.d.

ADMINISTRATION
P.O.
● Give drug without regard for meals.
● *Alert:* Serax tablets may contain tartrazine.

ACTION
May stimulate GABA receptors in the ascending reticular activating system.

Route	Onset	Peak	Duration
P.O.	Unknown	3 hr	Unknown

Half-life: 5 to 13 hours.

ADVERSE REACTIONS
CNS: *drowsiness, lethargy,* dizziness, vertigo, headache, syncope, tremor, slurred speech, changes in EEG patterns.
CV: edema.
GI: nausea.
Hepatic: *hepatic dysfunction.*
Skin: rash.
Other: altered libido.

INTERACTIONS
Drug-drug. *CNS depressants:* May increase CNS depression. Use together cautiously.
Digoxin: May increase digoxin level and risk of toxicity. Monitor patient closely.
Drug-herb. *Kava:* May increase sedation. Discourage use together.
Drug-lifestyle. *Alcohol use:* May cause additive CNS effects. Discourage use together.

EFFECTS ON LAB TEST RESULTS
● May increase liver function test values.

CONTRAINDICATIONS & CAUTIONS
● Contraindicated in patients hypersensitive to drug; in pregnant women, especially in the first trimester; and in those with psychoses.

● Use cautiously in elderly patients and in those with history of drug abuse or in whom a decrease in blood pressure might lead to cardiac problems.

NURSING CONSIDERATIONS
● Monitor hepatic, renal, and hematopoietic function periodically in patients receiving repeated or prolonged therapy.
● *Alert:* Use of this drug may lead to abuse and addiction. Don't stop drug abruptly because withdrawal symptoms may occur.
● *Look alike–sound alike:* Don't confuse oxazepam with oxaprozin.

PATIENT TEACHING
● Warn patient to avoid hazardous activities that require alertness or good coordination until effects of drug are known.
● Tell patient to avoid use of alcohol while taking drug.
● Notify patient that smoking may decrease drug's effectiveness.
● Warn patient not to stop drug abruptly because withdrawal symptoms may occur.
● Warn woman of childbearing age to avoid use during pregnancy.

✳ NEW DRUG

paliperidone
pahl-ee-PEHR-ih-dohn

Invegra

Pharmacologic class: benzisoxazole derivative
Pregnancy risk category C

AVAILABLE FORMS
Tablets (extended-release): 3 mg, 6 mg, 9 mg

INDICATIONS & DOSAGES
➤ **Schizophrenia**
Adults: 6 mg P.O. once daily in the morning; may increase or decrease dose by 3-mg increments to a range of 3 mg to 12 mg daily; don't exceed 12 mg per day.
Adjust-a-dose: In patients with creatinine clearance of 50 to 80 ml/minute, maximum dosage is 6 mg once daily; for patients with creatinine clearance of 10 to 49 ml/minute, maximum dosage is 3 mg once daily.

ADMINISTRATION
P.O.
● Don't crush or break tablets.

ACTION
May antagonize both central dopamine
(D_2) and serotonin type 2 receptors; also
alpha-1, alpha-2, and histamine-1 receptors. Drug is a major active metabolite of
risperidone.

Route	Onset	Peak	Duration
P.O.	Unknown	24 hr	Unknown

Half-life: 23 hours.

ADVERSE REACTIONS
CNS: *akathisia, headache, parkinsonism,
somnolence,* anxiety, asthenia, dizziness,
dystonia, extrapyramidal disorder, fatigue,
hypertonia, pyrexia, tremor, dyskinesia,
hyperkinesia.
CV: abnormal T waves, hypertension,
orthostatic hypotension, palpitations, sinus
arrhythmia, tachycardia, **AV BLOCK,**
bundle branch block, **PROLONGED QTC
INTERVAL.**
EENT: blurred vision.
GI: abdominal pain, dry mouth, dyspepsia,
nausea, salivary hypersecretion.
Metabolic: blood insulin increases, hyperprolactinemia.
Musculoskeletal: back pain, extremity
pain.
Respiratory: cough.

INTERACTIONS
Drug-drug. *Drugs that prolong QTc
intervals, such as antiarrhythmics (quinidine, procainamide, amiodarone, sotalol),
antipsychotics (chlorpromazine, thioridazine), quinolone antibiotics (moxifloxacin):* May further prolong QTc
interval. Avoid using together.
Levodopa, dopamine agonists: May antagonize effects of these drugs. Use cautiously
together.
Central-acting drugs: May worsen CNS
side effects. Use cautiously together.
Anticholinergics: May worsen side effects.
Use cautiously together.
Antihypertensives: May worsen orthostatic
hypotension. Avoid using together.

Drug-lifestyle. *Alcohol use:* May worsen
CNS side effects. Discourage use together.

EFFECTS ON LAB TEST RESULTS
● May increase insulin and prolactin
levels.

CONTRAINDICATIONS & CAUTIONS
● Contraindicated in patients hypersensitive to paliperidone or risperidone.
● *Alert:* Contraindicated in dementia-
related psychosis.
● Contraindicated in patients with congenital long QT syndrome or history of cardiac
arrhythmias.
● Contraindicated in patients with pre-
existing severe GI narrowing (esophageal
motility disorders, small bowel inflammatory disease, short gut syndrome).
● Use cautiously in patients with a history of seizures or diabetes; those at risk
for aspiration pneumonia; and those with
bradycardia, hypokalemia, hypomagnesemia, CV disease, cerebrovascular
disease, dehydration, or hypovolemia.
● Use cautiously in patients taking antihypertensives and drugs that lower the
seizure threshold.
● Use cautiously in patients with history of
suicide attempts.

PATIENT TEACHING
● Tell patient that remains of the tablet may
appear in feces.
● Tell patient to swallow whole with liquids and not to chew, crush, or break
tablets.
● Instruct the patient not to perform activities that require mental alertness until
effects of drug are known.
● Warn patient to use caution in performing excessively strenuous activities
because his body temperature may be
disrupted.
● Advise patient that drug may lower blood
pressure and to change positions slowly.
● Instruct patient to contact prescriber
before taking any other drugs to avoid
potential interactions.
● Advise patient to avoid alcohol while
taking this medication.
● Advise patient to contact prescriber if
she becomes pregnant or wants to breast-
feed.

paroxetine hydrochloride
pah-ROX-a-teen

Paxil, Paxil CR

Pharmacologic class: SSRI
Pregnancy risk category D

AVAILABLE FORMS
Suspension: 10 mg/5 ml
Tablets: 10 mg, 20 mg, 30 mg, 40 mg
Tablets (controlled-release): 12.5 mg,
25 mg, 37.5 mg

INDICATIONS & DOSAGES
➤ **Depression**
Adults: Initially, 20 mg P.O. daily, preferably in morning, as indicated. If patient doesn't improve, increase dose by
10 mg daily at intervals of at least 1 week
to a maximum of 50 mg daily. If using
controlled-release form, initially, 25 mg
P.O. daily. Increase dose by 12.5 mg daily
at weekly intervals to a maximum of
62.5 mg daily.
Elderly patients: Initially, 10 mg P.O. daily,
preferably in morning, as indicated. If
patient doesn't improve, increase dose by
10 mg daily at weekly intervals, to a maximum of 40 mg daily. If using controlled-
release form, start therapy at 12.5 mg P.O.
daily. Don't exceed 50 mg daily.
➤ **Obsessive-compulsive disorder**
Adults: Initially, 20 mg P.O. daily, preferably in morning. Increase dose by 10 mg
daily at weekly intervals. Recommended
daily dose is 40 mg. Maximum daily dose
is 60 mg.
➤ **Panic disorder**
Adults: Initially, 10 mg P.O. daily. Increase
dose by 10 mg at no less than weekly
intervals to maximum of 60 mg daily. Or,
12.5 mg Paxil CR P.O. as a single daily
dose, usually in the morning, with or
without food; increase dose at intervals of
at least 1 week by 12.5 mg daily, up to a
maximum of 75 mg daily.
Adjust-a-dose: In elderly or debilitated
patients and in those with severe renal or
hepatic impairment, the first dose of Paxil
CR is 12.5 mg daily; increase if indicated.
Dosage shouldn't exceed 50 mg daily.

➤ **Social anxiety disorder**
Adults: Initially, 20 mg P.O. daily, preferably in morning. Dosage range is 20
to 60 mg daily. Adjust dosage to maintain patient on lowest effective dose. Or,
12.5 mg Paxil CR P.O. as a single daily
dose, usually in morning, with or without
food. Increase dosage at weekly intervals
in increments of 12.5 mg daily, up to a
maximum of 37.5 mg daily.
➤ **Generalized anxiety disorder**
Adults: 20 mg P.O. daily initially, increasing by 10 mg per day weekly up to 50 mg
daily.
Adjust-a-dose: For debilitated patients or
those with renal or hepatic impairment
taking immediate-release form, initially,
10 mg P.O. daily, preferably in morning.
If patient doesn't respond after full antidepressant effect has occurred, increase
dose by 10 mg per day at weekly intervals
to a maximum of 40 mg daily. If using
controlled-release form, start therapy at
12.5 mg daily. Don't exceed 50 mg daily.
➤ **Posttraumatic stress disorder**
Adults: Initially, 20 mg P.O. daily. Increase
dose by 10 mg daily at intervals of at least
1 week. Maximum daily dose is 50 mg P.O.
➤ **Premenstrual dysphoric disorder
(PMDD)**
Adults: Initially, 12.5 mg Paxil CR P.O. as
a single daily dose, usually in morning,
with or without food, daily or during the
luteal phase of the menstrual cycle. Dose
changes should occur at intervals of at
least 1 week. Maximum dose is 25 mg P.O.
daily.
➤ **Premature ejaculation ♦**
Adults: 10 to 40 mg P.O. daily. Or, 20 mg
P.O. as needed 3 to 4 hours before planned
intercourse.
➤ **Diabetic neuropathy ♦**
Adults: 40 mg P.O. daily.

ADMINISTRATION
P.O.
● Give drug without regard for food.
● Don't split or crush controlled-release
tablets.

ACTION
Thought to be linked to drug's inhibition of
CNS neuronal uptake of serotonin.

Route	Onset	Peak	Duration
P.O.	Unknown	2–8 hr	Unknown
P.O. (controlled-release)	Unknown	6–10 hr	Unknown

Half-life: About 24 hours.

ADVERSE REACTIONS

CNS: *asthenia, dizziness, headache, insomnia, somnolence, tremor, nervousness,* **suicidal behavior,** anxiety, paresthesia, confusion, agitation.
CV: palpitations, vasodilation, orthostatic hypotension.
EENT: lump or tightness in throat.
GI: *dry mouth, nausea, constipation, diarrhea,* flatulence, vomiting, dyspepsia, dysgeusia, increased or decreased appetite, abdominal pain.
GU: *ejaculatory disturbances, sexual dysfunction,* urinary frequency, other urinary disorders.
Musculoskeletal: myopathy, myalgia, myasthenia.
Skin: *diaphoresis,* rash, pruritus.
Other: *decreased libido,* yawning.

INTERACTIONS

Drug-drug. *Amphetamines, buspirone, dextromethorphan, dihydroergotamine, lithium salts, meperidine, other SSRIs or SSNRIs (duloxetine, venlafaxine),* **tramadol,** *trazodone, tricyclic antidepressants, tryptophan:* May increase the risk of serotonin syndrome. Avoid combining drugs that increase the availability of serotonin in the CNS; monitor patient closely if used together.
Cimetidine: May decrease hepatic metabolism of paroxetine, leading to risk of adverse reactions. Dosage adjustments may be needed.
Digoxin: May decrease digoxin level. Use together cautiously.
MAO inhibitors, such as phenelzine, selegiline, tranylcypromine: May cause serotonin syndrome. Avoid using within 14 days of MAO inhibitor therapy.
Phenobarbital, phenytoin: May alter pharmacokinetics of both drugs. Dosage adjustments may be needed.

Procyclidine: May increase procyclidine level. Watch for excessive anticholinergic effects.
Sumatriptan: May cause weakness, hyperreflexia, and incoordination. Monitor patient closely.
Theophylline: May decrease theophylline clearance. Monitor theophylline level.
Thioridazine: May prolong QTc interval and increase risk of serious ventricular arrhythmias, such as torsades de pointes, and sudden death. Avoid using together.
Tricyclic antidepressants: May inhibit tricyclic antidepressant metabolism. Dose of tricyclic antidepressant may need to be reduced. Monitor patient closely.
Triptans: May cause serotonin syndrome (restlessness, hallucinations, loss of coordination, fast heartbeat, rapid changes in blood pressure, increased body temperature, overactive reflexes, nausea, vomiting, and diarrhea). Use cautiously, especially at the start of therapy and at dosage increases.
Warfarin: May cause bleeding. Use together cautiously.
Drug-herb. *St. John's wort:* May increase sedative-hypnotic effects. Discourage use together.
Drug-lifestyle. *Alcohol use:* May alter psychomotor function. Discourage use together.

EFFECTS ON LAB TEST RESULTS
None reported.

CONTRAINDICATIONS & CAUTIONS
• Contraindicated in patients hypersensitive to drug, within 14 days of MAO inhibitor therapy, and in those taking thioridazine.
• Contraindicated in children and adolescents younger than age 18 for major depressive disorders.
• Use cautiously in patients with history of seizure disorders or mania and in those with other severe, systemic illness.
• Use cautiously in patients at risk for volume depletion and monitor them appropriately.
• Using drug in the first trimester may increase the risk of congenital fetal malformations; using drug in the third trimester

may cause neonatal complications at birth. Consider the risk versus benefit of therapy.

NURSING CONSIDERATIONS
• Patients taking drug may be at increased risk for developing suicidal behavior, but this hasn't been definitively attributed to use of the drug.
• Patients taking Paxil CR for PMDD should be periodically reassessed to determine the need for continued treatment.
• If signs or symptoms of psychosis occur or increase, expect prescriber to reduce dosage. Record mood changes. Monitor patient for suicidal tendencies, and allow only a minimum supply of drug.
• *Alert:* Drug may increase the risk of suicidal thinking and behavior in children, adolescents, and young adults ages 18 to 24 during the first 2 months of treatment, especially in those with major depressive disorder or other psychiatric disorder.
• Monitor patient for complaints of sexual dysfunction. In men, they include anorgasmy, erectile difficulties, delayed ejaculation or orgasm, or impotence; in women, they include anorgasmia or difficulty with orgasm.
• *Alert:* Don't stop drug abruptly. Withdrawal or discontinuation syndrome may occur if drug is stopped abruptly. Symptoms include headache, myalgia, lethargy, and general flulike symptoms. Taper drug slowly over 1 to 2 weeks.
• *Alert:* Combining triptans with an SSRI or an SSNRI may cause serotonin syndrome. Signs and symptoms may include restlessness, hallucinations, loss of coordination, fast heartbeat, rapid changes in blood pressure, increased body temperature, overactive reflexes, nausea, vomiting, and diarrhea. Serotonin syndrome may be more likely to occur when starting or increasing the dose of triptan, SSRI, or SSNRI.
• *Look alike–sound alike:* Don't confuse paroxetine with paclitaxel, or Paxil with Doxil, paclitaxel, Plavix, or Taxol.

PATIENT TEACHING
• Tell patient that drug may be taken with or without food, usually in morning.
• Tell patient not to break, crush, or chew controlled-release tablets.

• Warn patient to avoid activities that require alertness and good coordination until effects of drug are known.
• Advise woman of childbearing age to contact prescriber if she becomes pregnant or plans to become pregnant during therapy or if she's currently breast-feeding.
• Tell patient to avoid alcohol and to consult prescriber before taking other prescription or OTC drugs or herbal medicines.
• Instruct patient not to stop taking drug abruptly.

SAFETY ALERT!

pentobarbital sodium
pen-toe-BAR-bi-tal

Nembutal Sodium†*

Pharmacologic class: barbiturate
Pregnancy risk category D
Controlled substance schedule II

AVAILABLE FORMS
Injection: 50 mg/ml*

INDICATIONS & DOSAGES
➤ **Insomnia**
Adults: 150 to 200 mg deep I.M. Or, 100 mg I.V. initially in 70-kg patient, with further small doses up to total of 500 mg.
Adjust-a-dose: For debilitated, elderly, pediatric, or smaller patients, dosage may be decreased. For heavier patients, dosage may be increased.
➤ **Preoperative sedation**
Adults: 150 to 200 mg I.M.
Children: 2 to 6 mg/kg P.O., P.R., or I.M. Maximum dose is 100 mg.

ADMINISTRATION
I.V.
• I.V. barbiturates may cause severe respiratory depression, laryngospasm, or hypotension. Reserve their use for emergencies, under close supervision, with resuscitation equipment nearby.
• To minimize deterioration, use injection solution within 30 minutes of opening container. Don't use cloudy solution.

Reactions may be *common*, uncommon, *life-threatening*, or COMMON AND LIFE-THREATENING.
Interaction may have a *rapid onset* or *delayed onset*.

- Don't mix in syringe or in solutions or lines with other drugs.
- Give slowly at no more than 50 mg/ minute.
- Parenteral solution is alkaline. Local tissue reactions and injection site pain may occur. Monitor site for extravasation. Assess patency of site before and during administration.
- **Incompatibilities:** Other I.V. drugs or solutions.

I.M.

- Give deep I.M. injection with no more than 5 ml of drug at any one site. Superficial injection may cause pain, sterile abscess, and sloughing.

ACTION

May interfere with transmission of impulses from the thalamus to the cortex of the brain and alter cerebellar function.

Route	Onset	Peak	Duration
I.V.	Immediate	Immediate	15 min
I.M.	10–25 min	Unknown	Unknown

Half-life: 35 to 50 hours.

ADVERSE REACTIONS

CNS: *drowsiness, lethargy, hangover,* paradoxical excitement in elderly patients, somnolence, physical and psychological dependence.
GI: nausea, vomiting.
Hematologic: worsening porphyria.
Respiratory: *respiratory depression.*
Skin: rash, urticaria, *Stevens-Johnson syndrome.*
Other: *angioedema.*

INTERACTIONS

Drug-drug. *CNS depressants including opioid analgesics:* May cause excessive CNS and respiratory depression. Use together cautiously.
Corticosteroids, doxycycline, estrogens and hormonal contraceptives, oral anticoagulants, theophylline, verapamil: May enhance metabolism of these drugs. Watch for decreased effect.
Griseofulvin: May decrease absorption of griseofulvin. Monitor effectiveness of griseofulvin.

MAO inhibitors, valproic acid: May inhibit metabolism of barbiturates; may prolong CNS depression. Reduce barbiturate dosage.
Metoprolol, propranolol: May reduce effects of these drugs. May need to increase beta-blocker dose.
Rifampin: May decrease barbiturate level. Watch for decreased effect of pentobarbital.
Drug-lifestyle. *Alcohol use:* May impair coordination, increase CNS effects, and cause death. Strongly discourage alcohol use with these drugs.

EFFECTS ON LAB TEST RESULTS
None reported.

CONTRAINDICATIONS & CAUTIONS

- Contraindicated in patients hypersensitive to barbiturates and in those with porphyria, bronchopneumonia, or other severe pulmonary insufficiency, and in severe liver or renal dysfunction.
- Use cautiously in elderly or debilitated patients and in patients with acute or chronic pain, mental depression, suicidal tendencies, history of drug abuse, or hepatic impairment.

NURSING CONSIDERATIONS

- Assess mental status before starting therapy and reduce doses in elderly patients; these patients may be more sensitive to drug's adverse CNS effects.
- Take precautions to prevent hoarding by patients who are depressed, suicidal, or drug-dependent or who have a history of drug abuse.
- Watch for signs of barbiturate toxicity: coma, pupillary constriction, cyanosis, clammy skin, and hypotension. Overdose can be fatal.
- Inspect patient's skin. Skin eruptions may precede fatal reactions. If skin reactions occur, stop drug and call prescriber. In some patients, high temperature, stomatitis, headache, or rhinitis may precede skin reactions.
- Drug has no analgesic effect and may cause restlessness or delirium in patients with pain.
- Long-term use for insomnia isn't recommended; drug loses its effectiveness

in promoting sleep after 14 days of continuous use. Long-term high dosage may cause drug dependence, and patient may experience withdrawal symptoms if drug is suddenly stopped. Withdraw barbiturates gradually.
• EEG patterns show a change in low-voltage, fast activity; changes persist after therapy.
• *Alert:* Nembutal may contain tartrazine.
• *Look alike–sound alike:* Don't confuse pentobarbital with phenobarbital.

PATIENT TEACHING
• Inform patient that morning hangover is common after hypnotic dose, which suppresses REM sleep. Patient may experience increased dreaming after drug is stopped.
• Caution patient to avoid performing activities that require mental alertness or physical coordination.
• Tell patient to avoid alcohol use while taking drug.
• Because drug may decrease the effect of hormonal contraceptives, instruct patient to also use a barrier contraceptive.

---

perphenazine
per-FEN-uh-zeen

Pharmacologic class: phenothiazine
Pregnancy risk category C

AVAILABLE FORMS
Oral concentrate: 16 mg/5 ml
Tablets: 2 mg, 4 mg, 8 mg, 16 mg

INDICATIONS & DOSAGES
➤ **Psychosis in nonhospitalized patients**
Adults and children older than age 12:
Initially, 4 to 8 mg P.O. t.i.d.; reduce as soon as possible to minimum effective dose.
➤ **Psychosis in hospitalized patients**
Adults and children older than age 12:
Initially, 8 to 16 mg P.O. b.i.d., t.i.d., or q.i.d.; increase to 64 mg daily, as needed.
➤ **Severe nausea and vomiting**
Adults: 8 to 16 mg P.O. daily in divided doses to maximum of 24 mg.

ADMINISTRATION
P.O.
• Dilute liquid concentrate with fruit juice, milk, carbonated beverage, or semisolid food just before giving. Don't use colas, black coffee, grape juice, apple juice, or tea because turbidity or precipitation may result.
• Protect drug from light. Slight yellowing of concentrate is common and doesn't affect potency. Discard markedly discolored solutions.

ACTION
May exert antipsychotic effects by blocking postsynaptic dopamine receptors in the brain.

Route	Onset	Peak	Duration
P.O.	Unknown	Unknown	Unknown

Half-life: 9 to 12 hours.

ADVERSE REACTIONS
CNS: *extrapyramidal reactions, tardive dyskinesia,* **seizures, neuroleptic malignant syndrome,** sedation, pseudoparkinsonism, dizziness, drowsiness.
CV: *orthostatic hypotension,* tachycardia, ECG changes.
EENT: *blurred vision,* ocular changes, nasal congestion.
GI: *dry mouth, constipation,* nausea, vomiting, diarrhea.
GU: *urine retention,* dark urine, menstrual irregularities, inhibited ejaculation.
Hematologic: *leukopenia, agranulocytosis, thrombocytopenia,* eosinophilia, hemolytic anemia.
Hepatic: cholestatic jaundice.
Metabolic: weight gain.
Skin: *mild photosensitivity reactions,* allergic reactions, sterile abscess.
Other: gynecomastia.

INTERACTIONS
Drug-drug. *Antacids:* May inhibit absorption of oral phenothiazines. Separate antacid and phenothiazine doses by at least 2 hours.
Barbiturates: May decrease phenothiazine effect. Monitor patient.
CNS depressants: May increase CNS depression. Use together cautiously.

Fluoxetine, paroxetine, sertraline, tricyclic antidepressants: May increase phenothiazine level. Monitor patient for increased adverse effects.

Lithium: May increase neurologic adverse effects. Monitor patient closely.

Drug-herb. *St. John's wort:* May cause photosensitivity reactions. Advise patient to avoid excessive sunlight exposure.

Drug-lifestyle. *Alcohol use:* May increase CNS depression, particularly psychomotor skills. Strongly discourage alcohol use.

Sun exposure: May increase risk of photosensitivity reactions. Advise patient to avoid excessive sunlight exposure.

EFFECTS ON LAB TEST RESULTS

● May decrease hemoglobin level and hematocrit.

● May increase liver function test values and eosinophil count. May decrease WBC, granulocyte, and platelet counts.

● May cause false-positive results for urinary porphyrin, urobilinogen, amylase, and 5-hydroxyindoleacetic acid tests and for urine pregnancy tests that use human chorionic gonadotropin.

CONTRAINDICATIONS & CAUTIONS

● Contraindicated in patients hypersensitive to drug and in those with CNS depression, blood dyscrasia, bone marrow depression, liver damage, or subcortical damage; also contraindicated in those experiencing coma or receiving large doses of CNS depressants.

● Use cautiously in elderly or debilitated patients and in those taking other CNS depressants or anticholinergics.

● Use cautiously in patients with alcohol withdrawal, psychotic depression, suicidal tendency, severe adverse reactions to other phenothiazines, renal impairment, CV disease, or respiratory disorders.

NURSING CONSIDERATIONS

● Obtain baseline blood pressure measurements before starting therapy and monitor pressure regularly. Watch for orthostatic hypotension, especially with parenteral administration.

● Monitor patient for tardive dyskinesia, which may occur after prolonged use. It may not appear until months or years later and may disappear spontaneously or persist for life, despite ending drug.

● *Alert:* Watch for evidence of neuroleptic malignant syndrome (extrapyramidal effects, hyperthermia, autonomic disturbance), which is rare but deadly.

● Monitor therapy with weekly bilirubin tests during 1st month, periodic blood tests (CBC and liver function tests), and ophthalmic tests (long-term use).

● Withhold dose and notify prescriber if jaundice, symptoms of blood dyscrasia (fever, sore throat, infection, cellulitis, weakness), or persistent extrapyramidal reactions (longer than a few hours) develop.

● Don't withdraw drug abruptly unless severe adverse reactions occur.

● After abrupt withdrawal of long-term therapy, gastritis, nausea, vomiting, dizziness, tremor, feeling of warmth or cold, diaphoresis, tachycardia, headache, or insomnia may occur.

PATIENT TEACHING

● Tell patient which beverages he may use to dilute oral concentrate.

● Warn patient to avoid activities that require alertness or good coordination until effects of drug are known. Drowsiness and dizziness usually subside after a few weeks.

● Tell patient to avoid alcohol while taking drug.

● Advise patient to report signs of urine retention or constipation.

● Tell patient to use sunblock and wear protective clothing to avoid oversensitivity to the sun.

● Advise patient to relieve dry mouth with sugarless gum or hard candy.

phenobarbital
(phenobarbitone)
fee-noe-BAR-bi-tal

Solfoton

phenobarbital sodium
Luminal Sodium

Pharmacologic class: barbiturate
Pregnancy risk category D
Controlled substance schedule IV

AVAILABLE FORMS
Elixir: 20 mg/5 ml*
Injection: 30 mg/ml, 60 mg/ml, 130 mg/ml
Tablets: 15 mg, 30 mg, 60 mg, 100 mg

INDICATIONS & DOSAGES
➤ **Anticonvulsant, febrile seizures**
Adults: 60 to 100 mg P.O. daily. For acute
seizures, 200 to 320 mg I.M. or I.V., repeat
in 6 hours as necessary.
Children: 3 to 6 mg/kg P.O. daily, usually
divided every 12 hours. Drug can be given
once daily, usually at bedtime. Or, 10 to
15 mg/kg daily I.V. or I.M.
➤ **Status epilepticus**
Adults: 200 to 600 mg I.V.
Children: 15 to 20 mg/kg I.V. over 10 to
15 minutes.
➤ **Sedation**
Adults: 30 to 120 mg P.O., I.V., or I.M.
daily in two or three divided doses. Maximum dose is 400 mg/24 hours.
Children: 8 to 32 mg P.O.
➤ **Short-term treatment of insomnia**
Adults: 100 to 200 mg P.O. or 100 to
320 mg I.M. or I.V. at bedtime.
➤ **Preoperative sedation**
Adults: 100 to 200 mg I.M. 60 to 90 min-
utes before surgery.
Children: 1 to 3 mg/kg I.V. or I.M. 60 to
90 minutes before surgery.
➤ **Prevention and treatment of
hyperbilirubinemia ◆**
Neonates: 7 mg/kg P.O. daily from days 1
to 5 of life. Or, 5 mg/kg I.M. on day 1 of
life, then 5 mg/kg P.O. on days 2 to 7 of
life.

➤ **To lower serum bilirubin or
serum lipid levels in the treatment of
chronic cholestasis ◆**
Adults: 90 to 180 mg P.O. daily in two or
three divided doses.
Children younger than age 12: 3 to 12 mg/
kg P.O. daily in two to three divided doses.

ADMINISTRATION
P.O.
• Give drug without regard for food.
I.V.
• I.V. route is used for emergency treat-
ment only.
• Dilute drug in half-normal or normal
saline, D_5W, lactated Ringer's, or Ringer's
solution.
• If solution contains precipitate, don't use.
• Give slowly (no more than 60 mg/
minute) under close supervision. Have
resuscitation equipment available.
• Monitor respirations closely.
• Inadvertent intra-arterial injection can
cause spasm of the artery and severe pain
and may lead to gangrene.
• Up to 30 minutes may be required for
maximum effect; allow time for anticonvulsant effect to develop to avoid overdose.
• **Incompatibilities:** Acidic solutions,
amphotericin B, chlorpromazine, dimenhydrinate, diphenhydramine, ephedrine,
hydralazine, hydrocortisone sodium succinate, hydromorphone, insulin, kanamycin,
levorphanol, meperidine, morphine, norepinephrine, pentazocine lactate, phenytoin,
prochlorperazine mesylate, promethazine
hydrochloride, ranitidine hydrochloride,
streptomycin, vancomycin.
I.M.
• Give I.M. injection deeply into large
muscles. Superficial injection may cause
pain, sterile abscess, and tissue sloughing.

ACTION
As a barbiturate, may depress CNS and
increase seizure threshold. As a sedative, may interfere with transmission of
impulses from thalamus to cortex of brain.

Route	Onset	Peak	Duration
P.O.	1 hr	8–12 hr	10–12 hr
I.V.	5 min	30 min	4–10 hr
I.M.	> 5 min	> 30 min	4–10 hr

Half-life: 5 to 7 days.

ADVERSE REACTIONS

CNS: *drowsiness, lethargy, hangover,* paradoxical excitement in elderly patients, somnolence, changes in EEG patterns, physical and psychological dependence, pain.
CV: *bradycardia,* hypotension, syncope.
GI: nausea, vomiting.
Hematologic: exacerbation of porphyria.
Respiratory: *respiratory depression, apnea.*
Skin: rash, *erythema multiforme, Stevens-Johnson syndrome,* urticaria, swelling, thrombophlebitis, necrosis, nerve injury at injection site.
Other: injection site pain, *angioedema.*

INTERACTIONS

Drug-drug. *Chloramphenicol, MAO inhibitors:* May potentiate barbiturate effect. Monitor patient for increased CNS and respiratory depression.
CNS depressants including opioid analgesics: Excessive CNS depression. Monitor patient closely.
Corticosteroids, doxycycline, estrogens and hormonal contraceptives, oral anticoagulants, tricyclic antidepressants: May enhance metabolism of these drugs. Watch for decreased effect.
Diazepam: May increase effects of both drugs. Use together cautiously.
Griseofulvin: May decrease absorption of griseofulvin. Monitor effectiveness of griseofulvin.
Mephobarbital, primidone: May cause excessive phenobarbital level. Monitor patient closely.
Metoprolol, propranolol: May reduce the effects of these drugs. Consider an increased beta-blocker dose.
Rifampin: May decrease barbiturate level. Watch for decreased effect.
Valproic acid: May increase phenobarbital level. Watch for toxicity.

Warfarin: May increase warfarin metabolism and decrease effect. Monitor patient for decreased warfarin effect.
Drug-herb. *Evening primrose oil:* May increase anticonvulsant dosage requirement. Discourage use together.
Drug-lifestyle. *Alcohol use:* May impair coordination, increase CNS effects, and lead to death. Strongly discourage use together.

EFFECTS ON LAB TEST RESULTS
● May decrease bilirubin level.
● May cause false-positive phentolamine test result.

CONTRAINDICATIONS & CAUTIONS
● Contraindicated in patients hypersensitive to barbiturates and in those with history of manifest or latent porphyria.
● Contraindicated in patients with hepatic or renal dysfunction, respiratory disease with dyspnea or obstruction, or nephritis.
● Use cautiously in patients with acute or chronic pain, depression, suicidal tendencies, history of drug abuse, fever, hyperthyroidism, diabetes mellitus, severe anemia, blood pressure alterations, CV disease, shock, or uremia, and in elderly or debilitated patients.

NURSING CONSIDERATIONS
● *Alert:* Watch for signs of barbiturate toxicity, such as coma, cyanosis, asthmatic breathing, clammy skin, and hypotension. Overdose can be fatal.
● Therapeutic level is 15 to 40 mcg/ml.
● Elderly patients are more sensitive to drug's effects; drug may produce paradoxical excitement.
● Don't stop drug abruptly because this may worsen seizures. Call prescriber immediately if adverse reactions develop.
● First withdrawal symptoms occur within 8 to 12 hours and include anxiety, muscle twitching, tremor of hands and fingers, progressive weakness, dizziness, visual distortion, nausea, vomiting, insomnia, and orthostatic hypotension. Seizures and delirium may occur within 16 hours and last up to 5 days after abruptly stopping drug.

- Use for insomnia isn't recommended, and treatment shouldn't last longer than 14 days.
- Some products contain tartrazine; use cautiously in patients with aspirin sensitivity.
- EEG patterns show a change in low-voltage fast activity. Changes persist after therapy ends.
- Drug may decrease bilirubin level in neonates, patients with epilepsy, and those with congenital nonhemolytic, unconjugated hyperbilirubinemia.
- The physiologic effects of drug may impair the absorption of cyanocobalamin Co 57.
- *Look alike–sound alike:* Don't confuse phenobarbital with pentobarbital.

PATIENT TEACHING

- Ensure that patient is aware that drug is available in different milligram strengths and sizes. Advise him to check prescription and refills closely.
- Inform patient that full therapeutic effects aren't seen for 2 to 3 weeks, except when loading dose is used.
- Advise patient to avoid driving and other potentially hazardous activities that require mental alertness until drug's CNS effects are known.
- Warn patient and parents not to stop drug abruptly.
- Tell woman using hormonal contraceptives to consider a nonhormonal form of birth control because drug may decrease effectiveness.

physostigmine salicylate (eserine salicylate)
fis-oh-STIG-meen

Antilirium

Pharmacologic class: cholinesterase inhibitor
Pregnancy risk category C

AVAILABLE FORMS
Injection: 1 mg/ml

INDICATIONS & DOSAGES
➤ **Reversal of drug-induced anti-cholinergic effects**
Adults: 0.5 to 2 mg slow I.V. or I.M. not to exceed 1 mg/minute I.V. repeated every 20 minutes as needed until patient responds or develops adverse cholinergic effects. Give additional 1 to 4 mg I.V. or I.M. every 30 to 60 minutes if life-threatening problems, such as coma, seizures, and arrhythmias, recur.
Children: Only for life-threatening situations. Give 0.02 mg/kg I.M. or slow I.V. at 0.5 mg/minute or slower, and repeat every 5 to 10 minutes until patient responds, adverse anticholinergic reactions develop, or a total dose of 2 mg has been given. Or, give 0.03 mg/kg or 0.9 mg/m^2, as needed.

ADMINISTRATION
I.V.
- Use only clear solution. Darkening may indicate loss of potency.
- Position patient to ease breathing. Keep atropine injection available.
- Give drug at controlled rate; use direct injection at no more than 1 mg/minute in adults or 0.5 mg/minute in children.
- Monitor vital signs frequently, especially respirations. Provide respiratory support, as needed.
- **Incompatibilities:** None reported.
I.M.
- Use only clear solution. Darkening may indicate loss of potency.

ACTION
Inhibits acetylcholinesterase, blocking destruction of acetylcholine from the parasympathetic and somatic efferent nerves. Acetylcholine accumulates, promoting increased stimulation of the receptors.

Route	Onset	Peak	Duration
I.V.	3–5 min	5 min	45 min–1 hr
I.M.	3–5 min	20–30 min	45 min–1 hr

Half-life: 1 to 2 hours.

ADVERSE REACTIONS
CNS: *restlessness, excitability,* **seizures,** muscle weakness.

Reactions may be *common,* uncommon, *life-threatening,* or COMMON AND LIFE-THREATENING.
Interaction may have a *rapid onset* or **delayed onset.**

CV: *bradycardia,* hypotension, palpitations, irregular pulse.
EENT: miosis, lacrimation.
GI: *diarrhea, excessive salivation,* nausea, vomiting, epigastric pain.
GU: urinary urgency.
Respiratory: *bronchospasm, bronchial constriction, respiratory paralysis,* dyspnea.
Skin: diaphoresis.

INTERACTIONS
Drug-drug. *Anticholinergics, atropine, local and general anesthetics, procainamide, quinidine:* May reverse cholinergic effects. Observe patient for lack of drug effect.
Ganglionic blockers: May decrease blood pressure. Avoid using together.
Neuromuscular blockers (succinylcholine): May increase neuromuscular blockade, respiratory depression. Use together cautiously.
Drug-herb. *Jaborandi tree, pill-bearing spurge:* May have additive effect. Ask patient about use of herbal remedies, and advise caution.

EFFECTS ON LAB TEST RESULTS
None reported.

CONTRAINDICATIONS & CAUTIONS
• Contraindicated in patients with mechanical obstruction of the intestine or urogenital tract; in patients with asthma, gangrene, diabetes, CV disease, or vagotonia; and in patients receiving choline esters or depolarizing neuromuscular blockers.
• Use cautiously in pregnant patients and those with epilepsy, parkinsonism, or bradycardia.

NURSING CONSIDERATIONS
• *Alert:* Watch closely for adverse reactions, particularly CNS disturbances. Raise side rails of bed if patient becomes restless or hallucinates. Adverse reactions may indicate drug toxicity.
• Effectiveness is typically immediate and dramatic but may be short-lived. Patient may need repeated dosages.
• Drug contains benzyl alcohol and has been associated with fatal "gasping syndrome" in premature infants.

• Drug contains sulfites, which may cause an allergic reaction in susceptible people.

PATIENT TEACHING
• Inform patient of need for drug, explain its use and adverse reactions, and answer any questions or concerns.
• Tell patient to report adverse reactions promptly.
• Instruct patient to report discomfort at I.V. site.

prochlorperazine
proe-klor-PER-a-zeen

Compazine, Compro

prochlorperazine edisylate
Compazine, Compazine Syrup

prochlorperazine maleate
Compazine, Compazine Spansule, Nu-Prochlor†

Pharmacologic class: dopamine antagonist
Pregnancy risk category C

AVAILABLE FORMS
prochlorperazine
Injection: 5 mg/ml
Suppositories: 2.5 mg, 5 mg, 25 mg
Tablets: 5 mg, 10 mg
prochlorperazine edisylate
Injection: 5 mg/ml
Syrup: 5 mg/5 ml
prochlorperazine maleate
Capsules (extended-release): 10 mg, 15 mg, 30 mg
Tablets: 5 mg, 10 mg, 25 mg

INDICATIONS & DOSAGES
➤ To control preoperative nausea
Adults: 5 to 10 mg I.M. 1 to 2 hours before induction of anesthesia; repeat once in 30 minutes, if needed. Or, 5 to 10 mg I.V. 15 to 30 minutes before induction of anesthesia; repeat once, if needed.
➤ Severe nausea and vomiting
Adults: 5 to 10 mg P.O., t.i.d. or q.i.d.; 15 mg sustained-release form P.O. on rising; 10 mg sustained-release form P.O. every 12 hours; 25 mg P.R., b.i.d.; or 5 to

10 mg I.M., repeated every 3 to 4 hours, as needed. Maximum I.M. dose is 40 mg daily. Or, 2.5 to 10 mg I.V. at no more than 5 mg/minute.

Children who weigh 18 to 39 kg (39 to 86 lb): 2.5 mg P.O. or P.R., t.i.d.; or 5 mg P.O. or P.R., b.i.d. Maximum, 15 mg daily. Or, 0.132 mg/kg by deep I.M. injection. Control is usually achieved with one dose.

Children who weigh 14 to 17 kg (30 to 38 lb): 2.5 mg P.O. or P.R., b.i.d. or t.i.d. Maximum, 10 mg daily. Or, 0.132 mg/kg by deep I.M. injection. Control is usually achieved with one dose.

Children who weigh 9 to 13 kg (20 to 29 lb): 2.5 mg P.O. or P.R. once daily or b.i.d. Maximum, 7.5 mg daily. Or, 0.132 mg/kg by deep I.M. injection. Control is usually achieved with one dose.

➤ **To manage symptoms of psychotic disorders**
Adults and children age 12 and older: 5 to 10 mg P.O., t.i.d. or q.i.d.
Children ages 2 to 12: Give 2.5 mg P.O. or P.R., b.i.d. or t.i.d. Don't exceed 10 mg on day 1. Increase dosage gradually to maximum, if needed. In children ages 2 to 5, maximum is 20 mg daily. In children ages 6 to 12, maximum is 25 mg daily.

➤ **To manage symptoms of severe psychosis**
Adults and children age 12 and older: 10 to 20 mg I.M., repeated in 1 to 4 hours, if needed. Rarely, patients may receive 10 to 20 mg every 4 to 6 hours. Start oral therapy after symptoms are controlled.
Children ages 2 to 12: Give 0.13 mg/kg I.M.

➤ **Nonpsychotic anxiety**
Adults: 5 to 10 mg P.O., t.i.d., or q.i.d. Or, 15 mg extended-release capsule once daily. Or, 10 mg extended-release capsule every 12 hours. Don't exceed 20 mg daily, and don't give for longer than 12 weeks.

ADMINISTRATION
P.O.
● Dilute oral solution with tomato juice, fruit juice, milk, coffee, carbonated beverage, tea, water, or soup. Or, mix with pudding.
● To prevent contact dermatitis, avoid getting concentrate solution on hands or clothing.

I.V.
● Add 20 mg of drug per liter of D_5W and normal saline solution, 15 to 30 minutes before induction of anesthesia.
● Infuse slowly; rate shouldn't exceed 5 mg/minute. Maximum parenteral dose is 40 mg daily.
● To prevent contact dermatitis, avoid getting injection solution on hands or clothing.
● **Incompatibilities:** Aldesleukin, allopurinol, amifostine, aminophylline, amphotericin B, ampicillin sodium, aztreonam, calcium gluconate, chloramphenicol sodium succinate, chlorothiazide, dexamethasone sodium phosphate, dimenhydrinate, etoposide, filgrastim, fludarabine, foscarnet, furosemide, gemcitabine, heparin sodium, hydrocortisone sodium succinate, hydromorphone, ketorolac, solutions containing methylparabens, midazolam hydrochloride, morphine, penicillin G potassium, penicillin G sodium, pentobarbital, phenobarbital sodium, phenytoin sodium, piperacillin sodium and tazobactam sodium, solutions containing propylparabens, thiopental, vitamin B complex with C.

I.M.
● For I.M. use, inject deeply into upper outer quadrant of gluteal region.
● Don't give by subcutaneous route or mix in syringe with another drug.
● To prevent contact dermatitis, avoid getting injection solution on hands or clothing.
● Store in light-resistant container. Slight yellowing doesn't affect potency; discard extremely discolored solutions.

Rectal
● Protect from light.

ACTION
Acts on the chemoreceptor trigger zone to inhibit nausea and vomiting; in larger doses, it partially depresses vomiting center.

Route	Onset	Peak	Duration
P.O.	30–40 min	Unknown	3–12 hr
P.O. (extended-release)	30–40 min	Unknown	10–12 hr
I.V.	Unknown	Unknown	Unknown
I.M.	10–20 min	Unknown	3–4 hr
P.R.	1 hr	Unknown	3–4 hr

Half-life: Unknown.

ADVERSE REACTIONS
CNS: *extrapyramidal reactions,* dizziness, EEG changes, pseudoparkinsonism, sedation.
CV: *orthostatic hypotension,* ECG changes, tachycardia.
EENT: *blurred vision, ocular changes.*
GI: *constipation, dry mouth,* increased appetite.
GU: *urine retention,* dark urine, inhibited ejaculation, menstrual irregularities.
Hematologic: *agranulocytosis, transient leukopenia.*
Hepatic: cholestatic jaundice.
Metabolic: weight gain.
Skin: *mild photosensitivity reactions,* allergic reactions, exfoliative dermatitis.
Other: gynecomastia, hyperprolactinemia.

INTERACTIONS
Drug-drug. *Antacids:* May inhibit absorption of oral phenothiazines. Separate antacid and phenothiazine doses by at least 2 hours.
Anticholinergics, including antidepressants and antiparkinsonians: May increase anticholinergic activity and may aggravate parkinsonian symptoms. Use together cautiously.
Barbiturates: May decrease phenothiazine effect. Monitor patient for decreased antiemetic effect.
Drug-herb. *Dong quai, St. John's wort:* May increase risk of photosensitivity. Advise patient to avoid excessive sun exposure.
Kava: May increase risk of dystonic reactions. Discourage use together.
Drug-lifestyle. *Alcohol use:* May increase CNS depression, particularly psychomotor skills. Strongly discourage use together.

EFFECTS ON LAB TEST RESULTS
● May decrease WBC and granulocyte counts.
● May cause false-positive results for urinary porphyrins, urobilinogen, amylase, and 5-hydroxyindoleacetic acid, and false-positive results in urine pregnancy tests using human chorionic gonadotropin. May cause abnormal liver function test results.

CONTRAINDICATIONS & CAUTIONS
● Contraindicated in patients hypersensitive to phenothiazines and in patients with CNS depression, including those in a coma.
● Contraindicated during pediatric surgery, when using spinal or epidural anesthetic or adrenergic blockers, and in children younger than age 2.
● Use cautiously in patients with impaired CV function, glaucoma, seizure disorders, and Parkinson disease; in those who have been exposed to extreme heat; and in children with acute illness.

NURSING CONSIDERATIONS
● Watch for orthostatic hypotension, especially when giving drug I.V.
● Monitor CBC and liver function studies during long-term therapy.
● *Alert:* Use drug only when vomiting can't be controlled by other measures or when only a few doses are needed. If more than four doses are needed in 24 hours, notify prescriber.

PATIENT TEACHING
● Teach patient what to use to dilute oral solution.
● Advise patient to wear protective clothing when exposed to sunlight.
● Tell patient to call prescriber if more than four doses are needed within 24 hours.

promethazine hydrochloride
proe-METH-a-zeen

Phenadoz, Phenergan*

Pharmacologic class: phenothiazine
Pregnancy risk category C

AVAILABLE FORMS
Injection: 25 mg/ml, 50 mg/ml
Suppositories: 12.5 mg, 25 mg, 50 mg
Syrup: 6.25 mg/5 ml*
Tablets: 12.5 mg, 25 mg, 50 mg

INDICATIONS & DOSAGES
➤ **Motion sickness**
Adults: 25 mg P.O. or P.R. taken 30 minutes to 1 hour before departure. May repeat dose 8 to 12 hours later p.r.n.
Children older than age 2: 12.5 to 25 mg or 0.5 mg/kg P.O. or P.R. 30 minutes to 1 hour before departure. May repeat dose 8 to 12 hours later p.r.n.
➤ **Nausea and vomiting**
Adults: 12.5 to 25 mg P.O., I.M., or P.R. every 4 to 6 hours p.r.n.
Children older than age 2: Give 12.5 to 25 mg P.O. or P.R. every 4 to 6 hours p.r.n. Or, 6.25 to 12.5 mg I.M. every 4 to 6 hours p.r.n.
➤ **Rhinitis, allergy symptoms**
Adults: 25 mg P.O. or P.R. at bedtime; or, 12.5 mg P.O. or P.R. t.i.d. and at bedtime.
Children older than age 2: Give 25 mg P.O. or P.R. at bedtime; or, 6.25 to 12.5 mg P.O. or P.R. t.i.d. Alternatively, 0.5 mg/kg at bedtime or 0.125 mg/kg p.r.n.
➤ **Nighttime sedation**
Adults: 25 to 50 mg P.O., I.V., I.M., or P.R. at bedtime.
Children older than age 2: Give 12.5 to 25 mg P.O., I.M., or P.R. at bedtime.
➤ **Adjunct to analgesics for routine preoperative or postoperative sedation**
Adults: 25 to 50 mg I.V., I.M., P.O. or P.R.
Children older than age 2: Give 0.5 to 1.1 mg/kg P.O., I.M., or P.R.

ADMINISTRATION
P.O.
• Reduce GI distress by giving drug with food or milk.

I.V.
• If solution is discolored or contains a precipitate, discard.
• Give injection through a free-flowing I.V. line.
• Don't give at a concentration above 25 mg/ml or a rate above 25 mg/minute.
• **Incompatibilities:** Aldesleukin, allopurinol, aminophylline, amphotericin B, cephalosporins, chloramphenicol sodium succinate, chloroquine phosphate, chlorothiazide, diatrizoate, dimenhydrinate, doxorubicin liposomal, foscarnet, furosemide, heparin sodium, hydrocortisone sodium succinate, iodipamide meglumine (52%), iothalamate, ketorolac, methohexital, morphine, nalbuphine, penicillin G potassium and sodium, pentobarbital sodium, phenobarbital sodium, phenytoin sodium, thiopental, vitamin B complex.
I.M.
• I.M. injection is the preferred parenteral route. Inject deep I.M. into large muscle mass. Rotate injection sites.
• Don't give subcutaneously.
Rectal
• If suppository is too soft, place wrapped in refrigerator for 15 minutes or run under cold water.

ACTION
Phenothiazine derivative that competes with histamine for H_1-receptor sites on effector cells. Prevents, but doesn't reverse, histamine-mediated responses. At high doses, drug also has local anesthetic effects.

Route	Onset	Peak	Duration
P.O.	15–60 min	Unknown	< 12 hr
I.V.	3–5 min	Unknown	< 12 hr
I.M., P.R.	20 min	Unknown	< 12 hr

Half-life: Unknown.

ADVERSE REACTIONS
CNS: *drowsiness, sedation,* confusion, sleepiness, dizziness, disorientation, extrapyramidal symptoms.
CV: hypotension, hypertension.
EENT: *dry mouth,* blurred vision.
GI: nausea, vomiting.
GU: urine retention.

Reactions may be *common*, uncommon, *life-threatening*, or COMMON AND LIFE-THREATENING.
Interaction may have a *rapid onset* or *delayed onset*.

Hematologic: *leukopenia, agranulocytosis, thrombocytopenia.*
Metabolic: hyperglycemia.
Respiratory: *respiratory depression, apnea.*
Skin: photosensitivity, rash.

INTERACTIONS
Drug-drug. *Anticholinergics, tricyclic antidepressants:* May increase anticholinergic effects. Avoid using together.
CNS depressants: May increase sedation. Use together cautiously. If used together, reduce opiate dose by at least 25% to 50%, and reduce barbiturate dose by at least 50%.
Epinephrine: May block or reverse effects of epinephrine. Use other pressor drugs instead.
Levodopa: May decrease antiparkinsonian action of levodopa. Avoid using together.
Lithium: May reduce GI absorption or enhance renal elimination of lithium. Avoid using together.
MAO inhibitors: May increase extrapyramidal effects. Avoid using together.
Quinolones: May cause life-threatening arrhythmias. Avoid using together.
Drug-herb. *Yohimbe:* May increase risk of herb toxicity. Ask patient about use of herbal remedies, and recommend caution.
Drug-lifestyle. *Alcohol use:* May increase sedation. Discourage use together.
Sun exposure: May cause photosensitivity reactions. Advise patient to avoid extensive sunlight exposure and to use sunblock.

EFFECTS ON LAB TEST RESULTS
● May increase hemoglobin level and hematocrit.
● May decrease WBC, platelet, and granulocyte counts.
● May prevent, reduce, or mask positive result in diagnostic skin test. May cause false-positive or false-negative pregnancy test result. May interfere with blood grouping in the ABO system.

CONTRAINDICATIONS & CAUTIONS
● Contraindicated in patients hypersensitive to drug, those who have experienced adverse reactions to phenothiazines, breast-feeding women, children younger

than age 2, comatose patients, and acutely ill or dehydrated children.
● Use cautiously in patients with asthma or pulmonary, hepatic, or CV disease and in those with intestinal obstruction, prostatic hyperplasia, bladder-neck obstruction, angle-closure glaucoma, seizure disorders, CNS depression, and stenosing or peptic ulcerations.

NURSING CONSIDERATIONS
● Monitor patient for neuroleptic malignant syndrome: altered mental status, autonomic instability, muscle rigidity, and hyperpyrexia.
● Stop drug 4 days before diagnostic skin testing because antihistamines can prevent, reduce, or mask positive skin test response.
● Drug is used as an adjunct to analgesics, usually to increase sedation; it has no analgesic activity.
● Drug may be mixed with meperidine in same syringe.
● In patients scheduled for a myelogram, stop drug 48 hours before procedure. Don't resume drug until 24 hours after procedure because of the risk of seizures.

PATIENT TEACHING
● Tell patient to take oral form with food or milk.
● When treating motion sickness, tell patient to take first dose 30 to 60 minutes before travel; dose may be repeated in 8 to 12 hours, if necessary. On succeeding days of travel, patient should take dose upon arising and with evening meal.
● Warn patient to avoid alcohol and hazardous activities that require alertness until CNS effects of drug are known.
● Inform patient that sugarless gum, hard candy, or ice chips may relieve dry mouth.
● Warn patient about possible photosensitivity reactions. Advise use of a sunblock.

SAFETY ALERT!

propofol
PRO-puh-fole

Diprivan

Pharmacologic class: phenol
derivative
Pregnancy risk category B

AVAILABLE FORMS
Injection: 10 mg/ml in 20-ml ampules;
50-ml prefilled syringes; 50-ml and 100-ml
infusion vials

INDICATIONS & DOSAGES
➤ **To induce anesthesia**
*Adults younger than age 55 classified as
American Society of Anesthesiologists
(ASA) Physical Status (PS) category I or
II:* Give 2 to 2.5 mg/kg. Give in 40-mg
boluses every 10 seconds until desired
response is achieved.
*Children ages 3 to 16 classified as ASA
I or II:* Give 2.5 to 3.5 mg/kg over 20 to
30 seconds.
Adjust-a-dose: In geriatric, debilitated,
hypovolemic, or ASA PS III or IV patients,
give half the usual induction dose, in
20-mg boluses, every 10 seconds. For
cardiac anesthesia, give 20 mg (0.5 to
1.5 mg/kg) every 10 seconds until desired
response is achieved. For neurosurgical patients, give 20 mg (1 to 2 mg/kg) every
10 seconds until desired response is
achieved.
➤ **To maintain anesthesia**
Healthy adults younger than age 55: Give
0.1 to 0.2 mg/kg/minute (6 to 12 mg/kg/
hour). Or, give in 20- to 50-mg intermittent
boluses, p.r.n.
*Healthy children ages 2 months to 16
years:* Give 125 to 300 mcg/kg/minute (7.5
to 18 mg/kg/hour).
Adjust-a-dose: In geriatric, debilitated,
hypovolemic, or ASA PS III or IV patients,
give half the usual maintenance dose (0.05
to 0.1 mg/kg/minute or 3 to 6 mg/kg/hour).
For cardiac anesthesia with secondary
opioid, 100 to 150 mcg/kg/minute; low
dose with primary opioid, 50 to 100 mcg/
kg/minute. For neurosurgical patients,
100 to 200 mcg/kg/minute (6 to 12 mg/
kg/hour).
➤ **Monitored anesthesia care**
Healthy adults younger than age 55:
Initially, 100 to 150 mcg/kg/minute (6
to 9 mg/kg/hour) for 3 to 5 minutes or
a slow injection of 0.5 mg/kg over 3 to
5 minutes. For maintenance dose, give
infusion of 25 to 75 mcg/kg/minute (1.5
to 4.5 mg/kg/hour), or incremental 10- or
20-mg boluses.
Adjust-a-dose: In geriatric, debilitated, or
ASA PS III or IV patients, give 80% of
usual adult maintenance dose. Don't use
rapid bolus.
➤ **To sedate intubated intensive care
unit (ICU) patients**
Adults: Initially, 5 mcg/kg/minute (0.3 mg/
kg/hour) for 5 minutes. Increments of 5 to
10 mcg/kg/minute (0.3 to 0.6 mg/kg/hour)
over 5 to 10 minutes may be used until
desired sedation is achieved. Maintenance
rate, 5 to 50 mcg/kg/minute (0.3 to 3
mg/kg/hour).

ADMINISTRATION
I.V.
● Maintain sterile technique when handling
the solution. Drug can support the growth
of microorganisms; don't use if solution
might be contaminated.
● Protect drug from light. Shake well.
● Dilute only with D_5W. Don't dilute to
less than 2 mg/ml.
● Don't use if emulsion shows evidence of
separation.
● Don't infuse through a filter with a pore
size smaller than 5 microns. Give via
larger veins in arms to decrease injection
site pain.
● Titrate drug daily to maintain minimum
effective level. Allow 3 to 5 minutes
between dosage adjustments to assess
effects.
● Discard tubing and unused portions of
drug after 12 hours.
● **Incompatibilities:** Other I.V. drugs,
blood and plasma.

Reactions may be *common,* uncommon, ***life-threatening***, or COMMON AND LIFE-THREATENING.
Interaction may have a *rapid onset* or ***delayed onset***.

ACTION

Unknown. Rapid-acting I.V. sedative-hypnotic.

Route	Onset	Peak	Duration
I.V.	< 40 sec	Unknown	10–15 min

Half-life: Initial (distribution) phase, about 2 to 10 minutes; second (redistribution) phase, 21 to 70 minutes; terminal (elimination) phase, 1½ to 31 hours.

ADVERSE REACTIONS

CNS: dystonic or choreiform movement.
CV: *bradycardia,* *hypotension,* hypertension, decreased cardiac output.
Metabolic: hyperlipemia.
Respiratory: APNEA, *respiratory acidosis.*
Skin: rash.
Other: *burning or stinging at injection site.*

INTERACTIONS

Drug-drug. *Inhaled anesthetics (such as enflurane, halothane, isoflurane), opioids (alfentanil, fentanyl, meperidine, morphine), sedatives (such as barbiturates, benzodiazepines, chloral hydrate, droperidol):* May increase anesthetic and sedative effects and further decrease blood pressure and cardiac output. Monitor patient closely.
Drug-herb. *St. John's wort:* May prolong anesthetic effects. Advise patient to stop using herb 5 days before surgery.

EFFECTS ON LAB TEST RESULTS

• May increase lipid levels.

CONTRAINDICATIONS & CAUTIONS

• Contraindicated in patients hypersensitive to drug or its components (including egg lecithin, soybean oil, and glycerol), in pregnant women (because it may cause fetal depression), and in those unable to undergo general anesthesia or sedation.
• Use cautiously in patients who are hemodynamically unstable or who have seizures, disorders of lipid metabolism, or increased intracranial pressure.
• Because drug appears in breast milk, avoid using in breast-feeding women.

NURSING CONSIDERATIONS

• If drug is used for prolonged sedation in ICU, urine may turn green.
• For general anesthesia or monitored anesthesia care sedation, trained staff not involved in the surgical or diagnostic procedure should give drug. For ICU sedation, persons skilled in managing critically ill patients and trained in cardiopulmonary resuscitation and airway management should give drug.
• Continuously monitor vital signs.
• *Alert:* The FDA issued an alert after receiving reports of chills, fever, and body aches in several clusters of patients shortly after patients received propofol for sedation or general anesthesia. Various lots of the drug were tested, but no toxins, bacteria, or other signs of contamination were found. The FDA advises all health care providers to carefully follow the handling and use sections of the prescribing information for this drug. They recommend that all patients be evaluated for possible reactions following use of the drug, and that anyone experiencing signs of acute febrile reactions be evaluated for possible bacterial sepsis. They ask that any adverse events following the use of propofol be reported to MedWatch.
• Monitor patient at risk for hyperlipidemia for elevated triglyceride levels.
• Drug contains 0.1 g of fat (1.1 kcal)/ml. Reduce other lipid products if given together.
• Drug contains ethylenediaminetetraacetic acid, a strong metal chelator. Consider supplemental zinc during prolonged therapy.
• When giving drug in the ICU, assess patient's CNS function daily to determine minimum dose needed.
• Stop drug gradually to prevent abrupt awakening and increased agitation.
• *Look alike–sound alike:* Don't confuse Diprivan with Ditropan or Dipivefrin.

PATIENT TEACHING

• Advise patient that performance of activities requiring mental alertness may be impaired for some time after drug use.

SAFETY ALERT!

propranolol hydrochloride
proe-PRAN-oh-lol

Inderal, Inderal LA, InnoPran XL, Novopranol†

Pharmacologic class: beta blocker
Pregnancy risk category C

AVAILABLE FORMS
Capsules (extended-release): 60 mg, 80 mg, 120 mg, 160 mg
Injection: 1 mg/ml
Oral solution: 4 mg/ml, 8 mg/ml, 80 mg/ml (concentrate)
Tablets: 10 mg, 20 mg, 40 mg, 60 mg, 80 mg, 90 mg

INDICATIONS & DOSAGES
➤ **Angina pectoris**
Adults: Total daily doses of 80 to 320 mg P.O. when given b.i.d., t.i.d., or q.i.d. Or, one 80-mg extended-release capsule daily. Dosage increased at 3- to 7-day intervals.
➤ **To decrease risk of death after MI**
Adults: 180 to 240 mg P.O. daily in divided doses beginning 5 to 21 days after MI has occurred. Usually given t.i.d. or q.i.d.
➤ **Supraventricular, ventricular, and atrial arrhythmias; tachyarrhythmias caused by excessive catecholamine action during anesthesia, hyperthyroidism, or pheochromocytoma**
Adults: 1 to 3 mg by slow I.V. push, not to exceed 1 mg/minute. After 3 mg have been given, another dose may be given in 2 minutes; subsequent doses, no sooner than every 4 hours. Usual maintenance dose is 10 to 30 mg P.O. t.i.d. or q.i.d.
➤ **Hypertension**
Adults: Initially, 80 mg P.O. daily in two divided doses or extended-release form once daily. Increase at 3- to 7-day intervals to maximum daily dose of 640 mg. Usual maintenance dose is 120 to 240 mg daily or 120 to 160 mg daily as extended-release. For InnoPran XL, dose is 80 mg P.O. once daily at bedtime. Give consistently with or without food. Adjust to maximum of 120 mg daily if needed. Full effects are seen in about 2 to 3 weeks.
Children: 0.5 mg/kg (conventional tablets) P.O. b.i.d. Increase every 3 to 5 days to a maximum dose of 16 mg/kg daily. Usual dose is 2 to 4 mg/kg daily in two equally divided doses.
➤ **To prevent frequent, severe, uncontrollable, or disabling migraine or vascular headache**
Adults: Initially, 80 mg P.O. daily in divided doses or 1 extended-release capsule daily. Usual maintenance dose is 160 to 240 mg daily, t.i.d. or q.i.d.
➤ **Essential tremor**
Adults: 40 mg (tablets or oral solution) P.O. b.i.d. Usual maintenance dose is 120 to 320 mg daily in three divided doses.
➤ **Hypertrophic subaortic stenosis**
Adults: 20 to 40 mg P.O. t.i.d. or q.i.d.; or 80 to 160 mg extended-release capsules once daily.
➤ **Adjunct therapy in pheochromocytoma**
Adults: 60 mg P.O. daily in divided doses with an alpha blocker 3 days before surgery.

ADMINISTRATION
P.O.
• Give drug consistently with meals. Food may increase absorption of propranolol.
• Compliance may be improved by giving drug twice daily or as extended-release capsules. Check with prescriber.
• Check blood pressure and apical pulse before giving drug. If hypotension or extremes in pulse rate occur, withhold drug and notify prescriber.
I.V.
• For direct injection, give into a large vessel or into the tubing of a free-flowing, compatible I.V. solution; don't give by continuous I.V. infusion.
• Drug is compatible with D_5W, half-normal saline solution, normal saline solution, and lactated Ringer solution.
• Infusion rate shouldn't exceed 1 mg/minute.
• Double-check dose and route. I.V. doses are much smaller than oral doses.
• Monitor blood pressure, ECG, central venous pressure, and heart rate and rhythm frequently, especially during I.V. administration. If patient develops severe

hypotension, notify prescriber; a vasopressor may be prescribed.
● For overdose, give I.V. isoproterenol, I.V. atropine, or glucagon; refractory cases may require a pacemaker.
● **Incompatibilities:** Amphotericin B, diazoxide.

ACTION
Reduces cardiac oxygen demand by blocking catecholamine-induced increases in heart rate, blood pressure, and force of myocardial contraction. Drug depresses renin secretion and prevents vasodilation of cerebral arteries.

Route	Onset	Peak	Duration
P.O.	30 min	60–90 min	12 hr
P.O. (extended)	Unknown	6–14 hr	24 hr
I.V.	Immediate	1 min	5 min

Half-life: About 4 hours; 8 hours for InnoPran XL.

ADVERSE REACTIONS
CNS: *fatigue, lethargy,* fever, vivid dreams, hallucinations, mental depression, light-headedness, dizziness, insomnia.
CV: hypotension, **bradycardia, heart failure, intensification of AV block,** intermittent claudication.
GI: abdominal cramping, constipation, diarrhea, nausea, vomiting.
Hematologic: *agranulocytosis.*
Respiratory: *bronchospasm.*
Skin: rash.

INTERACTIONS
Drug-drug. *Aminophylline:* May antagonize beta-blocking effects of propranolol. Use together cautiously.
Cardiac glycosides: May reduce the positive inotrope effect of the glycoside. Monitor patient for clinical effect.
Cimetidine: May inhibit metabolism of propranolol. Watch for increased beta-blocking effect.
Diltiazem, verapamil: May cause hypotension, bradycardia, and increased depressant effect on myocardium. Use together cautiously.
Epinephrine: May cause severe vasoconstriction. Monitor blood pressure and observe patient carefully.

Glucagon, isoproterenol: May antagonize propranolol effect. May be used therapeutically and in emergencies.
Haloperidol: May cause cardiac arrest. Avoid using together.
Insulin, oral antidiabetics: May alter requirements for these drugs in previously stabilized diabetics. Monitor patient for hypoglycemia.
Phenothiazines (chlorpromazine, thioridazine): May increase risk of serious adverse reactions of either drug. Use with thioridazine is contraindicated. If chlorpromazine must be used, monitor patient's pulse and blood pressure; decrease propranolol dose as needed.
Propafenone: May increase propranolol level. Monitor cardiac function, and adjust propranolol dose as needed.
Drug-herb. *Betel palm:* May decrease temperature-elevating effects and enhanced CNS effects. Discourage use together.
Ma huang: May decrease antihypertensive effects. Discourage use together.
Drug-lifestyle. *Alcohol:* May increase propranolol level. Discourage alcohol use.
Cocaine use: May increase angina-inducing potential of cocaine. Inform patient of this interaction.

EFFECTS ON LAB TEST RESULTS
● May increase BUN, transaminase, alkaline phosphatase, potassium, and LDH levels.
● May decrease granulocyte count.

CONTRAINDICATIONS & CAUTIONS
● Contraindicated in patients with bronchial asthma, sinus bradycardia and heart block greater than first-degree, cardiogenic shock, and overt and decompensated heart failure (unless failure is secondary to a tachyarrhythmia that can be treated with propranolol).
● Use cautiously in patients with hepatic or renal impairment, nonallergic bronchospastic diseases, or hepatic disease and in those taking other antihypertensives.
● Use cautiously in patients who have diabetes mellitus because drug masks some symptoms of hypoglycemia.

• In patients with thyrotoxicosis, use drug cautiously because it may mask the signs and symptoms.
• Elderly patients may experience enhanced adverse reactions and may need dosage adjustment.
• Use cautiously in pregnant women because drug may be associated with small placenta and congenital anomalies.

NURSING CONSIDERATIONS
• Drug masks common signs and symptoms of shock and hypoglycemia.
• *Alert:* Don't stop drug before surgery for pheochromocytoma. Before any surgical procedure, tell anesthesiologist that patient is receiving propranolol.
• *Look alike–sound alike:* Don't confuse propranolol with Pravachol. Don't confuse Inderal with Inderide, Isordil, Adderall, or Imuran.

PATIENT TEACHING
• Caution patient to continue taking this drug as prescribed, even when he's feeling well.
• Instruct patient to take drug with food.
• *Alert:* Tell patient not to stop drug suddenly because this can worsen chest pain and trigger a heart attack.

---

quetiapine fumarate
kwe-TIE-ah-peen

Seroquel, Seroquel XR

Pharmacologic class:
dibenzothiazepine derivative
Pregnancy risk category C

AVAILABLE FORMS
Tablets: 25 mg, 50 mg, 100 mg, 200 mg, 300 mg
Tablets (extended-release): 200 mg, 300 mg, 400 mg

INDICATIONS & DOSAGES
➤ **Schizophrenia**
Adults: Initially, 25 mg P.O. b.i.d., with increases in increments of 25 to 50 mg b.i.d. or t.i.d. on days 2 and 3, as tolerated. Target range is 300 to 400 mg daily divided into two or three doses by day 4. Further

dosage adjustments, if indicated, should occur at intervals of not less than 2 days. Dosage can be increased or decreased by 25 to 50 mg b.i.d. Effect generally occurs at 150 to 750 mg daily. Safety of dosages over 800 mg daily hasn't been evaluated.
   Or, 300 mg/day extended-release tablets P.O. once daily, preferably in the evening. Titrate within a dose range of 400 to 800 mg/day, depending on the response and tolerance of the individual. Increase at intervals as short as 1 day and in increments of 300 mg/day.
Adjust-a-dose: Elderly patients: Titrate on immediate-release formula, starting at 25 mg/day. Use slow titration and regular monitoring; may be switched to extended-release formulation when stabilized on 200 mg/day. In patients with hepatic impairment, initial dose is 25 mg daily. Increase daily in increments of 25 to 50 mg daily to an effective dose; may be switched to extended-release formulation when stabilized on 200 mg/day. For debilitated patients and those with hypotension, consider lower dosages and slower adjustment.
➤ **Monotherapy and adjunct therapy with lithium or divalproex for the short-term treatment of acute manic episodes associated with bipolar I disorder**
Adults: Initially, 50 mg P.O. b.i.d. Increase dosage in increments of 100 mg daily in two divided doses up to 200 mg P.O. b.i.d. on day 4. May increase dosage in increments no greater than 200 mg daily up to 800 mg daily by day 6. Usual dose is 400 to 800 mg daily.
Adjust-a-dose: Elderly patients: Titrate on immediate-release formula, starting at 25 mg/day. Use slow titration and regular monitoring. In patients with hepatic impairment, initial dose is 25 mg daily. Increase daily in increments of 25 to 50 mg to an effective dose. For debilitated patients and those with hypotension, consider lower dosages and slower adjustment.
➤ **Depression associated with bipolar disorder**
Adults: Initially, 50 mg P.O. once daily at bedtime; increase on day 2 to 100 mg; increase on day 3 to 200 mg; increase on day 4 to maintenance dose of 300 mg.

Adjust-a-dose: Elderly patients: Titrate on immediate-release formula, starting at 25 mg/day. Use slow titration and regular monitoring. In patients with hepatic impairment, initial dose is 25 mg daily. Increase daily in increments of 25 to 50 mg to an effective dose. For debilitated patients and those with hypotension, consider lower dosages and slower adjustment.

ADMINISTRATION
P.O.
● Don't break or crush extended-release tablets.
● Give drug without regard for food; give extended-release tablets without food or with a light meal (about 300 calories).
● Schizophrenic patients who are currently being treated with divided doses of the immediate-release form may be switched to extended-release tablets at the equivalent total daily dose taken once daily. Individual dosage adjustments may be necessary. Those requiring less than 200 mg/dose should remain on the immediate-release form.

ACTION
Blocks dopamine and serotonin 5-HT$_2$ receptors. Its action may be mediated through this antagonism.

Route	Onset	Peak	Duration
P.O.	Unknown	1½ hr	Unknown
P.O. extended-release	Unknown	6 hr	Unknown

Half-life: 6 hours, extended-release 7 to 12 hours.

ADVERSE REACTIONS
CNS: *dizziness, headache, somnolence, neuroleptic malignant syndrome, seizures,* hypertonia, dysarthria, asthenia.
CV: orthostatic hypotension, tachycardia, palpitations, peripheral edema.
EENT: ear pain, pharyngitis, rhinitis.
GI: dry mouth, dyspepsia, abdominal pain, constipation, anorexia.
Hematologic: *leukopenia.*
Metabolic: *weight gain,* hyperglycemia.
Musculoskeletal: back pain.
Respiratory: increased cough, dyspnea.

Skin: rash, diaphoresis.
Other: flulike syndrome.

INTERACTIONS
Drug-drug. *Antihypertensives:* May increase effects of antihypertensives. Monitor blood pressure.
Carbamazepine, glucocorticoids, phenobarbital, phenytoin, rifampin, thioridazine: May increase quetiapine clearance. May need to adjust quetiapine dosage.
CNS depressants: May increase CNS effects. Use together cautiously.
Dopamine agonists, levodopa: May antagonize the effects of these drugs. Monitor patient.
Erythromycin, fluconazole, itraconazole, ketoconazole: May decrease quetiapine clearance. Use together cautiously.
Lorazepam: May decrease lorazepam clearance. Monitor patient for increased CNS effects.
Drug-lifestyle. *Alcohol use:* May increase CNS effects. Discourage use together.

EFFECTS ON LAB TEST RESULTS
● May increase liver enzyme, cholesterol, triglyceride, and glucose levels. May decrease T$_4$ and thyroid-stimulating hormone levels.
● May decrease WBC count.

CONTRAINDICATIONS & CAUTIONS
● Contraindicated in patients hypersensitive to drug or its ingredients.
● Use cautiously in patients with CV disease, cerebrovascular disease, conditions that predispose to hypotension, a history of seizures or conditions that lower the seizure threshold, and conditions in which core body temperature may be elevated.
● Use cautiously in patients at risk for aspiration pneumonia.

NURSING CONSIDERATIONS
● Dispense lowest appropriate quantity of drug to reduce risk of overdose.
● *Alert:* Drug isn't indicated for use in elderly patients with dementia-related psychosis because of increased risk of death from CV disease or infection.
● *Alert:* Watch for evidence of neuroleptic malignant syndrome (extrapyramidal

effects, hyperthermia, autonomic disturbance), which is rare but deadly.
• Monitor patient for tardive dyskinesia, which may occur after prolonged use. It may not appear until months or years later and may disappear spontaneously or persist for life, despite ending drug.
• Hyperglycemia may occur in patients taking drug. Monitor patients with diabetes regularly.
• Monitor patient for weight gain.
• *Alert:* Monitor patient for symptoms of metabolic syndrome (significant weight gain and increased body mass index, hypertension, hyperglycemia, hypercholesterolemia, and hypertriglyceridemia).
• Drug use may cause cataract formation. Obtain baseline ophthalmologic examination and reassess every 6 months.
• *Alert:* Drug may increase the risk of suicidal thinking and behavior in young adults ages 18 to 24 during the first 2 months of treatment.

PATIENT TEACHING
• Warn patient about risk of dizziness when standing up quickly. The risk is greatest during the 3- to 5-day period of first dosage adjustment, when resuming treatment, and when increasing dosages.
• Tell patient to avoid becoming overheated or dehydrated.
• Warn patient to avoid activities that require mental alertness until effects of drug are known, especially during first dosage adjustment or dosage increases.
• Remind patient to have an eye examination at start of therapy and every 6 months during therapy to check for cataracts.
• Tell patient to notify prescriber about other prescription or OTC drugs he's taking or plans to take.
• Tell woman of childbearing age to notify prescriber about planned, suspected, or known pregnancy. Advise her not to breast-feed during therapy.
• Advise patient to avoid alcohol while taking drug.
• Tell patient to take drug with or without food.
• Tell patient not to crush, chew, or break extended-release tablets.

• Tell patient to take extended-release tablets without food or with a light meal.

SAFETY ALERT!

ramelteon
rah-MELL-tee-on

Rozerem

Pharmacologic class: melatonin receptor agonist
Pregnancy risk category C

AVAILABLE FORMS
Tablets: 8 mg

INDICATIONS & DOSAGES
➤ **Insomnia characterized by trouble falling asleep**
Adults: 8 mg P.O. within 30 minutes of bedtime.

ADMINISTRATION
P.O.
• Don't give drug with or immediately after a high-fat meal.
• Give drug within 30 minutes of bedtime.

ACTION
Acts on receptors believed to maintain the circadian rhythm underlying the normal sleep-wake cycle.

Route	Onset	Peak	Duration
P.O.	Rapid	$\frac{1}{2}$–$1\frac{1}{2}$ hr	Unknown

Half-life: Parent compound, 1 to $2\frac{1}{2}$ hours; metabolite M-II, 2 to 5 hours.

ADVERSE REACTIONS
CNS: complex sleep-related behaviors, depression, dizziness, fatigue, headache, somnolence, worsened insomnia.
GI: diarrhea, impaired taste, nausea.
Musculoskeletal: arthralgia, myalgia.
Respiratory: upper respiratory tract infection.
Other: *anaphylaxis, angioedema,* flulike symptoms.

Reactions may be *common*, uncommon, *life-threatening*, or COMMON AND LIFE-THREATENING.
Interaction may have a *rapid onset* or *delayed onset*.

INTERACTIONS
Drug-drug. *CNS depressants:* May cause excessive CNS depression. Use together cautiously.
Fluconazole (strong CYP2C9 inhibitor), ketoconazole (strong CYP3A4 inhibitor), weak CYP1A2 inhibitors: May increase ramelteon level. Use together cautiously.
Fluvoxamine (strong CYP1A2 inhibitor): May increase ramelteon level. Avoid use together.
Rifampin (strong CYP enzyme inducer): May decrease ramelteon level. Monitor patient for lack of effect.
Drug-food. *Food (especially high-fat meals):* May delay time to peak drug effect. Tell patient to take drug on an empty stomach.
Drug-lifestyle. *Alcohol use:* May cause excessive CNS depression. Discourage alcohol use.

EFFECTS ON LAB TEST RESULTS
● May increase prolactin level. May alter blood cortisol and testosterone levels.

CONTRAINDICATIONS & CAUTIONS
● Contraindicated in those hypersensitive to drug or its components. Don't use in patients taking fluvoxamine or in those with severe hepatic impairment, severe sleep apnea, or severe COPD.
● Use cautiously in patients with depression or moderate hepatic impairment.

NURSING CONSIDERATIONS
● *Alert:* Anaphylaxis and angioedema may occur as early as the first dose. Monitor patient closely.
● Thoroughly evaluate the cause of insomnia before starting drug.
● Assess patient for behavioral or cognitive disorders.
● Drug doesn't cause physical dependence.

PATIENT TEACHING
● *Alert:* Warn patient that drug may cause allergic reactions, facial swelling, and complex sleep-related behaviors, such as driving, eating, and making phone calls while asleep. Advise patient to report these adverse effects.
● Instruct patient to take dose within 30 minutes of bedtime.

● Tell patient not to take drug with or after a heavy meal.
● Caution against performing activities that require mental alertness or physical coordination after taking drug.
● Caution patient to avoid alcohol while taking drug.
● Tell patient to consult prescriber if insomnia worsens or behavior changes.
● Urge woman to consult prescriber if menses stops, libido decreases, or galactorrhea or fertility problems develop.

---

risperidone
ris-PEER-i-dohn

Risperdal, Risperdal Consta, Risperdal M-Tab

Pharmacologic class: benzisoxazole derivative
Pregnancy risk category C

AVAILABLE FORMS
Injection: 12.5 mg, 25 mg, 37.5 mg, 50 mg
Solution: 1 mg/ml
Tablets: 0.25 mg, 0.5 mg, 1 mg, 2 mg, 3 mg, 4 mg
Tablets (orally disintegrating): 0.5 mg, 1 mg, 2 mg, 3 mg, 4 mg

INDICATIONS & DOSAGES
➤ **Schizophrenia**
Adults: Drug may be given once or twice daily. Initial dosing is generally 2 mg/day. Increase dosage at intervals not less than 24 hours, in increments of 1 to 2 mg/day, as tolerated, to a recommended dose of 4 to 8 mg/day. Periodically reassess to determine the need for maintenance treatment with an appropriate dose.
Adolescents ages 13 to 17: Start treatment with 0.5 mg once daily, given as a single daily dose in either the morning or evening. Adjust dose, if indicated, at intervals not less than 24 hours, in increments of 0.5 or 1 mg/day, as tolerated, to a recommended dose of 3 mg/day. There are no data to support use beyond 8 weeks.

➤ **12-week parenteral therapy for schizophrenia**

Adults: Establish tolerance to oral risperidone before giving I.M. Give 25 mg deep I.M. into the buttock every 2 weeks, alternating injections between the two buttocks. Adjust dose no sooner than every 4 weeks. Maximum, 50 mg I.M. every 2 weeks. Continue oral antipsychotic for 3 weeks after first I.M. injection, then stop oral therapy.

Adjust-a-dose: Patients with hepatic or renal impairment: Titrate slowly to 2 mg P.O.; if tolerated, give 25 mg I.M. every 2 weeks, or give initial dose of 12.5 mg I.M. Continue oral form of risperidone (or another antipsychotic drug) with the first injection and for 3 subsequent weeks to maintain therapeutic drug levels.

➤ **Monotherapy or combination therapy with lithium or valproate for 3-week treatment of acute manic or mixed episodes from bipolar I disorder**

Adults: 2 to 3 mg P.O. once daily. Adjust dose by 1 mg daily. Dosage range is 1 to 6 mg daily.

Adjust-a-dose: In elderly or debilitated patients, hypotensive patients, or those with severe renal or hepatic impairment, start with 0.5 mg P.O. b.i.d. Increase dosage by 0.5 mg b.i.d. Increase in dosages above 1.5 mg b.i.d. should occur at least 1 week apart. Subsequent switches to once-daily dosing may be made after patient is on a twice-daily regimen for 2 to 3 days at the target dose.

Children and adolescents ages 10 to 17: Give 0.5 mg P.O. as a single daily dose in either the morning or evening. Adjust dose, if indicated, at intervals not less than 24 hours, in increments of 0.5 or 1 mg/day, as tolerated, to a recommended dose of 2.5 mg/day.

➤ **Irritability, including aggression, self-injury, and temper tantrums, associated with an autistic disorder**

Adolescents and children age 5 and older who weigh 20 kg (44 lb) or more: Initially, 0.5 mg P.O. once daily or divided b.i.d. After 4 days, increase dose to 1 mg. Increase dosage further in 0.5-mg increments at intervals of at least 2 weeks.

Children age 5 and older who weigh less than 20 kg: Initially, 0.25 mg P.O. once daily or divided b.i.d. After 4 days, increase dose to 0.5 mg. Increase dosage further in 0.25-mg increments at intervals of at least 2 weeks. Increase cautiously in children who weigh less than 15 kg (33 lb).

ADMINISTRATION

P.O.
● Give drug without regard for meals.
● Open package for orally disintegrating tablets (ODTs) immediately before giving by peeling off foil backing with dry hands. Don't push tablets through the foil.
● Phenylalanine contents of ODTs are as follows: 0.5-mg tablet contains 0.14 mg phenylalanine; 1-mg tablet contains 0.28 mg phenylalanine; 2-mg tablet contains 0.56 mg phenylalanine; 3-mg tablet contains 0.63 mg phenylalanine; 4-mg tablet contains 0.84 mg phenylalanine.

I.M.
● Continue oral therapy for the first 3 weeks of I.M. injection therapy until injections take effect, then stop oral therapy.
● To reconstitute I.M. injection, inject premeasured diluent into vial and shake vigorously for at least 10 seconds. Suspension appears uniform, thick, and milky; particles are visible, but no dry particles remain. Use drug immediately, or refrigerate for up to 6 hours after reconstitution. If more than 2 minutes pass before injection, shake vigorously again. See manufacturer's package insert for more detailed instructions.
● Refrigerate I.M. injection kit and protect it from light. Drug can be stored at temperature less than 77° F (25° C) for no more than 7 days before administration.

ACTION

Blocks dopamine and 5-HT$_2$ receptors in the brain.

Route	Onset	Peak	Duration
P.O.	Unknown	1 hr	Unknown
I.M.	3 wk	4–6 wk	7 wk

Half-life: 3 to 20 hours.

ADVERSE REACTIONS

CNS: *akathisia, somnolence, dystonia, headache, insomnia, agitation, anxiety, pain, parkinsonism,* **neuroleptic malignant syndrome, suicide attempt,** dizziness, fever, hallucination, mania, impaired concentration, abnormal thinking and dreaming, tremor, hypoesthesia, fatigue, depression, nervousness.

CV: tachycardia, chest pain, orthostatic hypotension, peripheral edema, syncope, hypertension.

EENT: *rhinitis,* sinusitis, pharyngitis, abnormal vision, ear disorder (I.M.).

GI: *constipation, nausea, vomiting, dyspepsia, abdominal pain,* anorexia, dry mouth, increased saliva, diarrhea.

GU: urinary incontinence, increased urination, abnormal orgasm, vaginal dryness.

Metabolic: *weight gain, hyperglycemia,* weight loss.

Musculoskeletal: arthralgia, back pain, leg pain, myalgia.

Respiratory: coughing, dyspnea, upper respiratory infection.

Skin: rash, dry skin, photosensitivity reactions, acne, injection site pain (I.M.).

Other: tooth disorder, toothache, injury, decreased libido.

INTERACTIONS

Drug-drug. *Antihypertensives:* May enhance hypotensive effects. Monitor blood pressure.

Carbamazepine: May increase risperidone clearance and decrease effectiveness. Monitor patient closely.

Clozapine: May decrease risperidone clearance, increasing toxicity. Monitor patient closely.

CNS depressants: May cause additive CNS depression. Use together cautiously.

Dopamine agonists, levodopa: May antagonize effects of these drugs. Use together cautiously and monitor patient.

Fluoxetine, paroxetine: May increase the risk of risperidone's adverse effects, including serotonin syndrome. Monitor patient closely and adjust risperidone dose, as needed.

Drug-lifestyle. *Alcohol use:* May cause additive CNS depression. Discourage use together.

Sun exposure: May increase risk of photosensitivity reactions. Advise patient to avoid excessive sunlight exposure.

EFFECTS ON LAB TEST RESULTS

● May increase prolactin level. May decrease hemoglobin level and hematocrit.

CONTRAINDICATIONS & CAUTIONS

● Contraindicated in patients hypersensitive to drug and in breast-feeding women.
● Use cautiously in patients with prolonged QT interval, CV disease, cerebrovascular disease, dehydration, hypovolemia, history of seizures, or conditions that could affect metabolism or hemodynamic responses.
● Use cautiously in patients exposed to extreme heat.
● Use caution in patients at risk for aspiration pneumonia.
● Use I.M. injection cautiously in those with hepatic or renal impairment.

NURSING CONSIDERATIONS

● *Alert:* Obtain baseline blood pressure measurements before starting therapy, and monitor pressure regularly. Watch for orthostatic hypotension, especially during first dosage adjustment.
● *Alert:* Fatal cerebrovascular adverse events (stroke, transient ischemic attacks) may occur in elderly patients with dementia. Drug isn't safe or effective in these patients.
● Monitor patient for tardive dyskinesia, which may occur after prolonged use. It may not appear until months or years later and may disappear spontaneously or persist for life, despite stopping drug.
● *Alert:* Watch for evidence of neuroleptic malignant syndrome (extrapyramidal effects, hyperthermia, autonomic disturbance), which is rare but can be fatal.
● Life-threatening hyperglycemia may occur in patients taking atypical antipsychotics. Monitor patients with diabetes regularly.
● *Alert:* Monitor patient for symptoms of metabolic syndrome (significant weight gain and increased body mass index, hypertension, hyperglycemia, hypercholesterolemia, and hypertriglyceridemia).

• Periodically reevaluate drug's risks and benefits, especially during prolonged use.
• Monitor patient for weight gain.
• *Look alike–sound alike:* Don't confuse risperidone with reserpine.

PATIENT TEACHING
• Warn patient to avoid activities that require alertness until effects of drug are known.
• Warn patient to rise slowly, avoid hot showers, and use other precautions to avoid fainting when starting therapy.
• Advise patient to use caution in hot weather to prevent heatstroke.
• Tell patient to take drug with or without food.
• Instruct patient to keep the ODT in the blister pack until just before taking it. After opening the pack, dissolve the tablet on tongue without cutting or chewing. Use dry hands to peel apart the foil to expose the tablet; don't attempt to push it through the foil.
• Tell patient to use sunblock and wear protective clothing outdoors.
• Advise women not to become pregnant or to breast-feed for 12 weeks after the last I.M. injection.
• Advise patient to avoid alcohol during therapy.

---

rivastigmine tartrate
riv-ah-STIG-meen

Exelon, Exelon Patch

Pharmacologic class: cholinesterase inhibitor
Pregnancy risk category B

AVAILABLE FORMS
Capsules: 1.5 mg, 3 mg, 4.5 mg, 6 mg
Patch, transdermal: 4.6 mg/24 hours, 9.5 mg/24 hours
Solution: 2 mg/ml

INDICATIONS & DOSAGES
➤ **Mild to moderate Alzheimer dementia**
Adults: Initially, 1.5 mg P.O. b.i.d. with food. If tolerated, may increase to 3 mg b.i.d. after 2 weeks. After 2 weeks at this dose, may increase to 4.5 mg b.i.d. and 6 mg b.i.d., as tolerated. Effective dosage range is 6 to 12 mg daily; maximum, 12 mg daily. Or, 4.6 mg/24 hours transdermal patch. After 4 weeks, if tolerated, increase to 9.5 mg/24 hours transdermal patch.
➤ **Mild to moderate dementia associated with Parkinson disease**
Adults: Initially, 1.5 mg P.O. b.i.d. May increase, as tolerated, to 3 mg b.i.d., then 4.5 mg b.i.d., and finally to 6 mg b.i.d. after a minimum of 4 weeks at each dose. Or, 4.6 mg/24 hours transdermal patch. After 4 weeks, if tolerated, increase to 9.5 mg/24 hours transdermal patch.

ADMINISTRATION
P.O.
• Give drug with food in the morning and evening.
• Solution may be taken directly or mixed with small glass of water, cold fruit juice, or soda.
• Capsule and solution doses are interchangeable.
Transdermal
• Apply patch once daily to clean, dry, hairless skin on the upper or lower back, upper arm, or chest, in a place not rubbed by tight clothing.
• Change the site daily, and don't use the same site within 14 days.
• Press patch firmly into place until the edges stick well.

ACTION
Thought to increase acetylcholine level by inhibiting cholinesterase enzyme, which causes acetylcholine hydrolysis.

Route	Onset	Peak	Duration
P.O.	Unknown	1 hr	12 hr
Transdermal	Unknown	8 hr	24 hr

Half-life: 1½ hours (oral); 3 hours (transdermal).

ADVERSE REACTIONS
CNS: *headache, dizziness,* syncope, fatigue, asthenia, malaise, somnolence, tremor, insomnia, confusion, depression, anxiety, hallucinations, aggressive

---

reaction, vertigo, agitation, nervousness, delusions, paranoid reaction, pain.
CV: hypertension, chest pain, peripheral edema.
EENT: rhinitis, pharyngitis.
GI: *nausea, vomiting, diarrhea, anorexia, abdominal pain,* dyspepsia, constipation, flatulence, eructation.
GU: UTI, incontinence.
Metabolic: weight loss.
Musculoskeletal: back pain, arthralgia, bone fracture.
Respiratory: upper respiratory tract infection, cough, bronchitis.
Skin: increased sweating, rash.
Other: *accidental trauma,* flulike symptoms.

INTERACTIONS

Drug-drug. *Bethanechol, succinylcholine, other neuromuscular-blocking drugs or cholinergic antagonists:* May have synergistic effect. Monitor patient closely.
Drug-lifestyle. *Smoking:* May increase drug clearance. Discourage smoking.

EFFECTS ON LAB TEST RESULTS
None reported.

CONTRAINDICATIONS & CAUTIONS
• Contraindicated in patients hypersensitive to drug, other carbamate derivatives, or other components of the drug.

NURSING CONSIDERATIONS
• Expect significant GI adverse effects (such as nausea, vomiting, anorexia, and weight loss). These effects are less common during maintenance doses.
• Monitor patient for evidence of active or occult GI bleeding.
• Dramatic memory improvement is unlikely. As disease progresses, the benefits of drug may decline.
• Monitor patient for severe nausea, vomiting, and diarrhea, which may lead to dehydration and weight loss.
• Carefully monitor patient with a history of GI bleeding, NSAID use, arrhythmias, seizures, or pulmonary conditions for adverse effects.
• If adverse reactions, such as diarrhea, loss of appetite, nausea, or vomiting, occur with patch, stop use for several days,

then restart at the same or lower dose. If treatment is interrupted for more than several days, restart patch at the lowest dose and retitrate.
• Patients weighing less than 50 kg (110 lb) may experience more adverse reactions when using the transdermal patch.
• When switching from an oral form to the transdermal patch, patients on a total daily dose of less than 6 mg can be switched to 4.6 mg/24 hours. Patients taking 6 to 12 mg orally can switch to the 9.5 mg/ 24 hour patch. The patch should be applied on the day after the last oral dose.

PATIENT TEACHING
• Tell caregiver to give drug with food in the morning and evening.
• Advise patient that memory improvement may be subtle and that drug more likely slows future memory loss.
• Tell patient to report nausea, vomiting, or diarrhea.
• Tell patient to consult prescriber before using OTC drugs.
• Tell patient to apply patch once daily to clean, dry, hairless skin in a place not rubbed by tight clothing.
• Teach patient that the recommended sites for patch placement include the upper or lower back, upper arm, or chest.
• Tell patient to change the site daily and not to use the same site within 14 days.
• Tell patient to press the patch firmly into place until the edges stick well.

SAFETY ALERT!

secobarbital sodium
see-koe-BAR-bi-tal

Seconal Sodium

Pharmacologic class: barbiturate
Pregnancy risk category D
Controlled substance schedule II

AVAILABLE FORMS
Capsules: 100 mg

INDICATIONS & DOSAGES
➤ **Preoperative sedation**
Adults: 200 to 300 mg P.O. 1 to 2 hours before surgery.
Children: 2 to 6 mg/kg P.O. 1 to 2 hours before surgery. Maximum single dose is 100 mg P.O.
➤ **Insomnia**
Adults: 100 mg P.O. at bedtime.
Adjust-a-dose: In debilitated, elderly, and patients with renal or hepatic impairment, consider reducing dose.

ADMINISTRATION
P.O.
• Give drug without regard for food.

ACTION
Probably interferes with transmission of impulses from the thalamus to the cortex of the brain.

Route	Onset	Peak	Duration
P.O.	15 min	15–30 min	1–4 hr

Half-life: About 30 hours.

ADVERSE REACTIONS
CNS: *hangover, lethargy,* complex sleep-related behaviors, drowsiness, paradoxical anxiety, somnolence.
GI: nausea, vomiting.
Hematologic: worsening of porphyria.
Respiratory: *respiratory depression.*
Skin: rash, urticaria, *Stevens-Johnson syndrome,* tissue reactions.
Other: *anaphylaxis, angioedema,* physical and psychological dependence.

INTERACTIONS
Drug-drug. *Chloramphenicol, MAO inhibitors, valproic acid:* May inhibit metabolism of barbiturates; may cause prolonged CNS depression. Reduce barbiturate dosage.
CNS depressants, including opioid analgesics: May cause excessive CNS and respiratory depression. Use together cautiously.
Corticosteroids, doxycycline, estrogens and hormonal contraceptives, oral anticoagulants, theophylline, tricyclic antidepressants, verapamil: May enhance metabolism of these drugs. Watch for decreased effect.
Griseofulvin: May decrease absorption of griseofulvin. Monitor effectiveness of griseofulvin.
Metoprolol, propranolol: May reduce the effects of these drugs. May need to increase beta blocker dose.
Rifampin: May decrease barbiturate level. Watch for decreased effect.
Drug-lifestyle. *Alcohol use:* May impair coordination, increase CNS effects, and cause death. Strongly discourage alcohol use with these drugs.

EFFECTS ON LAB TEST RESULTS
None reported.

CONTRAINDICATIONS & CAUTIONS
• Contraindicated in patients hypersensitive to barbiturates and in those with marked liver or renal impairment, respiratory disease in which dyspnea or obstruction is evident, or porphyria.
• Use cautiously in elderly or debilitated patients and in patients with acute or chronic pain, depression, suicidal tendencies, history of drug abuse, or hepatic or renal impairment.

NURSING CONSIDERATIONS
• **Alert:** Monitor the patient closely. Anaphylaxis and angioedema may occur as early as the first dose.
• Assess mental status before starting therapy and reduce doses in elderly patients; these patients may be more sensitive to drug's adverse CNS effects. Also watch for paradoxical excitement in this population.
• Take precautions to prevent hoarding by patients who are depressed, suicidal, or drug-dependent or who have history of drug abuse.
• Watch for signs of toxicity: coma, pupillary constriction, cyanosis, clammy skin, and hypotension. Overdose can be fatal.
• Inspect patient's skin. Skin eruptions may precede fatal reactions to drug therapy. Stop drug when skin reactions occur, and notify prescriber. In some patients, high temperature, stomatitis, headache, or rhinitis may precede skin reactions.

- Long-term use isn't recommended; drug loses its effect of promoting sleep after 14 days of continued use.
- Drug changes EEG patterns, altering low-voltage fast activity; changes persist for a while after therapy.

PATIENT TEACHING
- **Alert:** Warn patient that drug may cause allergic reactions, facial swelling, and complex sleep-related behaviors, such as driving, eating, and making phone calls while asleep. Advise patient to report these adverse effects.
- Tell patient that morning hangover is common after use because drug suppresses REM sleep. Patient may have increased dreams after drug is stopped.
- Advise patient to avoid alcohol use while taking drug.
- Caution patient to avoid performing activities that require mental alertness or physical coordination.
- Tell patient using hormonal contraceptives to consider a different birth control method.

---

sertraline hydrochloride
SIR-trah-leen

Zoloft

Pharmacologic class: SSRI
Pregnancy risk category C

AVAILABLE FORMS
Capsules: 25 mg, 50 mg, 100 mg
Oral concentrate: 20 mg/ml
Tablets: 25 mg, 50 mg, 100 mg

INDICATIONS & DOSAGES
➤ **Depression**
Adults: 50 mg P.O. daily. Adjust dosage as needed and tolerated; dosage range is 50 to 200 mg daily.
➤ **Obsessive-compulsive disorder**
Adults: 50 mg P.O. once daily. If patient doesn't improve, increase dosage, up to 200 mg daily.
Children ages 6 to 17: Initially, 25 mg P.O. daily in children ages 6 to 12, or 50 mg P.O. daily in adolescents ages 13 to 17.

Increase dosage, as needed, up to 200 mg daily at intervals of no less than 1 week.
➤ **Panic disorder**
Adults: Initially, 25 mg P.O. daily. After 1 week, increase dose to 50 mg P.O. daily. If patient doesn't improve, increase dose to maximum of 200 mg daily.
➤ **Posttraumatic stress disorder**
Adults: Initially, 25 mg P.O. once daily. Increase dosage to 50 mg P.O. once daily after 1 week. Increase at weekly intervals to a maximum of 200 mg daily. Maintain patient on lowest effective dose.
➤ **Premenstrual dysphoric disorder**
Adults: Initially, 50 mg daily P.O. either continuously or only during the luteal phase of the menstrual cycle. If patient doesn't respond, dose may be increased 50 mg per menstrual cycle, up to 150 mg daily for use throughout the menstrual cycle or 100 mg daily for luteal-phase doses. If a 100-mg daily dose has been established with luteal-phase dose, use a 50-mg daily adjustment for 3 days at the beginning of each luteal phase.
➤ **Social anxiety disorder**
Adults: Initially, 25 mg P.O. once daily. Increase dosage to 50 mg P.O. once daily after 1 week of therapy. Dose range is 50 to 200 mg daily. Adjust to the lowest effective dosage and periodically reassess patient to determine the need for long-term treatment.
➤ **Premature ejaculation ♦**
Adults: 25 to 50 mg P.O. daily or as needed.
Adjust-a-dose: For patients with hepatic disease, use lower or less-frequent doses.

ADMINISTRATION
P.O.
- Give drug without regard for food.
- Don't use oral concentrate dropper, which is made of rubber, for a patient with latex allergy.
- Mix oral concentrate with 4 oz (118 ml) of water, ginger ale, lemon-lime soda, lemonade, or orange juice only, and give immediately.

ACTION
Thought to be linked to drug's inhibition of CNS neuronal uptake of serotonin.

Route	Onset	Peak	Duration
P.O.	Unknown	4–8 hr	Unknown

Half-life: 26 hours.

ADVERSE REACTIONS
CNS: *fatigue, headache, tremor, dizziness, insomnia, somnolence,* **suicidal behavior,** paresthesia, hypesthesia, nervousness, anxiety, agitation, hypertonia, twitching, confusion.
CV: palpitations, chest pain, hot flashes.
GI: *dry mouth, nausea, diarrhea, loose stools, dyspepsia,* vomiting, constipation, thirst, flatulence, anorexia, abdominal pain, increased appetite.
GU: *male sexual dysfunction.*
Musculoskeletal: myalgia.
Skin: rash, pruritus, diaphoresis.

INTERACTIONS
Drug-drug. *Amphetamines, buspirone, dextromethorphan, dihydroergotamine, lithium salts, meperidine, other SSRIs or SSNRIs (duloxetine, venlafaxine), sumatriptan,* **tramadol,** *trazodone, tricyclic antidepressants, tryptophan:* May increase the risk of serotonin syndrome. Avoid combinations of drugs that increase the availability of serotonin in the CNS; monitor patient closely if used together.
Benzodiazepines, tolbutamide: May decrease clearance of these drugs. Significance unknown; monitor patient for increased drug effects.
Cimetidine: May decrease clearance of sertraline. Monitor patient closely.
Disulfiram: Oral concentrate contains alcohol, which may react with drug. Avoid using together.
MAO inhibitors, such as phenelzine, selegiline, tranylcypromine: May cause serotonin syndrome. Avoid using within 14 days of MAO inhibitor therapy.
Pimozide: May increase pimozide level. Avoid using together.
Triptans: May cause serotonin syndrome (restlessness, hallucinations, loss of coordination, fast heartbeat, rapid changes in blood pressure, increased body temperature, hyperreflexia, nausea, vomiting, and diarrhea). Use cautiously, with close monitoring, especially at the start of treatment and during dosage adjustments.

Warfarin, other highly protein-bound drugs: May increase level of sertraline or other highly protein-bound drug. May increase PT, or INR may increase by 8%. Monitor patient closely; monitor PT and INR.
Drug-herb. *St. John's wort:* May cause additive effects and serotonin syndrome. Discourage use together.

EFFECTS ON LAB TEST RESULTS
● May increase ALT and AST levels.

CONTRAINDICATIONS & CAUTIONS
● Contraindicated in patients hypersensitive to drug or its components.
● Contraindicated in patients taking pimozide or MAO inhibitors or within 14 days of MAO inhibitor therapy.
● Use cautiously in patients at risk for suicide and in those with seizure disorders, major affective disorder, or diseases or conditions that affect metabolism or hemodynamic responses.
● Use in third trimester of pregnancy may cause neonatal complications at birth. Consider the risk versus benefit of treatment during this time.

NURSING CONSIDERATIONS
● Give sertraline once daily, either in morning or evening, with or without food.
● Make dosage adjustments at intervals of no less than 1 week.
● Record mood changes. Monitor patient for suicidal tendencies and allow only a minimum supply of drug.
● *Alert:* Drug may increase the risk of suicidal thinking and behavior in children and adolescents with major depressive disorder or other psychiatric disorder.
● *Alert:* Drug may increase the risk of suicidal thinking and behavior in young adults ages 18 to 24 during the first 2 months of treatment.
● Don't use the oral concentrate dropper, which is made of rubber, for a patient with latex allergy.
● *Alert:* Combining triptans with an SSRI or an SSNRI may cause serotonin syndrome. Signs and symptoms may include restlessness, hallucinations, loss of coordination, fast heart beat, rapid changes in blood pressure, increased body

---

Reactions may be *common,* uncommon, *life-threatening,* or COMMON AND LIFE-THREATENING.
Interaction may have a *rapid onset* or **delayed onset.**

temperature, overactive reflexes, nausea, vomiting, and diarrhea. Serotonin syndrome may be more likely to occur when starting or increasing the dose of triptan, SSRI, or SSNRI.

PATIENT TEACHING
● Advise patient to use caution when performing hazardous tasks that require alertness.
● Tell patient to avoid alcohol and to consult prescriber before taking OTC drugs.
● Advise patient to mix the oral concentrate with 4 oz ($\frac{1}{2}$ cup) of water, ginger ale, lemon-lime soda, lemonade, or orange juice only, and to take the dose right away.
● Instruct patient to avoid stopping drug abruptly.

---

sildenafil citrate
sill-DEN-ah-fill

Viagra

Pharmacologic class: phosphodiesterase type-5 inhibitor
Pregnancy risk category B

AVAILABLE FORMS
Tablets: 25 mg, 50 mg, 100 mg

INDICATIONS & DOSAGES
➤ **Erectile dysfunction**
Adults younger than age 65: About 1 hour before sexual activity, 50 mg P.O., p.r.n. Dosage range is 25 to 100 mg based on effectiveness and tolerance. Maximum is one dose daily.
Elderly patients (age 65 and older): 25 mg P.O., as needed, about 1 hour before sexual activity. Dosage may be adjusted based on patient response. Maximum is one dose daily.
Adjust-a-dose: For adults with hepatic or severe renal impairment, 25 mg P.O. about 1 hour before sexual activity. Dosage may be adjusted based on patient response. Maximum is one dose daily.

ADMINISTRATION
P.O.
● For most rapid absorption, give to patient on empty stomach.

ACTION
Increases effect of nitric oxide by inhibiting phosphodiesterase type 5 (PDE_5), which is responsible for degradation of cyclic guanosine monophosphate (cGMP) in the corpus cavernosum. When sexual stimulation causes local release of nitric oxide, inhibition of PDE_5 by sildenafil causes increased levels of cGMP in the corpus cavernosum, resulting in smooth muscle relaxation and inflow of blood to the corpus cavernosum.

Route	Onset	Peak	Duration
P.O.	15–30 min	30–120 min	4 hr

Half-life: 4 hours.

ADVERSE REACTIONS
CNS: *headache, seizures,* anxiety, dizziness, somnolence, vertigo.
CV: *MI, sudden cardiac death, ventricular arrhythmias, cerebrovascular hemorrhage, transient ischemic attack,* hypotension, flushing.
EENT: diplopia, temporary vision loss, decrease or loss of hearing, tinnitus, ocular redness or bloodshot appearance, increased intraocular pressure, retinal vascular disease, retinal bleeding, vitreous detachment or traction, paramacular edema, photophobia, altered color perception, blurred vision, burning, swelling, pressure, nasal congestion.
GI: *dyspepsia,* diarrhea.
GU: hematuria, prolonged erection, priapism, UTI.
Musculoskeletal: arthralgia, back pain.
Respiratory: respiratory tract infection.
Skin: rash.
Other: flulike syndrome.

INTERACTIONS
Drug-drug. *Beta blockers, loop and potassium-sparing diuretics:* May increase sildenafil metabolite level. Monitor patient.
Cytochrome P-450 inducers, rifampin: May reduce sildenafil level. Monitor effect.

Delavirdine, protease inhibitors: May increase sildenafil level, increasing risk of adverse events, including hypotension, visual changes, and priapism. Reduce initial sildenafil dose to 25 mg.

Hepatic isoenzyme inhibitors (such as cimetidine, erythromycin, itraconazole, ketoconazole): May reduce sildenafil clearance. Avoid using together.

Isosorbide, nitroglycerin: May cause severe hypotension. Use of nitrates in any form with sildenafil is contraindicated.

Drug-food. *High-fat meal:* May reduce absorption rate and peak level of drug. Advise patient to take drug on empty stomach.

Grapefruit: May increase drug level, while delaying absorption. Advise patient to avoid using together.

EFFECTS ON LAB TEST RESULTS
None reported.

CONTRAINDICATIONS & CAUTIONS
- Contraindicated in patients hypersensitive to drug or its components and in those taking organic nitrates.
- Use cautiously in patients age 65 and older; in patients with hepatic or severe renal impairment, retinitis pigmentosa, bleeding disorders, or active peptic ulcer disease; in those who have suffered an MI, a stroke, or life-threatening arrhythmia within last 6 months; in those with history of cardiac failure, coronary artery disease, uncontrolled high or low blood pressure, or anatomic deformation of the penis (such as angulation, cavernosal fibrosis, or Peyronie disease); and in those with conditions that may predispose them to priapism (such as sickle cell anemia, multiple myeloma, or leukemia).

NURSING CONSIDERATIONS
- *Alert:* Drug increases risk of cardiac events. Systemic vasodilatory properties cause transient decreases in supine blood pressure and cardiac output (about 2 hours after ingestion). Patients with underlying CV disease are at increased risk for cardiac effects related to sexual activity.
- *Alert:* Serious CV events, including MI, sudden cardiac death, ventricular arrhythmias, cerebrovascular hemorrhage, tran-

sient ischemic attack, and hypertension, may occur with drug use. Most, but not all, of these incidents involve CV risk factors. Many events occur during or shortly after sexual activity; a few occur shortly after drug use without sexual activity, and others occur hours to days after drug use and sexual activity.
- Drug isn't indicated for use in neonates, children, or women.

PATIENT TEACHING
- Advise patient that drug shouldn't be used with nitrates under any circumstances.
- Advise patient of potential cardiac risk of sexual activity, especially in presence of CV risk factors. Instruct patient to notify prescriber and refrain from further activity if such symptoms as chest pain, dizziness, or nausea occur when starting sexual activity.
- Warn patient that erections lasting longer than 4 hours and priapism (painful erections lasting longer than 6 hours) may occur, and tell him to seek immediate medical attention. Penile tissue damage and permanent loss of potency may result if priapism isn't treated immediately.
- Inform patient that drug doesn't protect against sexually transmitted diseases; advise patient to use protective measures such as condoms.
- Tell patient receiving HIV medications that he's at increased risk for sildenafil adverse events, including low blood pressure, visual changes, and priapism, and that he should promptly report such symptoms to his prescriber. Tell him not to exceed 25 mg of sildenafil in 48 hours.
- Instruct patient to take drug 30 minutes to 4 hours before sexual activity; maximum benefit can be expected less than 2 hours after ingestion.
- Advise patient that drug is most rapidly absorbed if taken on an empty stomach.
- Inform patient that impairment of color discrimination (blue, green) may occur and to avoid hazardous activities that rely on color discrimination.
- Instruct patient to notify prescriber of vision or hearing changes.
- Advise patient that drug is effective only in presence of sexual stimulation.

• Caution patient to take drug only as prescribed.

spironolactone
speer-on-oh-LAK-tone

Aldactone, Novospiroton†

Pharmacologic class: potassium-sparing diuretic; aldosterone receptor antagonist
Pregnancy risk category C

AVAILABLE FORMS
Tablets: 25 mg, 50 mg, 100 mg

INDICATIONS & DOSAGES
➤ **Edema**
Adults: Initially, 100 mg P.O. daily given as a single dose or in divided doses. Usual range is 25 to 200 mg P.O. daily.
Children: Give 3.3 mg/kg P.O. daily or in divided doses.
➤ **Hypertension**
Adults: 50 to 100 mg P.O. daily or in divided doses. Some practitioners use a lower dose range of 25 to 50 mg daily and add another antihypertensive to the regimen, rather than continually increasing this drug.
Children ♦: Give 1 to 3.3 mg/kg P.O. (up to 100 mg daily) as a single dose or divided b.i.d.
➤ **Diuretic-induced hypokalemia**
Adults: 25 to 100 mg P.O. daily.
➤ **To detect primary hyperaldosteronism**
Adults: 400 mg P.O. daily for 4 days (short test) or 3 to 4 weeks (long test). If hypokalemia and hypertension are corrected, a presumptive diagnosis of primary hyperaldosteronism is made.
➤ **To manage primary hyperaldosteronism**
Adults: 100 to 400 mg P.O. daily. Use lowest effective dose.
➤ **Heart failure, as adjunct to ACE inhibitor or loop diuretic, with or without cardiac glycoside) ♦**
Adults: 12.5 to 25 mg P.O. daily. May increase to 50 mg daily after 8 weeks.

➤ **Hirsutism ♦**
Women: 50 to 200 mg P.O. daily. Or, 50 mg P.O. b.i.d. days 4 to 21 of menstrual cycle.
➤ **Premenstrual syndrome ♦**
Adults: 25 mg P.O. q.i.d. starting on day 14 of the menstrual cycle.
➤ **Acne vulgaris ♦**
Adults: 100 mg P.O. daily.
➤ **Familial male precocious puberty ♦**
Boys: 2 mg/kg P.O. daily with 20 to 40 mg/kg testolactone P.O. daily for at least 6 months.

ADMINISTRATION
P.O.
• To enhance absorption, give drug with meals.
• Give drug in morning to prevent nocturia. If second dose is needed, give it with food in early afternoon.
• Protect tablets from light.

ACTION
Antagonizes aldosterone in the distal tubules, increasing sodium and water excretion.

Route	Onset	Peak	Duration
P.O.	1–2 days	2–3 days	2–3 days

Half-life: 1¼ to 2 hours.

ADVERSE REACTIONS
CNS: headache, drowsiness, lethargy, confusion, ataxia.
GI: diarrhea, gastric bleeding, ulceration, cramping, gastritis, vomiting.
GU: inability to maintain erection, menstrual disturbances.
Hematologic: *agranulocytosis.*
Metabolic: *hyperkalemia,* dehydration, hyponatremia, mild acidosis.
Skin: urticaria, hirsutism, maculopapular eruptions.
Other: *anaphylaxis,* gynecomastia, breast soreness, drug fever.

INTERACTIONS
Drug-drug. *ACE inhibitors, indomethacin, other potassium-sparing diuretics, potassium supplements:* May increase risk of hyperkalemia. Use together cautiously,

especially in patients with renal impairment. Monitor potassium level.

Anticoagulants: May decrease anticoagulant effects. Monitor PT and INR.

Aspirin and other salicylates: May block diuretic effect of spironolactone. Watch for diminished spironolactone response.

Digoxin: May alter digoxin clearance, increasing risk of toxicity. Monitor digoxin level.

Drug-herb. *Licorice:* May block ulcer-healing and aldosterone-like effects of herb; may increase risk of hypokalemia. Discourage use together.

Drug-food. *Potassium-rich foods, such as citrus fruits and tomatoes, salt substitutes containing potassium:* May increase risk of hyperkalemia. Urge caution.

EFFECTS ON LAB TEST RESULTS
● May increase BUN and potassium levels. May decrease sodium level.
● May decrease granulocyte count.
● May alter fluorometric determinations of plasma and urinary 17-hydroxycorticosteroid levels.

CONTRAINDICATIONS & CAUTIONS
● Contraindicated in patients hypersensitive to drug and in those with anuria, acute or progressive renal insufficiency, or hyperkalemia.
● Use cautiously in patients with fluid or electrolyte imbalances, impaired renal function, or hepatic disease, or in pregnant women.

NURSING CONSIDERATIONS
● Monitor electrolyte levels, fluid intake and output, weight, and blood pressure.
● Monitor elderly patients closely, who are more susceptible to excessive diuresis.
● Inform laboratory that patient is taking spironolactone because drug may interfere with tests that measure digoxin level.
● Drug is less potent than thiazide and loop diuretics and is useful as an adjunct to other diuretic therapy. Diuretic effect is delayed 2 to 3 days when used alone.
● Maximum antihypertensive response may be delayed for up to 2 weeks.
● Watch for hyperchloremic metabolic acidosis, especially in patients with hepatic cirrhosis.

● *Look alike–sound alike:* Don't confuse Aldactone with Aldactazide.

PATIENT TEACHING
● Instruct patient to take drug in morning to prevent need to urinate at night. If second dose is needed, tell him to take it with food in early afternoon.
● *Alert:* To prevent serious hyperkalemia, warn patient to avoid excessive ingestion of potassium-rich foods (such as citrus fruits, tomatoes, bananas, dates, and apricots), salt substitutes containing potassium, and potassium supplements.
● Caution patient not to perform hazardous activities if adverse CNS reactions occur.
● Advise men about possible breast tenderness or enlargement.

---

tacrine hydrochloride
TAY-krin

Cognex

Pharmacologic class: cholinesterase inhibitor
Pregnancy risk category C

AVAILABLE FORMS
Capsules: 10 mg, 20 mg, 30 mg, 40 mg

INDICATIONS & DOSAGES
➤ **Mild to moderate Alzheimer dementia**
Adults: Initially, 10 mg P.O. q.i.d. After 4 weeks, if patient tolerates treatment and has no increase in transaminase levels, increase dosage to 20 mg q.i.d. After an additional 4 weeks, increase to 30 mg q.i.d. If still tolerated, increase dosage to 40 mg q.i.d. after another 4 weeks.
Adjust-a-dose: For patients with ALT level three to five times the upper limit of normal (ULN), reduce dosage by 40 mg daily and monitor ALT level weekly until normal. If ALT is more than five times ULN, stop therapy and monitor patient for signs and symptoms of hepatitis. May rechallenge when ALT returns to normal if benefits outweigh risk. With rechallenge doses, monitor ALT weekly for 16 weeks,

---

then monthly for 2 months, and every 3 months thereafter.

ADMINISTRATION
P.O.
- Give drug between meals.
- If GI upset occurs, give drug with meals; doing so may decrease drug level by 30% to 40%.

ACTION
Reversibly inhibits the enzyme cholinesterase in the CNS, preventing or blocking the breakdown of acetylcholine and temporarily improving cognitive function in patients with mild to moderate Alzheimer disease.

Route	Onset	Peak	Duration
P.O.	Unknown	30 min–3 hr	Unknown

Half-life: 2 to 4 hours.

ADVERSE REACTIONS
CNS: *dizziness, headache,* agitation, ataxia, insomnia, abnormal thinking, somnolence, depression, anxiety, fatigue, confusion.
CV: chest pain.
EENT: rhinitis.
GI: *nausea, vomiting, diarrhea,* dyspepsia, loose stools, changes in stool color, anorexia, abdominal pain, flatulence, constipation.
Hepatic: LIVER TOXICITY.
Metabolic: weight loss.
Musculoskeletal: myalgia.
Respiratory: upper respiratory tract infection, cough.
Skin: rash, jaundice, facial flushing.

INTERACTIONS
Drug-drug. *Anticholinergics:* May lessen the effects of tacrine. Avoid using together.
Cholinergics such as bethanechol, anticholinesterases: May have additive effects. Monitor patient for toxicity.
Cimetidine, ciprofloxacin, fluvoxamine, ritonavir: May increase tacrine level. Monitor patient for adverse effects.
Succinylcholine: May enhance neuromuscular blockade and prolong duration of action. Monitor patient closely.

Theophylline: May increase theophylline level and prolong theophylline half-life. Carefully monitor theophylline level and adjust dosage.
Drug-food. *Any food:* May delay drug absorption. Give between meals.
Drug-lifestyle. *Smoking:* May decrease drug level. Ask patient if he smokes, and monitor him closely.

EFFECTS ON LAB TEST RESULTS
- May increase ALT and AST levels.

CONTRAINDICATIONS & CAUTIONS
- Contraindicated in patients hypersensitive to drug or to acridine derivatives.
- Contraindicated in patients for whom tacrine-related jaundice has previously been confirmed, with a total bilirubin level of more than 3 mg/dl.
- Use cautiously in patients with sick sinus syndrome or bradycardia, in patients at risk for peptic ulcers (including those taking NSAIDs or those with history of peptic ulcer), and in those with a history of hepatic disease.
- Use cautiously in patients with renal disease, asthma, prostatic hyperplasia, or other urine outflow impairment.

NURSING CONSIDERATIONS
- Monitor ALT level every other week from week 4 to week 16 of initial therapy, then decrease to once every 3 months. If ALT is modestly elevated (twice ULN range), begin weekly monitoring until ALT returns to normal. When dosage is increased, resume monitoring every other week.
- If drug is stopped for 4 weeks or longer, full dosage adjustment and monitoring schedule must be restarted.

PATIENT TEACHING
- Stress that drug doesn't alter the underlying degenerative disease but can stabilize or alleviate symptoms. Effect of therapy depends on regular drug administration.
- *Alert:* Remind caregiver that dosage adjustment is an integral part of safe drug use. Abruptly stopping or largely reducing the daily dosage by 80 mg or more may cause behavioral disturbances and a decline in cognitive function.

• Tell caregiver to give drug between meals whenever possible. If GI upset becomes a problem, drug may be taken with meals, although doing so may reduce levels by 30% to 40%.

• Advise patient and caregiver to immediately report significant adverse reactions or changes in status.

---

tadalafil
tah-DAL-ah-fill

Cialis

Pharmacologic class: phosphodiesterase type-5 inhibitor
Pregnancy risk category B

AVAILABLE FORMS
Tablets (film-coated): 2.5 mg, 5 mg, 10 mg, 20 mg

INDICATIONS & DOSAGES
➤ **Erectile dysfunction**
Adults: 10 mg P.O. as a single dose, as needed, before sexual activity. Range is 5 to 20 mg, based on effectiveness and tolerance. Maximum is one dose daily. Or 2.5 mg P.O. once daily without regard to timing of sexual activity. May increase to 5 mg P.O. daily.
Adjust-a-dose: If creatinine clearance is 31 to 50 ml/minute, starting dosage is 5 mg once daily and maximum is 10 mg once every 48 hours. If clearance is 30 ml/minute or less, maximum is 5 mg once daily. Patients with Child-Pugh category A or B shouldn't exceed 10 mg daily. Patients taking potent cytochrome P-450 inhibitors (such as erythromycin, itraconazole, ketoconazole, and ritonavir) shouldn't exceed one 10-mg dose every 72 hours.

ADMINISTRATION
P.O.
• Give drug without regard for food.

ACTION
Increases cGMP levels, prolongs smooth muscle relaxation, and promotes blood flow into the corpus cavernosum.

Route	Onset	Peak	Duration
P.O.	Immediate	½–6 hr	Unknown

Half-life: 17½ hours.

ADVERSE REACTIONS
CNS: dizziness, *headache.*
CV: flushing.
EENT: decrease or loss of hearing, nasal congestion, tinnitus.
GI: *dyspepsia.*
Musculoskeletal: back pain, limb pain, myalgia.

INTERACTIONS
Drug-drug. *Alpha blockers (except 0.4 mg tamsulosin daily), nitrates:* May enhance hypotensive effects. Use together is contraindicated.
Potent cytochrome P-450 inhibitors (such as erythromycin, itraconazole, ketoconazole, ritonavir): May increase tadalafil level. Don't exceed a 10-mg dose every 72 hours.
Rifampin and other cytochrome P-450 inducers: May decrease tadalafil level. Monitor patient closely.
Drug-food. *Grapefruit:* May increase drug level. Discourage use together.
Drug-lifestyle. *Alcohol use:* May increase risk of headache, dizziness, orthostatic hypotension, and increased heart rate. Discourage use together.

EFFECTS ON LAB TEST RESULTS
None reported.

CONTRAINDICATIONS & CAUTIONS
• Contraindicated in patients hypersensitive to drug or its components and in those taking nitrates or alpha blockers (other than tamsulosin 0.4 mg once daily).
• Drug isn't recommended for patients with Child-Pugh category C, unstable angina, angina that occurs during sexual intercourse, New York Heart Association class II or greater heart failure within past 6 months, uncontrolled arrhythmias, hypotension (lower than 90/50 mm Hg), uncontrolled hypertension (higher than 170/100 mm Hg), stroke within past 6 months, or an MI within past 90 days.
• Drug isn't recommended for patients whose cardiac status makes sexual activity

---

inadvisable or for those with hereditary degenerative retinal disorders.
• Use cautiously in patients taking potent cytochrome P-450 inhibitors (such as erythromycin, itraconazole, ketoconazole, and ritonavir) and in patients with bleeding disorders, significant peptic ulceration, or renal or hepatic impairment.
• Use cautiously in patients with conditions predisposing them to priapism (such as sickle cell anemia, multiple myeloma, and leukemia), anatomical penis abnormalities, or left ventricular outflow obstruction.
• Use cautiously in elderly patients, who may be more sensitive to drug effects.

NURSING CONSIDERATIONS
• **Alert:** Sexual activity may increase cardiac risk. Evaluate patient's cardiac risk before he starts taking drug.
• Before patient starts drug, assess him for underlying causes of erectile dysfunction.
• Transient decreases in supine blood pressure may occur.
• Prolonged erections and priapism may occur.

PATIENT TEACHING
• Warn patient that taking drug with nitrates could cause a serious drop in blood pressure, which increases the risk of heart attack or stroke.
• Tell patient to seek immediate medical attention if chest pain develops after taking the drug.
• Tell patient that drug doesn't protect against sexually transmitted diseases and that he should use protective measures.
• Urge patient to seek emergency medical care if his erection lasts more than 4 hours.
• Tell patient to take drug about 60 minutes before anticipated sexual activity. Explain that drug has no effect without sexual stimulation.
• Warn patient not to change dosage unless directed by prescriber.
• Caution patient against drinking large amounts of alcohol while taking drug.
• Instruct patient to notify prescriber of hearing changes.

temazepam
te-MAZ-e-pam

Restoril

Pharmacologic class:
benzodiazepine
Pregnancy risk category X
Controlled substance schedule IV

AVAILABLE FORMS
Capsules: 7.5 mg, 15 mg, 22.5 mg, 30 mg

INDICATIONS & DOSAGES
➤ **Insomnia**
Adults: 15 to 30 mg P.O. at bedtime.
Elderly or debilitated patients: 15 mg P.O. at bedtime until individualized response is determined.

ADMINISTRATION
P.O.
• Give drug 15 to 30 minutes before bedtime.
• Give drug without regard for food.

ACTION
Probably acts on the limbic system, thalamus, and hypothalamus of the CNS to produce hypnotic effects.

Route	Onset	Peak	Duration
P.O.	Unknown	1–2 hr	3–18 hr

Half-life: 10 to 17 hours.

ADVERSE REACTIONS
CNS: complex sleep-related behaviors, drowsiness, dizziness, lethargy, disturbed coordination, daytime sedation, confusion, nightmares, vertigo, euphoria, weakness, headache, fatigue, nervousness, anxiety, depression, minor changes in EEG patterns (usually low-voltage fast activity).
EENT: blurred vision.
GI: diarrhea, nausea, dry mouth.
Other: *anaphylaxis, angioedema,* physical and psychological dependence.

INTERACTIONS
Drug-drug. *CNS depressants:* May increase CNS depression. Use together cautiously.
Drug-herb. *Calendula, hops, kava, lemon balm, passion flower, skullcap, valerian:* May enhance sedative effect of drug. Discourage use together.
Drug-lifestyle. *Alcohol use:* May cause additive CNS effects. Discourage use together.

EFFECTS ON LAB TEST RESULTS
• May increase liver function test values.

CONTRAINDICATIONS & CAUTIONS
• Contraindicated in pregnant patients and those hypersensitive to drug or other benzodiazepines.
• Use cautiously in patients with chronic pulmonary insufficiency, impaired hepatic or renal function, severe or latent depression, suicidal tendencies, and history of drug abuse.

NURSING CONSIDERATIONS
• *Alert:* Monitor patient closely. Anaphylaxis and angioedema may occur as early as the first dose.
• Assess mental status before starting therapy and reduce doses in elderly patients; these patients may be more sensitive to drug's adverse CNS effects.
• Take precautions to prevent hoarding by patients who are depressed, suicidal, or drug-dependent or who have history of drug abuse.
• *Look alike–sound alike:* Don't confuse Restoril with Vistaril.

PATIENT TEACHING
• *Alert:* Warn patient that drug may cause allergic reactions, facial swelling, and complex sleep-related behaviors, such as driving, eating, and making phone calls while asleep. Advise patient to report these adverse effects.
• Tell patient to avoid alcohol during therapy.
• Caution patient to avoid performing activities that require mental alertness or physical coordination.
• Warn patient not to stop drug abruptly if taken for 1 month or longer.

• Tell patient that onset of drug's effects may take as long as 2 to 2¼ hours.

testosterone
Striant, Testopel Pellets

testosterone cypionate
Depo-Testosterone

testosterone enanthate
Delatestryl

testosterone propionate

Pharmacologic class: androgen
Pregnancy risk category X
Controlled substance schedule III

AVAILABLE FORMS
testosterone
Blister packs (buccal; extended-release): 30 mg
Pellets (subcutaneous implant): 75 mg
testosterone cypionate
Injection (in oil): 100 mg/ml, 200 mg/ml
testosterone enanthate
Injection (in oil): 200 mg/ml
testosterone propionate
Injection (in oil): 100 mg/ml

INDICATIONS & DOSAGES
➤ **Hypogonadism**
Men: 10 to 25 mg propionate I.M. two to three times weekly; or 50 to 400 mg cypionate or enanthate I.M. every 2 to 4 weeks. Or, 75 to 150 mg enanthate I.M. every 7 to 10 days. Or, 150 to 450 mg (2 to 6 pellets) implanted subcutaneously every 3 to 6 months. Or, apply 1 buccal system (30 mg) to the gum region just above the incisor tooth on either side of the mouth, b.i.d., morning and evening about 12 hours apart. Alternate sides of the mouth with each application.
➤ **Delayed puberty**
Men and boys: 50 to 200 mg enanthate I.M. every 2 to 4 weeks for 4 to 6 months.
➤ **Metastatic breast cancer**
Women 1 to 5 years after menopause: 50 to 100 mg propionate I.M. three times weekly; or 200 to 400 mg cypionate or enanthate I.M. every 2 to 4 weeks.

ADMINISTRATION
I.M.
● Store I.M. preparations at room temperature. If crystals appear, warm and shake bottle to disperse them.
● Inject deep into upper outer quadrant of gluteal muscle. Rotate injection sites; report soreness at site.
Subcutaneous
● In most men, the pellets are implanted in an area on the anterior abdominal wall.
Buccal
● The buccal system should be placed in the gum region just above the incisor tooth on either side of the mouth.
● Have the patient rotate sides of the mouth with each administration.
● Make sure the patient doesn't chew or swallow the buccal system.
● The buccal system should remain in place until the next dosing. Check placement after toothbrushing, mouthwash use, eating, and drinking.
● To remove the system, gently slide it downward from the gum toward the tooth.

ACTION
Stimulates target tissues to develop normally in androgen-deficient men. May have some antiestrogen properties, making it useful in treating certain estrogen-dependent breast cancers.

Route	Onset	Peak	Duration
I.M.	Unknown	10–100 min	Unknown
Subcut	Unknown	Unknown	3–6 mo
Buccal	Unknown	10–12 hr	2 4 hr

Half-life: 10 to 100 minutes.

ADVERSE REACTIONS
CNS: headache, anxiety, depression, paresthesia, sleep apnea.
CV: edema.
GI: nausea, gum or mouth irritation, bitter taste, gum pain, tenderness, or edema, taste perversion (with buccal application).
GU: amenorrhea, oligospermia, decreased ejaculatory volume, priapism.
Hematologic: polycythemia, *suppression of clotting factors.*
Hepatic: reversible jaundice, *cholestatic hepatitis.*

Metabolic: hypernatremia, *hyperkalemia,* hypercalcemia, hyperphosphatemia, hypercholesterolemia.
Skin: pain, induration at injection site, local edema, acne.
Other: androgenic effects in women, gynecomastia, hypersensitivity reactions, hypoestrogenic effects in women, excessive hormonal effects in men, male pattern baldness.

INTERACTIONS
Drug-drug. *Corticosteroids:* May increase risk of edema. Use together cautiously, especially in patients with cardiac or hepatic disease.
Hepatotoxic drugs: May increase risk of hepatotoxicity. Monitor liver function closely.
Insulin, oral antidiabetics: May decrease glucose level; may alter dosage requirements. Monitor glucose level in diabetic patients.
Oral anticoagulants: May increase sensitivity; may alter dosage requirements. Monitor PT and INR; decrease anticoagulant dose if necessary.
Oxyphenbutazone: May increase oxyphenbutazone level. Monitor patient.

EFFECTS ON LAB TEST RESULTS
● May increase sodium, potassium, phosphate, cholesterol, liver enzyme, calcium, and creatinine levels. May decrease thyroxine-binding globulin, total T_4 levels, serum creatinine, and 17-ketosteroid levels.
● May increase RBC count and resin uptake of T_3 and T_4.
● May cause abnormal glucose tolerance test results.

CONTRAINDICATIONS & CAUTIONS
● Contraindicated in patients hypersensitive to drug and in those with hypercalcemia or cardiac, hepatic, or renal decompensation.
● Contraindicated in men with breast or prostate cancer and in pregnant or breast-feeding women.
● Use cautiously in elderly patients

NURSING CONSIDERATIONS

• Unless contraindicated, use with high-calorie, high-protein diet. Give small, frequent meals to help avoid nausea.
• Don't give to woman of childbearing age until pregnancy is ruled out.
• Cypionate and enanthate are long-acting solutions.
• Monitor patient's liver function test results.
• In patients with metastatic breast cancer, hypercalcemia usually indicates progression of bone metastases. Report signs and symptoms of hypercalcemia.
• Report evidence of virilization in women. Androgenic effects include acne, edema, weight gain, increased hair growth, hoarseness, clitoral enlargement, decreased breast size, changes in libido, male pattern baldness, and oily skin or hair.
• Watch for hypoestrogenic effects in women (flushing; diaphoresis; vaginitis, including itching, drying, and burning; vaginal bleeding; menstrual irregularities).
• Watch for excessive hormonal effects in men and boys. In prepubertal boy, watch for premature epiphyseal closure, acne, priapism, growth of body and facial hair, and phallic enlargement. In postpubertal men, watch for testicular atrophy, oligospermia, decreased ejaculatory volume, impotence, gynecomastia, and epididymitis.
• Monitor patient's weight and blood pressure routinely.
• Monitor prepubertal boys by X-ray for rate of bone maturation.
• **Alert:** Therapeutic response in breast cancer is usually apparent within 3 months. If disease progresses, stop drug.
• Androgens may alter results of laboratory studies during therapy and for 2 to 3 weeks after therapy ends.
• **Look alike–sound alike:** Don't confuse testosterone with testolactone.
• **Alert:** Testosterone salts aren't interchangeable.

PATIENT TEACHING

• Make sure patient understands importance of using an effective nonhormonal contraceptive during therapy.

• Instruct patient to stop drug immediately and notify prescriber if pregnancy is suspected.
• Review signs and symptoms of virilization with woman, and instruct her to notify prescriber if they occur.
• Advise woman to wear cotton underwear and to wash after intercourse to decrease risk of vaginitis.
• Instruct man to notify prescriber about priapism, reduced ejaculatory volume, or gynecomastia.
• Warn diabetic patient to be alert for hypoglycemia and to notify prescriber if it occurs.
• Instruct boys using testosterone for delayed puberty to have X-rays of hand and wrist obtained every 6 months during treatment.
• Tell patient to report sudden weight gain.
• Warn patient that drug shouldn't be used to enhance athletic performance.
• Instruct patient how to use the buccal system.
• Advise patient to avoid dislodging buccal system and ensure that the system is in place after toothbrushing, use of mouthwash, and eating or drinking.
• Tell men not to chew or swallow buccal system.

testosterone transdermal
Androderm, AndroGel, Testim

Pharmacologic class: androgen
Pregnancy risk category X
Controlled substance schedule III

AVAILABLE FORMS
1% gel: 25 mg, 50 mg per unit dose; 1.25 g per nonaerosol metered pump
Transdermal system: 2.5 mg/day, 5 mg/day

INDICATIONS & DOSAGES
➤ **Primary or hypogonadotropic hypogonadism**
Men: One or two Androderm patches applied to back, abdomen, arm, or thigh nightly for total dosage of 5 mg daily. Dose may be increased to 7.5 mg once daily or decreased to 2.5 mg once daily, depending upon a.m. serum testosterone levels. Or,

initially, 50 mg applied every morning to shoulders, upper arms, or abdomen. Don't apply Testim to abdomen. Check testosterone level after about 2 weeks. If response is inadequate, may increase AndroGel to 75 mg daily. Then, adjust to 100 mg (either gel) if needed. Or, for AndroGel pump, 5 g (4 pumps) applied every morning to shoulders, upper arms, or abdomen. Check testosterone level after about 2 weeks. If response is inadequate, may increase to 7.5 g (6 pumps) daily or from 7.5 g to 10 g (8 pumps) daily.

ADMINISTRATION
Transdermal
● Wear gloves when handling patches. Fold used patches with adhesive sides together to discard.
● Apply patch to clean, dry, intact skin of the shoulders, upper arms, or abdomen only and not to scrotum or bony prominences.
Topical
● Fully prime the AndroGel pump by pumping three times before first use. Discard that gel.
● Wear gloves to apply gel to clean, dry, intact skin of the shoulders, upper arms, or abdomen only and not to scrotum or bony prominences. Testim shouldn't be applied to the abdomen.

ACTION
Releases testosterone, which stimulates target tissues to develop normally in androgen-deficient men.

Route	Onset	Peak	Duration
Transdermal, topical	Unknown	2–4 hr	2 hr after removal

Half-life: 10 to 100 minutes.

ADVERSE REACTIONS
CNS: *stroke,* asthenia, depression, headache.
GI: *GI bleeding.*
GU: prostatitis, prostate abnormalities, UTI.
Hepatic: *cholestatic hepatitis,* reversible jaundice.

Metabolic: hypernatremia, hyperkalemia, hypercalcemia, hyperphosphatemia, hypercholesterolemia.
Skin: *pruritus, blister under patch,* acne irritation, allergic contact dermatitis, burning.
Other: gynecomastia, breast tenderness, flulike syndrome.

INTERACTIONS
Drug-drug. *Corticosteroids:* May increase risk of edema. Use together cautiously, especially in patients with cardiac or hepatic disease.
Insulin: May alter insulin dosage requirements. Monitor glucose level.
Oral anticoagulants: May alter anticoagulant dosage requirements. Monitor PT and INR.
Oxyphenbutazone: May increase oxyphenbutazone level. Monitor patient.
Propranolol: May increase propranolol clearance. Monitor patient.

EFFECTS ON LAB TEST RESULTS
● May increase sodium, potassium, phosphate, cholesterol, liver enzyme, calcium, and creatinine levels and resin uptake of T_3 and T_4. May decrease total T_4 levels.
● May increase RBC count.

CONTRAINDICATIONS & CAUTIONS
● Contraindicated in patients hypersensitive to drug, in women, in men with known or suspected breast or prostate cancer, and in patients with CV, renal, or hepatic disease.
● Use cautiously in elderly men.

NURSING CONSIDERATIONS
● Periodically assess liver function test results, lipid profiles, hemoglobin level, hematocrit (with long-term use), and levels of prostatic acid phosphatase and prostate-specific antigen.
● Watch for excessive hormonal effects.

PATIENT TEACHING
● Tell patient to fully prime the AndroGel pump by pumping three times before first use and to discard that gel.
● Tell patient to apply gel or patch to clean, dry, intact skin of the shoulders, upper arms, or abdomen only and not to scrotum

or bony prominences. Testim shouldn't be applied to the abdomen. Tell him that he can first pump gel into his hand.
• Tell patient to wash his hands thoroughly with soap and water after applying.
• Instruct patient that patch must be changed every 24 hours.
• For best results, advise patient not to swim or shower for at least 5 hours after applying gel. Showering or swimming at least 1 hour after applying, if done infrequently, should have minimal effects on drug absorption.
• Tell patient that if the patch falls off, it may be reapplied. If patch falls off and can't be reapplied, and it has been worn at least 12 hours, a new patch may be applied at the next application time.
• Warn diabetic patient that drug may decrease glucose level and to be alert for hypoglycemia.
• Advise patient to report persistent erections, nausea, vomiting, changes in skin color, ankle swelling, or sudden weight gain to prescriber.
• Tell patient that drug may cause virilization in his female sexual partner, who should report acne or changes in body hair distribution.
• Tell patient that Androderm doesn't have to be removed during sexual intercourse or while showering.

---

thiamine hydrochloride (vitamin B₁)

Betaxin†, Thiamiject†, Thiamilate

Pregnancy risk category A; C if dose exceeds RDA

AVAILABLE FORMS
Injection: 100 mg/ml
Tablets: 50 mg ◊, 100 mg ◊, 250 mg ◊, 500 mg ◊
Tablets (enteric-coated): 20 mg ◊

INDICATIONS & DOSAGES
➤ **RDA**
Adult men: 1.2 mg.
Adult women: 1.1 mg.
Boys ages 14 to 18: Give 1.2 mg.
Girls ages 14 to 18: Give 1 mg.
Children ages 9 to 13: Give 0.9 mg.

Children ages 4 to 8: Give 0.6 mg.
Children ages 1 to 3: Give 0.5 mg.
Infants ages 6 months to 1 year: 0.3 mg.
Neonates and infants younger than age 6 months: 0.2 mg.
Pregnant women: 1.4 mg.
Breast-feeding women: 1.5 mg.
➤ **Beriberi**
Adults: Depending on severity, 5 to 30 mg I.M. t.i.d. for 2 weeks; then dietary correction and multivitamin supplement containing 5 to 30 mg thiamine daily for 1 month.
Children: Depending on severity, 10 to 25 mg I.V. or I.M. daily. For noncritically ill children, 10 to 50 mg P.O. daily in divided doses for several weeks with adequate diet.
➤ **Wet beriberi with myocardial failure**
Adults and children: 10 to 30 mg I.V. t.i.d.
➤ **Wernicke encephalopathy**
Adults: Initially, 100 mg I.V.; then 50 to 100 mg I.V. or I.M. daily until patient is consuming a regular balanced diet.

---

thioridazine hydrochloride
thye-oh-RYE-da-zeen

Pharmacologic class: phenothiazine
Pregnancy risk category C

AVAILABLE FORMS
Oral concentrate: 30 mg/ml, 100 mg/ml (3% to 4.2% alcohol)
Tablets: 10 mg, 15 mg, 25 mg, 50 mg, 100 mg, 150 mg, 200 mg

INDICATIONS & DOSAGES
➤ **Schizophrenia in patients who don't respond to treatment with at least two other antipsychotic drugs**
Adults: Initially, 50 to 100 mg P.O. t.i.d., increase gradually to 800 mg daily in divided doses, as needed.
Children ages 2 to 12: Initially, 0.5 mg/kg daily in divided doses. Increase gradually to optimal therapeutic effect; maximum dose is 3 mg/kg daily.

ADMINISTRATION
P.O.
- *Alert:* Different liquid formulations have different concentrations. Check dosage carefully.
- Prevent contact dermatitis by keeping drug away from skin and clothes. Wear gloves when preparing liquid forms.
- Dilute liquid concentrate with water or fruit juice just before giving.
- Shake suspension well before using.

ACTION
Unknown. A piperidine phenothiazine that probably blocks postsynaptic dopamine receptors in the brain.

Route	Onset	Peak	Duration
P.O.	Unknown	Unknown	Unknown

Half-life: 20 to 40 hours.

ADVERSE REACTIONS
CNS: *tardive dyskinesia, sedation,* **neuroleptic malignant syndrome,** EEG changes, dizziness.
CV: *orthostatic hypotension,* **prolonged QTc interval, torsades de pointes,** ECG changes, tachycardia.
EENT: *ocular changes, blurred vision,* retinitis pigmentosa.
GI: *dry mouth, constipation,* increased appetite.
GU: *urine retention,* dark urine, menstrual irregularities, inhibited ejaculation.
Hematologic: *transient leukopenia,* **agranulocytosis,** hyperprolactinemia.
Hepatic: cholestatic jaundice.
Metabolic: weight gain.
Skin: *mild photosensitivity reactions,* allergic reactions.
Other: gynecomastia, galactorrhea.

INTERACTIONS
Drug-drug. *Antacids:* May inhibit absorption of oral phenothiazines. Separate dosages by at least 2 hours.
Antiarrhythmics (amiodarone, bretylium, disopyramide, dofetilide, procainamide, quinidine, sotalol), duloxetine, fluoxetine, fluvoxamine, paroxetine, pimozide, pindolol, propranolol, other drugs that inhibit CYP2D6 enzyme, *quinolones:* May inhibit metabolism of thioridazine; may cause arrhythmias resulting from QTc interval prolongation. Use together is contraindicated.
Barbiturates: May decrease phenothiazine effect. Monitor patient.
Centrally acting antihypertensives: May decrease antihypertensive effect. Monitor blood pressure.
Lithium: May decrease phenothiazine effect and increase neurologic adverse effects. Monitor patient closely.
Other CNS depressants: May increase CNS depression. Use together cautiously.
Drug-herb. *St. John's wort:* May cause photosensitivity reactions. Advise patient to avoid excessive sunlight exposure.
Drug-lifestyle. *Alcohol use:* May increase CNS depression, particularly psychomotor skills. Strongly discourage use together.
Sun exposure: May increase risk of photosensitivity reactions. Advise patient to avoid excessive sunlight exposure.

EFFECTS ON LAB TEST RESULTS
- May increase liver enzyme levels.
- May decrease granulocyte and WBC counts.
- May cause false-positive results for urinary porphyrin, urobilinogen, amylase, and 5-hydroxyindoleacetic acid tests and for urine pregnancy tests that use human chorionic gonadotropin.

CONTRAINDICATIONS & CAUTIONS
- Contraindicated in patients hypersensitive to drug and in those with CNS depression, coma, or severe hypertensive or hypotensive cardiac disease.
- Contraindicated in patients taking fluvoxamine, propranolol, pindolol, fluoxetine, drugs that inhibit CYP2D6 enzyme, or drugs that prolong the QTc interval.
- Contraindicated in patients with reduced levels of CYP2D6 enzyme, those with congenital long QT interval syndrome, or those with history of cardiac arrhythmias.
- Use cautiously in elderly or debilitated patients and in patients with hepatic disease, CV disease, respiratory disorders, hypocalcemia, seizure disorders, or severe reactions to insulin or electroconvulsive therapy.

• Use cautiously in those exposed to extreme heat or cold (including antipyretic therapy) or organophosphate insecticides.

NURSING CONSIDERATIONS
• *Alert:* Before therapy, obtain baseline ECG and potassium level. Patients with a QTc interval greater than 450 msec shouldn't receive drug. Patients with a QTc interval greater than 500 msec should stop drug.
• *Alert:* Drug isn't used as first-line treatment of schizophrenia because of risk of life-threatening adverse reactions.
• Monitor patient for tardive dyskinesia, which may occur after prolonged use. It may not appear until months or years later and may disappear spontaneously or persist for life, despite ending drug.
• *Alert:* Watch for evidence of neuroleptic malignant syndrome (extrapyramidal effects, hyperthermia, autonomic disturbance), which is rare but commonly deadly.
• Monitor periodic blood tests (CBC and liver function tests) and ophthalmic tests (long-term use).
• Withhold dose and notify prescriber if jaundice, blood dyscrasia (fever, sore throat, infection, cellulitis, weakness), or persistent extrapyramidal reactions develop, especially in children or pregnant women.
• Don't stop drug abruptly unless required by severe adverse reactions.
• After abrupt withdrawal of long-term therapy, gastritis, nausea, vomiting, dizziness, tremor, feeling of warmth or cold, diaphoresis, tachycardia, headache, or insomnia may occur.
• *Look alike–sound alike:* Don't confuse thioridazine with Thorazine.

PATIENT TEACHING
• Tell patient to shake suspension before use.
• Warn patient to avoid activities that require alertness until effects of drug are known.
• Tell patient to watch for dizziness when standing quickly. Advise patient to change positions slowly.

• Instruct patient to report symptoms of dizziness, palpitations, or fainting to prescriber.
• Tell patient to avoid alcohol use.
• Have patient report signs of urine retention, constipation, or blurred vision.
• Tell patient that drug may discolor the urine.
• Advise patient to relieve dry mouth with sugarless gum or hard candy.
• Instruct patient to use sunblock and to wear protective clothing outdoors.

thiothixene
thye-oh-THIX-een

Navane

thiothixene hydrochloride
Navane*

Pharmacologic class: thioxanthene
Pregnancy risk category C

AVAILABLE FORMS
thiothixene
Capsules: 1 mg, 2 mg, 5 mg, 10 mg, 20 mg
thiothixene hydrochloride
Oral concentrate: 5 mg/ml*

INDICATIONS & DOSAGES
➤ **Mild to moderate psychosis**
Adults: Initially, 2 mg P.O. t.i.d. Increase gradually to 15 mg daily, as needed.
➤ **Severe psychosis**
Adults: Initially, 5 mg P.O. b.i.d. Increase gradually to 20 to 30 mg daily, as needed. Maximum dose is 60 mg daily.

ADMINISTRATION
P.O.
• Prevent contact dermatitis by keeping drug off skin and clothes. Wear gloves when preparing liquid forms.
• Dilute liquid concentrate with fruit juice, milk, or semisolid food just before giving.
• Slight yellowing of injection or concentrate is common and doesn't affect potency. Discard markedly discolored solutions.

ACTION

Unknown. Probably blocks dopamine receptors in the brain.

Route	Onset	Peak	Duration
P.O.	Unknown	Unknown	Unknown

Half-life: 20 to 40 hours.

ADVERSE REACTIONS

CNS: *extrapyramidal reactions, drowsiness, tardive dyskinesia,* **neuroleptic malignant syndrome,** restlessness, agitation, insomnia, sedation, EEG changes, pseudoparkinsonism, dizziness.
CV: *hypotension,* tachycardia, ECG changes.
EENT: *blurred vision,* ocular changes, nasal congestion.
GI: *dry mouth, constipation.*
GU: *urine retention,* menstrual irregularities, inhibited ejaculation.
Hematologic: *agranulocytosis, transient leukopenia,* leukocytosis.
Hepatic: jaundice.
Metabolic: weight gain.
Skin: *mild photosensitivity reactions,* allergic reactions, exfoliative dermatitis.
Other: gynecomastia.

INTERACTIONS

Drug-drug. *CNS depressants:* May increase CNS depression. Use together cautiously.
Drug-lifestyle. *Alcohol use:* May increase CNS depression. Discourage use together. *Sun exposure:* May increase risk of photosensitivity reactions. Advise patient to avoid excessive sunlight exposure.

EFFECTS ON LAB TEST RESULTS

• May increase liver enzyme levels.
• May increase or decrease WBC counts. May decrease granulocyte counts.
• May cause false-positive results for urinary porphyrin, urobilinogen, amylase, and 5-hydroxyindoleacetic acid tests and for urine pregnancy tests that use human chorionic gonadotropin.

CONTRAINDICATIONS & CAUTIONS

• Contraindicated in patients hypersensitive to drug and in those with CNS depression, circulatory collapse, coma, or blood dyscrasia.
• Use with caution in patients with history of seizure disorder and in those undergoing alcohol withdrawal.
• Use cautiously in elderly or debilitated patients and in those with CV disease (may cause sudden drop in blood pressure), hepatic disease, heat exposure, glaucoma, or prostatic hyperplasia.

NURSING CONSIDERATIONS

• Monitor patient for tardive dyskinesia, which may occur after prolonged use; it may not appear until months or years later, and may disappear spontaneously or persist for life, despite stopping drug.
• *Alert:* Watch for evidence of neuroleptic malignant syndrome (extrapyramidal effects, hyperthermia, autonomic disturbance), which is rare but deadly.
• Monitor periodic CBC, liver function tests, renal function tests, and ophthalmic tests for long-term use.
• Watch for orthostatic hypotension. Keep patient supine for 1 hour after drug administration, and tell him to change positions slowly.
• Withhold dose and notify prescriber if jaundice, blood dyscrasia (fever, sore throat, infection, cellulitis, weakness), or persistent extrapyramidal reactions develop, especially in pregnant women.
• Don't withdraw drug abruptly unless severe adverse reactions occur.
• After abrupt withdrawal of long-term therapy, gastritis, nausea, vomiting, dizziness, tremor, feeling of warmth or cold, diaphoresis, tachycardia, headache, or insomnia may occur.
• *Look alike–sound alike:* Don't confuse Navane with Nubain or Norvasc.

PATIENT TEACHING

• Warn patient to avoid activities that require alertness until effects of drug are known.
• Tell patient to watch for dizziness upon standing quickly. Advise him to change positions slowly.
• Instruct patient to dilute liquid appropriately.
• Tell patient to avoid alcohol use during therapy.

- Have patient report signs of urine retention, constipation, or blurred vision.
- Instruct patient to use sunblock and to wear protective clothing outdoors.

---

topiramate
toe-PIE-rah-mate

Topamax

Pharmacologic class: sulfamate-substituted monosaccharide
Pregnancy risk category C

AVAILABLE FORMS
Capsules, sprinkles: 15 mg, 25 mg
Tablets: 25 mg, 50 mg, 100 mg, 200 mg

INDICATIONS & DOSAGES
➤ **Initial monotherapy for partial-onset or primary generalized tonic-clonic seizures**
Adults and children age 10 or older: Recommended daily dose is 400 mg P.O. divided b.i.d. (morning and evening). To achieve this dosage, adjust as follows: 1st week, 25 mg P.O. b.i.d.; 2nd week, 50 mg P.O. b.i.d.; 3rd week, 75 mg P.O. b.i.d.; 4th week, 100 mg P.O. b.i.d.; 5th week, 150 mg P.O. b.i.d.; and 6th week, 200 mg P.O. b.i.d.
➤ **Adjunct treatment for partial-onset or primary generalized tonic-clonic seizures**
Adults: Initially, 25 to 50 mg P.O. daily; increase gradually by 25 to 50 mg/week until an effective daily dose is reached. Adjust to recommended daily dose of 200 to 400 mg P.O. in two divided doses for adults with partial seizures or 400 mg P.O. in two divided doses for adults with primary generalized tonic-clonic seizures.
Children ages 2 to 16: Initially, 1 to 3 mg/kg daily given at bedtime for 1 week. Increase at 1- or 2-week intervals by 1 to 3 mg/kg daily in two divided doses to achieve optimal response. Recommended daily dose is 5 to 9 mg/kg in two divided doses.
➤ **Lennox-Gastaut syndrome**
Children ages 2 to 16: Initially, 1 to 3 mg/kg daily given at bedtime for 1 week. Increase at 1- or 2-week intervals by

1 to 3 mg/kg daily in two divided doses to achieve optimal response. Recommended daily dose is 5 to 9 mg/kg, in two divided doses.
➤ **To prevent migraine headache**
Adults: Initially, 25 mg P.O. daily in evening for 1st week. Then, 25 mg P.O. b.i.d. in morning and evening for 2nd week. For 3rd week, 25 mg P.O. in morning and 50 mg P.O. in evening. For 4th week, 50 mg P.O. b.i.d. in morning and evening.
Adjust-a-dose: If creatinine clearance is less than 70 ml/minute, reduce dosage by 50%. For hemodialysis patients, supplemental doses may be needed to avoid rapid drops in drug level during prolonged dialysis treatment.

ADMINISTRATION
P.O.
- Give drug without regard for food.
- Crushed or broken tablets have a bitter taste.
- Capsules may be opened and contents sprinkled on a teaspoon of soft food. Patient should swallow immediately without chewing.

ACTION
Unknown. May block a sodium channel, potentiate the activity of GABA, and inhibit kainate's ability to activate an amino acid receptor.

Route	Onset	Peak	Duration
P.O.	Unknown	2 hr	Unknown

Half-life: 21 hours.

ADVERSE REACTIONS
CNS: *ataxia, confusion, difficulty with memory, dizziness, fatigue, nervousness, paresthesia, psychomotor slowing, somnolence, speech disorders, tremor,* **generalized tonic-clonic seizures, suicide attempts,** abnormal coordination, aggressive reaction, agitation, apathy, asthenia, depression, depersonalization, difficulty with concentration, attention, or language, emotional lability, euphoria, fever, hallucination, hyperkinesia, hypertonia, hypoesthesia, hypokinesia, insomnia, malaise, mood problems, personality disorder, psychosis, stupor, vertigo.

CV: chest pain, edema, palpitations, vasodilation.
EENT: *abnormal vision, diplopia, nystagmus,* conjunctivitis, epistaxis, eye pain, hearing problems, pharyngitis, sinusitis, tinnitus.
GI: *anorexia, nausea,* abdominal pain, constipation, diarrhea, dry mouth, dyspepsia, flatulence, gastroenteritis, gingivitis, taste perversion, vomiting.
GU: amenorrhea, dysuria, dysmenorrhea, hematuria, impotence, intermenstrual bleeding, leukorrhea, menstrual disorder, menorrhagia, urinary frequency, renal calculi, urinary incontinence, UTI, vaginitis.
Hematologic: *leukopenia,* anemia.
Metabolic: *decreased weight,* increased weight.
Musculoskeletal: arthralgia, back or leg pain, muscle weakness, myalgia, rigors.
Respiratory: *upper respiratory tract infection,* bronchitis, coughing, dyspnea.
Skin: acne, alopecia, increased sweating, pruritus, rash.
Other: body odor, breast pain, decreased libido, flulike syndrome, hot flashes, lymphadenopathy.

INTERACTIONS

Drug-drug. *Carbamazepine:* May decrease topiramate level. Monitor patient.
Carbonic anhydrase inhibitors (acetazolamide, dichlorphenamide): May cause renal calculus formation. Avoid using together.
CNS depressants: May cause CNS depression and other adverse cognitive and neuropsychiatric events. Use together cautiously.
Hormonal contraceptives: May decrease efficacy. Report changes in menstrual patterns. Advise patient to use another contraceptive method.
Phenytoin: May decrease topiramate level and increase phenytoin level. Monitor levels.
Valproic acid: May decrease valproic acid and topiramate level. Monitor patient.
Drug-lifestyle. *Alcohol use:* May cause CNS depression and other adverse cognitive and neuropsychiatric events. Discourage use together.

EFFECTS ON LAB TEST RESULTS
● May increase liver enzyme levels. May decrease bicarbonate and hemoglobin levels and hematocrit.
● May decrease WBC count.

CONTRAINDICATIONS & CAUTIONS
● Contraindicated in patients hypersensitive to drug or its components.
● Use cautiously in breast-feeding or pregnant women and in those with hepatic impairment.
● Use cautiously with other drugs that predispose patients to heat-related disorders, including other carbonic anhydrase inhibitors and anticholinergics.

NURSING CONSIDERATIONS
● If needed, withdraw anticonvulsant (including topiramate) gradually to minimize risk of increased seizure activity.
● Monitoring topiramate level isn't necessary.
● Drug may infrequently cause oligohidrosis and hyperthermia, mainly in children. Monitor patient closely, especially in hot weather.
● Drug may cause hyperchloremic, non-anion gap metabolic acidosis from renal bicarbonate loss. Factors that may predispose patients to acidosis, such as renal disease, severe respiratory disorders, status epilepticus, diarrhea, surgery, ketogenic diet, or drugs, may add to topiramate's bicarbonate-lowering effects.
● Measure baseline and periodic bicarbonate levels. If metabolic acidosis develops and persists, consider reducing the dose, gradually stopping the drug, or alkali treatment.
● Drug is rapidly cleared by dialysis. A prolonged period of dialysis may cause low drug level and seizures. A supplemental dose may be needed.
● Stop drug if patient experiences acute myopia and secondary angle-closure glaucoma.
● *Look alike–sound alike:* Don't confuse Topamax with Toprol-XL, Tegretol, or Tegretol-XR.

PATIENT TEACHING
• Tell patient to drink plenty of fluids during therapy to minimize risk of forming kidney stones.
• Advise patient not to drive or operate hazardous machinery until CNS effects of drug are known. Drug can cause sleepiness, dizziness, confusion, and concentration problems.
• Tell woman of childbearing age that drug may decrease effectiveness of hormonal contraceptives. Advise woman using hormonal contraceptives to report change in menstrual patterns.
• Tell patient to avoid crushing or breaking tablets because of bitter taste.
• Inform patient that drug can be taken without regard to food.
• Tell patient that capsules may either be swallowed whole or carefully opened and contents sprinkled on a teaspoonful of soft food. Tell patient to swallow immediately without chewing.
• Tell patient to notify prescriber immediately if he experiences changes in vision.

---

trazodone hydrochloride
TRAYZ-oh-dohn

Pharmacologic class: triazolopyridine derivative
Pregnancy risk category C

AVAILABLE FORMS
Tablets: 50 mg, 100 mg, 150 mg, 300 mg

INDICATIONS & DOSAGES
➤ **Depression**
Adults: Initially, 150 mg P.O. daily in divided doses; then increased by 50 mg daily every 3 to 4 days, as needed. Dose ranges from 150 to 400 mg daily. Maximum, 600 mg daily for inpatients and 400 mg daily for outpatients.
➤ **Insomnia ♦**
Adults: 25 to 75 mg P.O. in conjunction with an SSRI.

ADMINISTRATION
P.O.
• Give drug after meals or a light snack for optimal absorption and to decrease risk of dizziness.

ACTION
Unknown. Inhibits CNS neuronal uptake of serotonin; not a tricyclic derivative.

Route	Onset	Peak	Duration
P.O.	Unknown	1–2 hr	Unknown

Half-life: First phase, 3 to 6 hours; second phase, 5 to 9 hours.

ADVERSE REACTIONS
CNS: *drowsiness, dizziness,* nervousness, fatigue, confusion, tremor, weakness, hostility, anger, nightmares, vivid dreams, headache, insomnia, syncope.
CV: orthostatic hypotension, tachycardia, hypertension, shortness of breath, ECG changes.
EENT: blurred vision, tinnitus, nasal congestion.
GI: dry mouth, dysgeusia, constipation, nausea, vomiting, anorexia.
GU: urine retention, priapism possibly leading to impotence, hematuria.
Hematologic: anemia.
Skin: rash, urticaria, diaphoresis.
Other: decreased libido.

INTERACTIONS
Drug-drug. *Amphetamines, buspirone, dextromethorphan, dihydroergotamine, lithium salts, meperidine, SSRIs or SSNRIs (duloxetine, venlafaxine), sumatriptan, tramadol, tricyclic antidepressants, tryptophan:* May increase the risk of serotonin syndrome. Avoid combining drugs that increase the availability of serotonin in the CNS; monitor patient closely if used together.
Antihypertensives: May increase hypotensive effect of trazodone. Antihypertensive dosage may need to be decreased.
Clonidine, CNS depressants: May enhance CNS depression. Avoid using together.
CYP3A4 inducers (carbamazepine): May reduce trazodone level. Monitor patient closely; may need to increase trazodone dose.
CYP3A4 inhibitors (ketoconazole): May slow the clearance of trazodone and increase trazodone level. May cause nausea, hypotension, and fainting. Consider decreasing trazodone dose.

Digoxin, phenytoin: May increase levels of these drugs. Watch for toxicity.
MAO inhibitors: Effects unknown. Use together with extreme caution.
Protease inhibitors (amprenavir, atazanavir, fosamprenavir, indinavir, lopinavir and ritonavir, nelfinavir, ritonavir, saquinavir): May increase trazodone levels and adverse effects. Monitor patient and adjust trazodone dose, as needed.
Drug-herb. *Ginkgo biloba:* May cause sedation. Discourage use together.
St. John's wort: May cause serotonin syndrome. Discourage use together.
Drug-lifestyle. *Alcohol use:* May enhance CNS depression. Discourage use together.

EFFECTS ON LAB TEST RESULTS
● May increase ALT and AST levels. May decrease hemoglobin level.

CONTRAINDICATIONS & CAUTIONS
● Contraindicated in patients hypersensitive to drug.
● Use cautiously in patients with cardiac disease or in the initial recovery phase of MI and in patients at risk for suicide.

NURSING CONSIDERATIONS
● Record mood changes. Monitor patient for suicidal tendencies and allow only minimum supply of drug.
● *Alert:* Drug may increase the risk of suicidal thinking and behavior in children, adolescents, and young adults ages 18 to 24 during the first 2 months of treatment, especially those with major depressive disorder or other psychiatric disorder.
● *Look alike–sound alike:* Don't confuse trazodone hydrochloride with tramadol hydrochloride.

PATIENT TEACHING
● *Alert:* Tell patient to report a persistent, painful erection (priapism) right away because he may need immediate intervention.
● Warn patient to avoid activities that require alertness and good coordination until effects of drug are known. Drowsiness and dizziness usually subside after first few weeks.

● Teach caregivers how to recognize signs and symptoms of suicidal tendency or suicidal thoughts.

triazolam
trye-AY-zoe-lam

Apo-Triazo†, Halcion

Pharmacologic class:
benzodiazepine
Pregnancy risk category X
Controlled substance schedule IV

AVAILABLE FORMS
Tablets: 0.125 mg, 0.25 mg

INDICATIONS & DOSAGES
➤ **Insomnia**
Adults: 0.125 to 0.5 mg P.O. at bedtime.
Elderly or debilitated patients: 0.125 mg P.O. at bedtime; increase, as needed, to 0.25 mg P.O. at bedtime.

ADMINISTRATION
P.O.
● Give drug without regard for food, but avoid giving with grapefruit or grapefruit juice.

ACTION
Unknown. Probably acts on the limbic system, thalamus, and hypothalamus of the CNS to produce hypnotic effects.

Route	Onset	Peak	Duration
P.O.	Unknown	1–2 hr	1½–5½ hr

Half-life: 1½ to 5½ hours.

ADVERSE REACTIONS
CNS: complex sleep-related behaviors, drowsiness, amnesia, ataxia, depression, dizziness, headache, lack of coordination, mental confusion, nervousness, physical or psychological dependence, rebound insomnia.
GI: nausea, vomiting.
Other: *anaphylaxis, angioedema.*

INTERACTIONS
Drug-drug. *Cimetidine, erythromycin, fluoxetine, fluvoxamine, isoniazid, nefazodone, ranitidine:* May increase triazolam level. Avoid using with azole antifungals or nefazodone. Watch for increased sedation if used with other drugs.
CNS depressants: May cause excessive CNS depression. Use together cautiously.
Diltiazem: May increase CNS depression and prolonged effects of triazolam. Reduce triazolam dose.
Fluconazole, itraconazole, ketoconazole , miconazole: May increase and prolong drug level, CNS depression, and psychomotor impairment. Avoid using together.
Drug-herb. *Calendula, hops, kava, lemon balm, passion flower, skullcap, valerian:* May enhance sedative effect of drug. Discourage use together.
Drug-food. *Grapefruit:* May delay onset and increase drug effects. Discourage use together.
Drug-lifestyle. *Alcohol use:* May cause additive CNS effects. Discourage use together.
Smoking: May increase metabolism and clearance of drug. Advise patient who smokes to watch for decreased effectiveness of drug.

EFFECTS ON LAB TEST RESULTS
• May increase liver function test values.

CONTRAINDICATIONS & CAUTIONS
• Contraindicated in pregnant patients and those hypersensitive to benzodiazepines.
• Use cautiously in patients with impaired hepatic or renal function, chronic pulmonary insufficiency, sleep apnea, mental depression, suicidal tendencies, or history of drug abuse.
• Use cautiously in breast-feeding women.

NURSING CONSIDERATIONS
• *Alert:* Anaphylaxis and angioedema may occur as early as the first dose; monitor the patient closely.
• Assess mental status before starting therapy and reduce doses in elderly patients; these patients may be more sensitive to drug's adverse CNS effects.
• Monitor CBC, chemistry, and urinalysis.

• Take precautions to prevent hoarding or overdosing by patients who are depressed, suicidal, or drug-dependent or who have history of drug abuse.
• Minor changes in EEG patterns (usually low-voltage fast activity) may occur during and after therapy.
• *Look alike–sound alike:* Don't confuse Halcion with Haldol or halcinonide.

PATIENT TEACHING
• *Alert:* Warn patient that drug may cause allergic reactions, facial swelling, and complex sleep-related behaviors, such as driving, eating, and making phone calls while asleep. Advise patient to report these adverse effects.
• Warn patient not to take more than prescribed amount; overdose can occur at total daily dose of 2 mg (or four times highest recommended amount).
• Tell patient to avoid alcohol use while taking drug.
• Warn patient not to stop drug abruptly after taking for 2 weeks or longer.
• Caution patient to avoid performing activities that require mental alertness or physical coordination.
• Inform patient that drug doesn't tend to cause morning drowsiness.
• Tell patient that rebound insomnia may occur for 1 or 2 nights after stopping therapy.

---

trifluoperazine hydrochloride
trye-floo-oh-PER-eh-zeen

Pharmacologic class: phenothiazine
Pregnancy risk category NR

AVAILABLE FORMS
Tablets (regular and film-coated): 1 mg, 2 mg, 5 mg, 10 mg

INDICATIONS & DOSAGES
➤ **Anxiety states**
Adults: 1 to 2 mg P.O. b.i.d. Maximum, 6 mg daily. Don't give drug for longer than 12 weeks for anxiety.
➤ **Schizophrenia, other psychotic disorders**
Adults: In outpatients, 1 to 2 mg P.O. b.i.d. In hospitalized patients, 2 to 5 mg P.O.

---

b.i.d., gradually increased until therapeutic response occurs. Most patients respond to 15 to 20 mg P.O. daily, although some may need 40 mg daily or more.
Children ages 6 to 12: For hospitalized or closely supervised patients, 1 mg P.O. daily or b.i.d.; may increase gradually to 15 mg daily, if needed.

ADMINISTRATION
P.O.
● Give drug without regard for meals.

ACTION
Unknown. A piperazine phenothiazine that probably blocks dopamine receptors in the brain.

Route	Onset	Peak	Duration
P.O.	Unknown	Unknown	Unknown

Half-life: 20 to 40 hours.

ADVERSE REACTIONS
CNS: *extrapyramidal reactions, tardive dyskinesia,* **neuroleptic malignant syndrome,** pseudoparkinsonism, dizziness, drowsiness, insomnia, fatigue, headache.
CV: *orthostatic hypotension,* tachycardia, ECG changes.
EENT: *blurred vision,* ocular changes.
GI: *dry mouth, constipation,* nausea.
GU: *urine retention,* menstrual irregularities, inhibited ejaculation.
Hematologic: *transient leukopenia,* **agranulocytosis.**
Hepatic: cholestatic jaundice.
Metabolic: weight gain.
Skin: *photosensitivity reactions,* allergic reactions, rash.
Other: gynecomastia.

INTERACTIONS
Drug-drug. *Antacids:* May inhibit absorption of oral phenothiazines. Separate antacid and phenothiazine doses by at least 2 hours.
Barbiturates, lithium: May decrease phenothiazine effect. Monitor patient.
Centrally acting antihypertensives: May decrease antihypertensive effect. Monitor blood pressure.
CNS depressants: May increase CNS depression. Use together cautiously.

Propranolol: May increase propranolol and trifluoperazine levels. Monitor patient.
Warfarin: May decrease effect of oral anticoagulants. Monitor PT and INR.
Drug-herb. *St. John's wort:* May cause photosensitivity reactions. Advise patient to avoid excessive sunlight exposure.
Drug-lifestyle. *Alcohol use:* May increase CNS depression, particularly psychomotor skills. Strongly discourage alcohol use.
Sun exposure: May increase risk of photosensitivity reactions. Advise patient to avoid excessive sunlight exposure.

EFFECTS ON LAB TEST RESULTS
● May increase liver enzyme levels.
● May decrease WBC and granulocyte counts.
● May cause false-positive results for urinary porphyrin, urobilinogen, amylase, and 5-hydroxyindoleacetic acid tests and for urine pregnancy tests that use human chorionic gonadotropin.

CONTRAINDICATIONS & CAUTIONS
● Contraindicated in patients hypersensitive to phenothiazines and in those with CNS depression, coma, bone marrow suppression, or liver damage.
● Use cautiously in elderly or debilitated patients and in patients with CV disease (may decrease blood pressure), seizure disorder, glaucoma, or prostatic hyperplasia; also, use cautiously in those exposed to extreme heat.
● Use only in children who are hospitalized or under close supervision.

NURSING CONSIDERATIONS
● Watch for orthostatic hypotension. Keep patient supine for 1 hour after giving drug, and tell him to change positions slowly.
● Monitor patient for tardive dyskinesia, which may occur after prolonged use. It may not appear until months or years later and may disappear spontaneously or persist for life, despite ending drug.
● *Alert:* Watch for evidence of neuroleptic malignant syndrome (extrapyramidal effects, hyperthermia, autonomic disturbance), which is rare but deadly.
● Monitor periodic CBC and liver function tests and ophthalmic tests (long-term use).

• Withhold dose and notify prescriber if jaundice, signs and symptoms of blood dyscrasia (fever, sore throat, infection, cellulitis, weakness), or persistent extrapyramidal reactions (longer than a few hours) develop, especially in children or pregnant women.
• Don't withdraw drug abruptly unless severe adverse reactions occur.
• After abrupt withdrawal of long-term therapy, gastritis, nausea, vomiting, dizziness, tremor, feeling of warmth or cold, diaphoresis, tachycardia, headache, insomnia, anorexia, muscle rigidity, altered mental status, or evidence of autonomic instability may occur.
• *Look alike–sound alike:* Don't confuse trifluoperazine with triflupromazine.

PATIENT TEACHING
• Warn patient to avoid activities that require alertness until effects of drug are known.
• Tell patient to avoid alcohol while taking drug.
• Tell patient to report signs of urine retention or constipation.
• Tell patient to use sunblock and to wear protective clothing outdoors.
• Advise patient to relieve dry mouth with sugarless gum or hard candy.

valproate sodium
val-PROH-ayt

Depacon, Depakene

valproic acid
Depakene

divalproex sodium
Depakote, Depakote ER, Depakote Sprinkle, Epival†

Pharmacologic class: carboxylic acid derivative
Pregnancy risk category D

AVAILABLE FORMS
valproate sodium
Injection: 100 mg/ml
Syrup: 250 mg/5 ml
valproic acid
Capsules: 250 mg
Syrup: 200 mg/5 ml
Tablets (crushable): 100 mg
Tablets (enteric-coated): 200 mg, 500 mg
divalproex sodium
Capsules (sprinkle): 125 mg
Tablets (delayed-release): 125 mg, 250 mg, 500 mg
Tablets (extended-release): 250 mg, 500 mg

INDICATIONS & DOSAGES
➤ **Simple and complex absence seizures, mixed seizure types (including absence seizures)**
Adults and children: Initially, 15 mg/kg P.O. or I.V. daily; then increase by 5 to 10 mg/kg daily at weekly intervals up to maximum of 60 mg/kg daily. Don't use Depakote ER in children younger than age 10.
➤ **Complex partial seizures**
Adults and children age 10 and older: 10 to 15 mg/kg Depakote or Depakote ER P.O. or valproate sodium I.V. daily; then increase by 5 to 10 mg/kg daily at weekly intervals, up to 60 mg/kg daily.
➤ **Mania**
Adults: Initially, 750 mg Depakote daily P.O. in divided doses, or 25 mg/kg Depakote ER once daily. Adjust dosage based on patient's response; maximum dose for either form is 60 mg/kg daily.
➤ **To prevent migraine headache**
Adults: Initially, 250 mg delayed-release divalproex sodium P.O. b.i.d. Some patients may need up to 1,000 mg daily. Or, 500 mg Depakote ER P.O. daily for 1 week; then 1,000 mg P.O. daily.
Adjust-a-dose: For elderly patients, start at lower dosage. Increase dosage more slowly and with regular monitoring of fluid and nutritional intake, and watch for dehydration, somnolence, and other adverse reactions.

ADMINISTRATION
P.O.
• Give drug with food or milk to reduce adverse GI effects.
• Don't mix syrup with carbonated beverages; mixture may be irritating to oral mucosa.

Reactions may be *common*, uncommon, *life-threatening*, or COMMON AND LIFE-THREATENING.
Interaction may have a *rapid onset* or **delayed onset**.

• Don't give syrup to patients who need sodium restriction. Check with prescriber.
• Capsules may be swallowed whole or opened and contents sprinkled on a teaspoonful of soft food. Patient should swallow immediately without chewing.

I.V.
• I.V. use is indicated only in patients who can't take drug orally. Switch patient to oral form as soon as feasible; effects of I.V. use for longer than 14 days are unknown.
• Dilute valproate sodium injection with at least 50 ml of a compatible diluent. It's physically compatible and chemically stable in D_5W, normal saline, and lactated Ringer's solution for 24 hours.
• Infuse drug over 60 minutes at no more than 20 mg/minute and at the same frequency as oral dosage.
• Monitor drug level, and adjust dosage as needed.
• **Incompatibilities:** None reported.

ACTION

Unknown. Probably facilitates the effects of the inhibitory neurotransmitter GABA.

Route	Onset	Peak	Duration
P.O.	Unknown	15 min–4 hr	Unknown
I.V.	Unknown	1 hr	Unknown

Half-life: 6 to 16 hours.

ADVERSE REACTIONS

CNS: *asthenia, dizziness, headache, insomnia, nervousness, somnolence, tremor,* abnormal thinking, amnesia, ataxia, depression, emotional upset, fever.
CV: chest pain, edema, hypertension, hypotension, tachycardia.
EENT: *blurred vision, diplopia,* nystagmus, pharyngitis, rhinitis, tinnitus.
GI: *abdominal pain, anorexia, diarrhea, dyspepsia, nausea, vomiting, **pancreatitis,*** constipation, increased appetite.
Hematologic: *bone marrow suppression, hemorrhage, thrombocytopenia,* bruising, petechiae.
Hepatic: *hepatotoxicity.*
Metabolic: hyperammonemia, weight gain or loss.
Musculoskeletal: back and neck pain.
Respiratory: bronchitis, dyspnea.

Skin: *alopecia, flu syndrome, infection, **erythema multiforme, hypersensitivity reactions, Stevens-Johnson syndrome,*** rash, photosensitivity reactions, pruritus.

INTERACTIONS

Drug-drug. *Aspirin, chlorpromazine, cimetidine, erythromycin, felbamate:* May cause valproic acid toxicity. Use together cautiously and monitor drug level.
Benzodiazepines, other CNS depressants: May cause excessive CNS depression. Avoid using together.
Carbamazepine: May cause carbamazepine CNS toxicity; may decrease valproic acid level and cause loss of seizure control. Use together cautiously, if at all. Monitor patient for seizure activity and toxicity during therapy and for at least 1 month after stopping either drug.
Lamotrigine: May increase lamotrigine level; may decrease valproate level. Monitor levels closely.
Phenobarbital: May increase phenobarbital level; may increase clearance of valproate. Monitor patient closely.
Phenytoin: May increase or decrease phenytoin level; may decrease valproate level. Monitor patient closely.
Rifampin: May decrease valproate level. Monitor level of valproate.
Warfarin: May displace warfarin from binding sites. Monitor PT and INR.
Zidovudine: May decrease zidovudine clearance. Avoid using together.
Drug-lifestyle. *Alcohol use:* May cause excessive CNS depression. Discourage use together.

EFFECTS ON LAB TEST RESULTS

• May increase ammonia, ALT, AST, and bilirubin levels.
• May increase eosinophil count and bleeding time. May decrease platelet, RBC, and WBC counts.
• May cause false-positive results for urine ketone levels.

CONTRAINDICATIONS & CAUTIONS

• Contraindicated in patients hypersensitive to drug and in those with hepatic disease or significant hepatic dysfunction, and in patients with a urea cycle disorder (UCD).

• Safety and efficacy of Depakote ER in children younger than age 10 haven't been established.

NURSING CONSIDERATIONS
• Obtain liver function test results, platelet count, and PT and INR before starting therapy, and monitor these values periodically.
• Adverse reactions may not be caused by valproic acid alone because it's usually used with other anticonvulsants.
• When converting adults and children age 10 and older with seizures from Depakote to Depakote ER, make sure the extended-release dose is 8% to 20% higher than the regular dose taken previously. See manufacturer's package insert for more details.
• Divalproex sodium has a lower risk of adverse GI reactions.
• Never withdraw drug suddenly because sudden withdrawal may worsen seizures. Call prescriber at once if adverse reactions develop.
• *Alert:* Fatal hepatotoxicity may follow nonspecific symptoms, such as malaise, fever, and lethargy. If these symptoms occur during therapy, notify prescriber at once because patient who might be developing hepatic dysfunction must stop taking drug.
• Patients at high risk for hepatotoxicity include those with congenital metabolic disorders, mental retardation, or organic brain disease; those taking multiple anticonvulsants; and children younger than age 2.
• Notify prescriber if tremors occur; a dosage reduction may be needed.
• Monitor drug level. Therapeutic level is 50 to 100 mcg/ml.
• When converting patients from a brand-name drug to a generic drug, use caution because breakthrough seizures may occur.
• *Alert:* Sometimes fatal, hyperammonemic encephalopathy may occur when starting valproate therapy in patients with UCD. Evaluate patients with UCD risk factors before starting valproate therapy. Patients who develop symptoms of unexplained hyperammonemic encephalopathy during valproate therapy should stop drug, undergo prompt appropriate treatment, and be evaluated for underlying UCD.
• *Look alike–sound alike:* Don't confuse Depakote with Depakote ER.

PATIENT TEACHING
• Tell patient to take drug with food or milk to reduce adverse GI effects.
• Advise patient not to chew capsules; irritation of mouth and throat may result.
• Tell patient that capsules may be either swallowed whole or carefully opened and contents sprinkled on a teaspoonful of soft food. Tell patient to swallow immediately without chewing.
• Tell patient and parents that syrup shouldn't be mixed with carbonated beverages; mixture may be irritating to mouth and throat.
• Tell patient and parents to keep drug out of children's reach.
• Warn patient and parents not to stop drug therapy abruptly.
• Advise patient to avoid driving and other potentially hazardous activities that require mental alertness until drug's CNS effects are known.
• Instruct patient or parents to call prescriber if malaise, weakness, lethargy, facial swelling, loss of appetite, or vomiting occurs.
• Tell woman to call prescriber if she becomes pregnant or plans to become pregnant during therapy.

---

vardenafil hydrochloride
var-DEN-ah-fill

Levitra

Pharmacologic class: phosphodiesterase type-5 inhibitor
Pregnancy risk category B

AVAILABLE FORMS
Tablets (film-coated): 2.5 mg, 5 mg, 10 mg, 20 mg

INDICATIONS & DOSAGES
➤ **Erectile dysfunction**
Adults: 10 mg P.O. as a single dose, as needed, 1 hour before sexual activity. Dosage range is 5 to 20 mg, based on

effectiveness and tolerance. Maximum, one dose daily.

Elderly patients age 65 and older: Initially 5 mg as a single dose, as needed, 1 hour before sexual activity.

Adjust-a-dose: For patients with Child-Pugh category B, first dose is 5 mg daily, as needed. Don't exceed 10 mg daily in patients with hepatic impairment.

ADMINISTRATION
P.O.
● Give drug without regard for food.

ACTION
Increases cGMP levels, prolongs smooth muscle relaxation, and promotes blood flow into the corpus cavernosum.

Route	Onset	Peak	Duration
P.O.	Immediate	30–120 min	Unknown

Half-life: 4 to 5 hours.

ADVERSE REACTIONS
CNS: *headache,* dizziness.
CV: *flushing.*
EENT: decrease or loss of hearing, tinnitus, rhinitis, sinusitis.
GI: dyspepsia, nausea.
Musculoskeletal: back pain.
Other: flulike syndrome.

INTERACTIONS
Drug-drug. *Alpha blockers, nitrates:* May enhance hypotensive effects. Avoid using together.
Antiarrhythmics of class IA (quinidine, procainamide) and class III (amiodarone, sotalol): May prolong QTc interval. Avoid using together.
Erythromycin, indinavir, itraconazole, ketoconazole, ritonavir: May increase vardenafil level. Reduce dose of vardenafil. If taken with ritonavir, reduce and extend dosage interval to once every 72 hours.
Drug-food. *High-fat meals:* May reduce peak level of drug. Discourage use with a high-fat meal.

EFFECTS ON LAB TEST RESULTS
● May increase CK level.

CONTRAINDICATIONS & CAUTIONS
● Contraindicated in patients hypersensitive to drug or its components and in those taking nitrates or alpha blockers.
● Contraindicated in patients with unstable angina, hypotension (systolic less than 90 mm Hg), uncontrolled hypertension (over 170/110 mm Hg), stroke, life-threatening arrhythmia, an MI within past 6 months, severe cardiac failure, Child-Pugh category C, end-stage renal disease requiring dialysis, congenital QTc-interval prolongation, or hereditary degenerative retinal disorders.
● Use cautiously in patients with bleeding disorders or significant peptic ulceration.
● Use cautiously in those with anatomical penis abnormalities or conditions that predispose patient to priapism (such as sickle cell anemia, multiple myeloma, or leukemia).

NURSING CONSIDERATIONS
● *Alert:* Sexual activity may increase cardiac risk. Evaluate patient's cardiac risk before he starts taking drug.
● Before patient starts drug, assess for underlying causes of erectile dysfunction.
● Transient decreases in supine blood pressure may occur.
● Prolonged erections and priapism may occur.

PATIENT TEACHING
● Tell patient that drug doesn't protect against sexually transmitted diseases and that he should use protective measures.
● Advise patient that drug is absorbed most rapidly if taken on an empty stomach.
● Tell patient to notify prescriber about vision or hearing changes.
● Urge patient to seek immediate medical care if erection lasts more than 4 hours.
● Tell patient to take drug 60 minutes before anticipated sexual activity. Explain that drug has no effect without sexual stimulation.
● Warn patient not to change dosage unless directed by prescriber.

varenicline tartrate
vah-RENN-ih-kleen

Chantix

Pharmacologic class: nicotinic acetylcholine receptor partial agonist
Pregnancy risk category C

AVAILABLE FORMS
Tablets: 0.5 mg, 1 mg

INDICATIONS & DOSAGES
➤ **Smoking cessation**
Adults: Starting 1 week before patient stops smoking, give 0.5 mg P.O. once daily on days 1 through 3. Days 4 through 7, give 0.5 mg P.O. b.i.d. Day 8 through the end of week 12, give 1 mg P.O. b.i.d. If patient successfully stops smoking, give an additional 12-week course to help with long-term success.
Adjust-a-dose: In patient with renal impairment, 0.5 mg P.O. once daily. Adjust as needed to maximum of 0.5 mg b.i.d. In patient with end-stage renal disease who is undergoing dialysis, 0.5 mg once daily.

ADMINISTRATION
P.O.
● Give drug with full glass of water after a meal.

ACTION
Blocks the effects of nicotine by binding at alpha$_4$ beta$_2$ neuronal nicotinic acetylcholine receptors. Drug also provides some of nicotine's effects to ease withdrawal.

Route	Onset	Peak	Duration
P.O.	4 days	3–4 hr	24 hr

Half-life: 24 hours.

ADVERSE REACTIONS
CNS: *abnormal dreams, headache, insomnia,* altered attention or emotions, anxiety, asthenia, depression, dizziness, fatigue, irritability, lethargy, malaise, nightmares, restlessness, sensory disturbance, sleep disorder, somnolence.
CV: chest pain, edema, hot flush, hypertension.
EENT: altered taste, epistaxis.
GI: *nausea,* abdominal pain, constipation, diarrhea, dry mouth, dyspepsia, flatulence, gingivitis, vomiting.
GU: menstrual disorder, polyuria.
Metabolic: decreased appetite, increased appetite, thirst.
Musculoskeletal: arthralgia, back pain, muscle cramps, myalgia.
Respiratory: dyspnea, upper respiratory tract disorder.
Skin: rash.
Other: flulike illness.

INTERACTIONS
Drug-drug. *Nicotine-replacement therapy:* May increase nausea, vomiting, dizziness, dyspepsia, and fatigue. Monitor patient closely.

EFFECTS ON LAB TEST RESULTS
● May increase liver function test values.

CONTRAINDICATIONS & CAUTIONS
● Use cautiously in pregnant or breastfeeding women, elderly patients, and patients with severe renal impairment or pre-existing psychiatric illness.

NURSING CONSIDERATIONS
● Assess patient's readiness and motivation to stop smoking.
● *Alert:* Monitor patient for changes in behavior, agitation, depressed mood, suicidal ideation, suicidal behavior and worsening of pre-existing psychiatric illness and report immediately.
● Notify prescriber if patient develops intolerable nausea; dosage reduction may be needed.
● Temporarily monitor levels of drugs— such as theophylline, warfarin, and insulin—after patient stops smoking to be sure levels are still within therapeutic range.

PATIENT TEACHING
● Provide patient with educational materials and needed counseling.
● Instruct patient to choose a date to stop smoking and to begin treatment 1 week before this date.

- Advise patient to take each dose with a full glass of water after eating.
- Teach patient to gradually increase the dose over the 1st week to a target of 1 mg in the morning and 1 mg in the evening.
- Explain that nausea and insomnia are common and usually temporary. Urge him to contact the prescriber if adverse effects are persistently troubling; a dosage reduction may help.
- Urge patient to continue trying to abstain from smoking if he has early lapses after successfully quitting.
- Tell patient that dosages of other drugs he takes may need adjustment when he stops smoking.
- Advise patient to use caution when driving or operating machinery until effects of the drug are known.
- Instruct family to observe patient for changes in behavior and mood including agitation, depression, suicidal ideation or behavior and worsening of pre-existing psychiatric illness; report changes to healthcare provider immediately.
- If woman plans to become pregnant or to breast-feed, explain the risks of smoking and the risks and benefits of taking drug to aid smoking cessation.

venlafaxine hydrochloride
vin-lah-FACKS-in

Effexor, Effexor XR

Pharmacologic class: SSNRI
Pregnancy risk category C

AVAILABLE FORMS
Capsules (extended-release): 37.5 mg, 75 mg, 150 mg
Tablets: 25 mg, 37.5 mg, 50 mg, 75 mg, 100 mg

INDICATIONS & DOSAGES
➤ **Depression**
Adults: Initially, 75 mg P.O. daily in two or three divided doses with food. Increase as tolerated and needed by 75 mg daily every 4 days. For moderately depressed outpatients, usual maximum is 225 mg daily; in certain severely depressed patients, dose may be as high as 375 mg daily. For

extended-release capsules, 75 mg P.O. daily in a single dose. For some patients, it may be desirable to start at 37.5 mg P.O. daily for 4 to 7 days before increasing to 75 mg daily. Dosage may be increased by 75 mg daily every 4 days to maximum of 225 mg daily.
➤ **Generalized anxiety disorder**
Adults: Initially, 75 mg extended-release capsule P.O. daily in a single dose. For some patients, it may be desirable to start at 37.5 mg P.O. daily for 4 to 7 days before increasing to 75 mg daily. Dosage may be increased by 75 mg daily every 4 days to maximum of 225 mg daily.
➤ **Panic disorder**
Adults: Initially, 37.5 mg extended-release capsule P.O. daily for 1 week, then increase dose to 75 mg daily. If patient isn't responding, may increase dose by up to 75 mg/day in no less than weekly intervals, as needed, to a maximum dose of 225 mg daily.
➤ **Social anxiety disorder**
Adults: Initially, 75 mg extended-release capsule daily as a single dose. For some patients, it may be desirable to start at 37.5 mg P.O. daily for 4 to 7 days before increasing to 75 mg daily. Increase dosage as needed by 75 mg daily every 4 days. Maximum dose is 225 mg daily.
Adjust-a-dose: For patients with renal impairment, reduce daily amount by 25%. For those undergoing hemodialysis, reduce daily amount by 50% and withhold dose until dialysis is completed. For patients with hepatic impairment, reduce daily amount by 50%.
➤ **To prevent major depressive disorder relapse ◆**
Adults: 100 to 200 mg daily P.O. regular-release tablets or 75 to 225 mg daily P.O. extended-release capsules.

ADMINISTRATION
P.O.
- Give drug with food and a full glass of water.
- Give capsule whole; if patient can't swallow whole, open and sprinkle contents on spoonful of applesauce; mix and give immediately. Follow with a full glass of water.

ACTION

May increase the amount of norepineph-rine, serotonin, or both in the CNS by blocking their reuptake by the presynaptic neurons.

Route	Onset	Peak	Duration
P.O.	Unknown	1–2 hr	Unknown

Half-life: 5 hours.

ADVERSE REACTIONS

CNS: *asthenia, headache, somnolence, dizziness, nervousness, insomnia,* **suicidal behavior,** anxiety, tremor, abnormal dreams, paresthesia, agitation.
CV: hypertension, tachycardia, vasodila-tion.
EENT: blurred vision.
GI: *nausea, constipation, dry mouth, anorexia,* vomiting, diarrhea, dyspepsia, flatulence.
GU: *abnormal ejaculation,* impotence, urinary frequency, impaired urination.
Metabolic: weight loss.
Skin: *diaphoresis,* rash.
Other: yawning, chills, infection.

INTERACTIONS

Drug-drug. *MAO inhibitors, such as phenelzine, selegiline, tranylcypromine:* May cause serotonin syndrome. Avoid using within 14 days of MAO inhibitor therapy.
Tramadol, sibutramine, sumatriptan, trazodone: May cause serotonin syndrome. Monitor patient closely.
Triptans: May cause serotonin syndrome (restlessness, hallucinations, loss of co-ordination, fast heartbeat, rapid changes in blood pressure, increased body tem-perature, hyperreflexia, nausea, vomiting, and diarrhea). Use cautiously and with increased monitoring at the start of therapy and with dose increase.
Warfarin: May increase PT, PTT, or INR. Monitor these lab values and patient closely.
Drug-herb. *Yohimbe:* May cause additive stimulation. Urge caution.

EFFECTS ON LAB TEST RESULTS

None reported.

CONTRAINDICATIONS & CAUTIONS

• Contraindicated in patients hypersen-sitive to drug or within 14 days of MAO inhibitor therapy.
• Use cautiously in patients with renal impairment, diseases or conditions that could affect hemodynamic responses or metabolism, and in those with history of mania or seizures.
• Use in third trimester of pregnancy may be associated with neonatal complications at birth. Consider the risk versus benefit of treatment during this time.

NURSING CONSIDERATIONS

• *Alert:* Closely monitor patients being treated for depression for signs and symp-toms of clinical worsening and suicidal ideation, especially at the beginning of therapy and with dosage adjustments. Symptoms may include agitation, in-somnia, anxiety, aggressiveness, or panic attacks.
• *Alert:* Drug may increase the risk of suicidal thinking and behavior in children, adolescents, and young adults ages 18 to 24 during the first 2 months of treatment, especially those with major depressive disorder or other psychiatric disorder.
• Carefully monitor blood pressure. Drug therapy may cause sustained, dose-dependent increases in blood pressure. Greatest increases (averaging about 7 mm Hg above baseline) occur in patients taking 375 mg daily.
• Monitor patient's weight, particularly underweight, depressed patients.
• *Alert:* Combining triptans with an SSRI or an SSNRI may cause serotonin syn-drome. Signs and symptoms may include restlessness, hallucinations, loss of coor-dination, fast heartbeat, rapid changes in blood pressure, increased body tempera-ture, overactive reflexes, nausea, vomiting, and diarrhea. Serotonin syndrome may be more likely to occur when starting or increasing the dose of triptan, SSRI, or SSNRI.

PATIENT TEACHING

• If medication is to be stopped, inform patient who has received drug for 6 weeks or longer that drug will be stopped grad-ually by tapering dosage over a 2-week

---

Reactions may be *common,* uncommon, *life-threatening,* or COMMON AND LIFE-THREATENING.
Interaction may have a *rapid onset* or *delayed onset.*

period, as instructed by prescriber. Patient shouldn't abruptly stop taking the drug.
- *Alert:* Warn family members to closely monitor patient for signs of worsening condition or suicidal ideation.
- Warn patient to avoid hazardous activities that require alertness and good coordination until effects of drug are known.
- Tell patient to avoid alcohol and to consult prescriber before taking other prescription or OTC drugs.
- Advise woman of childbearing age to contact prescriber if she becomes pregnant or intends to become pregnant during therapy or if she's breast-feeding.
- Tell patient to take each dose with food and a full glass of water.
- Tell patient that if he can't swallow capsule whole, he may carefully open it and sprinkle contents on a spoonful of applesauce, mix, and take immediately. Follow with a full glass of water.

SAFETY ALERT!

zaleplon
ZAL-ah-plon

Sonata

Pharmacologic class:
pyrazolopyrimidine
Pregnancy risk category C
Controlled substance schedule IV

AVAILABLE FORMS
Capsules: 5 mg, 10 mg

INDICATIONS & DOSAGES
➤ **Insomnia**
Adults: 10 mg P.O. daily at bedtime; may increase to 20 mg as needed. Low-weight adults may respond to 5-mg dose. Limit use to 7 to 10 days. Reevaluate patient if drug is used for more than 2 to 3 weeks.
Elderly patients: Initially, 5 mg P.O. daily at bedtime; doses of more than 10 mg aren't recommended.
Adjust-a-dose: For debilitated patients, initially, 5 mg P.O. daily at bedtime; doses of more than 10 mg aren't recommended. For patients with mild to moderate hepatic impairment or those also taking cimetidine, 5 mg P.O. daily at bedtime.

ADMINISTRATION
P.O.
- Don't give drug after a high-fat or heavy meal.

ACTION
A hypnotic with chemical structure unrelated to benzodiazepines that interacts with the GABA-benzodiazepine receptor complex in the CNS. Modulation of this complex is thought to be responsible for sedative, anxiolytic, muscle relaxant, and anticonvulsant effects of benzodiazepines.

Route	Onset	Peak	Duration
P.O.	1 hr	1 hr	3–4 hr

Half-life: 1 hour.

ADVERSE REACTIONS
CNS: complex sleep-related behaviors, headache, amnesia, anxiety, asthenia, depersonalization, depression, difficulty concentrating, dizziness, fever, hallucinations, hypertonia, hypesthesia, malaise, migraine, nervousness, paresthesia, somnolence, tremor, vertigo.
CV: chest pain, peripheral edema.
EENT: abnormal vision, conjunctivitis, ear discomfort, epistaxis, eye discomfort, hyperacusis, smell alteration.
GI: abdominal pain, anorexia, colitis, constipation, dry mouth, dyspepsia, nausea.
GU: dysmenorrhea.
Musculoskeletal: arthritis, back pain, myalgia.
Respiratory: bronchitis.
Skin: photosensitivity reactions, pruritus, rash.
Other: *anaphylaxis, angioedema.*

INTERACTIONS
Drug-drug. *Carbamazepine, phenobarbital, phenytoin, rifampin, other CYP3A4 inducers:* May reduce zaleplon bioavailability and peak level by 80%. Consider using a different hypnotic.
Cimetidine: May increase zaleplon bioavailability and peak level by 85%. Use an initial zaleplon dose of 5 mg.

CNS depressants (imipramine, thioridazine): May cause additive CNS effects. Use together cautiously.

Drug-food. *High-fat foods, heavy meals:* May prolong absorption, delaying peak drug level by about 2 hours; may delay sleep onset. Advise patient to avoid taking with meals.

Drug-lifestyle. *Alcohol use:* May increase CNS effects. Discourage use together.

EFFECTS ON LAB TEST RESULTS
None reported.

CONTRAINDICATIONS & CAUTIONS
• Contraindicated in patients with severe hepatic impairment.
• Use cautiously in elderly, depressed, or debilitated patients, in breast-feeding women, and in patients with compromised respiratory function.

NURSING CONSIDERATIONS
• *Alert:* Monitor patient closely. Anaphylaxis and angioedema may occur as early as the first dose.
• Because drug works rapidly, give immediately before bedtime or after patient has gone to bed and has had difficulty falling asleep.
• Closely monitor patients who have compromised respiratory function caused by illness or who are elderly or debilitated because they are more sensitive to respiratory depression.
• Start treatment only after carefully evaluating patient because sleep disturbances may be a symptom of an underlying physical or psychiatric disorder.
• Adverse reactions are usually dose-related. Consult prescriber about dose reduction if adverse reactions occur.

PATIENT TEACHING
• *Alert:* Warn patient that drug may cause allergic reactions, facial swelling, and complex sleep-related behaviors, such as driving, eating, and making phone calls while asleep. Advise patient to report these adverse effects.
• Advise patient that drug works rapidly and should only be taken immediately before bedtime or after he has gone to bed and has had trouble falling asleep.

• Advise patient to take drug only if he will be able to sleep for at least 4 undisturbed hours.
• Caution patient that drowsiness, dizziness, light-headedness, and coordination problems occur most often within 1 hour after taking drug.
• Advise patient to avoid performing activities that require mental alertness until CNS adverse reactions are known.
• Advise patient to avoid alcohol use while taking drug and to notify prescriber before taking other prescription or OTC drugs.
• Tell patient not to take drug after a high-fat or heavy meal.
• Advise patient to report sleep problems that continue despite use of drug.
• Notify patient that dependence can occur and that drug is recommended for short-term use only.
• Warn patient not to abruptly stop drug because of the risk of withdrawal symptoms, including unpleasant feelings, stomach and muscle cramps, vomiting, sweating, shakiness, and seizures.
• Notify patient that insomnia may recur for a few nights after stopping drug but should resolve on its own.
• Warn patient that drug may cause changes in behavior and thinking, including outgoing or aggressive behavior, loss of personal identity, confusion, strange behavior, agitation, hallucinations, worsening of depression, or suicidal thoughts. Tell patient to notify prescriber immediately if these symptoms occur.

ziprasidone
zih-PRAZ-i-done

Geodon

Pharmacologic class: benzisoxazole derivative
Pregnancy risk category C

AVAILABLE FORMS
Capsules: 20 mg, 40 mg, 60 mg, 80 mg
I.M. injection: 20 mg/ml single-dose vials (after reconstitution)

INDICATIONS & DOSAGES
➤ **Symptomatic treatment of schizophrenia**
Adults: Initially, 20 mg b.i.d. with food. Dosages are highly individualized. Adjust dosage, if necessary, no more frequently than every 2 days; to allow for lowest possible doses, the interval should be several weeks to assess symptom response. Effective dosage range is usually 20 to 80 mg b.i.d. Maximum dosage is 100 mg b.i.d.
➤ **Rapid control of acute agitation in schizophrenic patients**
Adults: 10 to 20 mg I.M. as needed, up to a maximum dose of 40 mg daily. Doses of 10 mg may be given every 2 hours; doses of 20 mg may be given every 4 hours.
➤ **Acute bipolar mania, including manic and mixed episodes, with or without psychotic features**
Adults: 40 mg P.O. b.i.d., with food, on day 1. Increase to 60 to 80 mg P.O. b.i.d., with food, on day 2; then adjust dosage based on patient response from 40 to 80 mg b.i.d., with food.

ADMINISTRATION
P.O.
● Always give drug with food for optimal effect.
I.M.
● To prepare I.M. ziprasidone, add 1.2 ml of sterile water for injection to the vial and shake vigorously until drug is completely dissolved.
● Don't mix injection with other medicinal products or solvents other than sterile water for injection.
● Inspect parenteral drug products for particulate matter and discoloration before administration.
● The effects of giving I.M. for more than 3 consecutive days are unknown. If long-term therapy of drug is necessary, switch to P.O. as soon as possible.
● Store injection at controlled room temperature, 59° to 86° F (15° to 30° C) in dry form, and protect from light. After reconstituting, it may be stored away from light for up to 24 hours at 59° to 86° F (15° to 30° C) or up to 7 days refrigerated, 36° to 46° F (2° to 8° C).

ACTION
May inhibit dopamine and serotonin-2 receptors, causing reduction in schizophrenia symptoms.

Route	Onset	Peak	Duration
P.O.	1–3 days	6–8 hr	12 hr
I.M.	Unknown	1 hr	Unknown

Half-life: 2¼ to 7 hours.

ADVERSE REACTIONS
CNS: *dizziness, headache, somnolence, suicide attempt,* akathisia, dizziness, extrapyramidal symptoms, hypertonia, asthenia, dystonia (P.O.), anxiety, insomnia, agitation, cogwheel rigidity, paresthesia, personality disorder, psychosis, speech disorder (I.M.).
CV: *bradycardia, QT interval prolongation,* orthostatic hypotension, tachycardia (P.O.), hypertension, vasodilation (I.M.).
EENT: rhinitis, abnormal vision (P.O.).
GI: *nausea,* constipation, dyspepsia, diarrhea, dry mouth, anorexia, abdominal pain, *rectal hemorrhage,* vomiting, dyspepsia, tooth disorder (I.M.).
GU: dysmenorrhea, priapism (I.M.).
Metabolic: hyperglycemia.
Musculoskeletal: myalgia (P.O.), back pain (I.M.).
Respiratory: cough (P.O.).
Skin: rash (P.O.), injection site pain, furunculosis, sweating (I.M.).
Other: flulike syndrome (I.M.).

INTERACTIONS
Drug-drug. *Antiarrhythmics (amiodarone, bretylium, disopyramide, dofetilide, procainamide, quinidine, sotalol), arsenic trioxide, cisapride, dolasetron, droperidol, levomethadyl, mefloquine, pentamidine, phenothiazines, pimozide, quinolones, tacrolimus:* May increase the risk of life-threatening arrhythmias. Use together is contraindicated.
Antihypertensives: May enhance hypotensive effects. Monitor blood pressure.
Carbamazepine: May decrease ziprasidone level. May need to increase ziprasidone dose to achieve desired effect.
Drugs that decrease potassium or magnesium such as diuretics: May increase risk of arrhythmias. Monitor potassium

and magnesium levels if using these drugs together.

Itraconazole, ketoconazole: May increase ziprasidone level. May need to reduce ziprasidone dose to achieve desired effect.

EFFECTS ON LAB TEST RESULTS
None reported.

CONTRAINDICATIONS & CAUTIONS
● Contraindicated in patients hypersensitive to drug and in those with recent MI or uncompensated heart failure.

● Contraindicated in those with history of prolonged QT interval or congenital long QT interval syndrome and in those taking other drugs that prolong QT interval, such as dofetilide, sotalol, quinidine, other class IA and III antiarrhythmics, mesoridazine, thioridazine, chlorpromazine, droperidol, pimozide, sparfloxacin, gatifloxacin, moxifloxacin, halofantrine, mefloquine, pentamidine, arsenic trioxide, levomethadyl acetate, dolasetron mesylate, probucol, and tacrolimus.

P.O.
● Contraindicated in patients with a history of QT interval prolongation or congenital QT syndrome and in those taking other drugs that prolong QT interval.

● Use cautiously in patients with history of seizures, bradycardia, hypokalemia, or hypomagnesemia; in those with acute diarrhea; and in those with conditions that may lower the seizure threshold (such as Alzheimer dementia).

● Use cautiously in patients at risk for aspiration pneumonia.

● Don't use drug in breast-feeding women.
I.M.
● Contraindicated in schizophrenic patients already taking P.O. ziprasidone.

● Use cautiously in elderly and renally or hepatically impaired patients.

NURSING CONSIDERATIONS
● *Alert:* In elderly patients with dementia-related psychosis, drug isn't indicated for use because of increased risk of death from CV events or infection.

● *Alert:* Hyperglycemia may occur. Monitor patients with diabetes regularly. Patients with risk factors for diabetes should undergo fasting blood glucose testing at base-

line and periodically. Monitor all patients for symptoms of hyperglycemia, including excessive hunger or thirst, frequent urination, and weakness. Hyperglycemia may be reversible when drug is stopped.

● *Alert:* Monitor patient for symptoms of metabolic syndrome (significant weight gain and increased body mass index, hypertension, hyperglycemia, hypercholesterolemia, and hypertriglyceridemia).
P.O.
● Stop drug in patients with a QTc interval more than 500 msec.

● Dizziness, palpitations, or syncope may be symptoms of a life-threatening arrhythmia such as torsades de pointes. Provide CV evaluation and monitoring in patients who experience these symptoms.

● Don't give to patients with electrolyte disturbances, such as hypokalemia or hypomagnesemia, because these increase the risk of arrhythmia.

● Patient taking an antipsychotic may develop life-threatening neuroleptic malignant syndrome (hyperpyrexia, muscle rigidity, altered mental status, and autonomic instability) or tardive dyskinesia. Assess abnormal involuntary movement before starting therapy, at dosage changes, and periodically thereafter, to monitor patient for tardive dyskinesia.

● Monitor patient for abnormal body temperature regulation, especially if he is exercising strenuously, is exposed to extreme heat, is also receiving anticholinergics, or is subject to dehydration.

● Symptoms may not improve for 4 to 6 weeks.

PATIENT TEACHING
● Tell patient to take drug with food.

● Tell patient to immediately report to prescriber signs or symptoms of dizziness, fainting, irregular heartbeat, or relevant heart problems.

● Advise patient to report any recent episodes of diarrhea, abnormal movements, sudden fever, muscle rigidity, or change in mental status.

● Advise patient that symptoms may not improve for 4 to 6 weeks.

Reactions may be *common*, uncommon, *life-threatening*, or COMMON AND LIFE-THREATENING.
Interaction may have a *rapid onset* or **delayed onset**.

zolpidem tartrate
ZOL-pih-dem

Ambien, Ambien CR, Tolvalt ODT

Pharmacologic class: imidazo-pyridine
Pregnancy risk category C
Controlled substance schedule IV

AVAILABLE FORMS
Orally disintegrating tablet (ODT): 5 mg, 10 mg
Tablets: 5 mg, 10 mg
Tablets (extended-release): 6.25 mg, 12.5 mg

INDICATIONS & DOSAGES
➤ **Short-term management of insomnia**
Adults: 10 mg immediate-release or ODT, or 12.5 mg extended-release P.O. immediately before bedtime.
Elderly patients: 5 mg immediate-release or ODT, or 6.25 mg extended-release P.O. immediately before bedtime. Maximum daily dose is 10 mg immediate-release or 6.25 mg extended-release.
Adjust-a-dose: For debilitated patients and those with hepatic insufficiency, 5 mg P.O. immediately before bedtime. Maximum daily dose is 10 mg immediate-release and 6.25 mg extended-release.

ADMINISTRATION
P.O.
• For rapid sleep onset, drug should be taken with or immediately after meals.
• For ODTs, the tablet is placed in the mouth, allowed to disintegrate, and then swallowed. Tablet may be taken with or without water. Don't crush, break, or split tablet.
• Don't crush, break, or divide extended-release tablets.

ACTION
Although drug interacts with one of three identified GABA-benzodiazepine receptor complexes, it isn't a benzodiazepine. It exhibits hypnotic activity and minimal muscle relaxant and anticonvulsant properties.

Route	Onset	Peak	Duration
P.O.	Rapid	30–120 min	Unknown

Half-life: 2½ hours.

ADVERSE REACTIONS
CNS: *headache,* amnesia, change in dreams, complex sleep-related behaviors, daytime drowsiness, depression, dizziness, hangover, lethargy, light-headedness, nervousness, sleep disorder.
CV: palpitations.
EENT: pharyngitis, sinusitis.
GI: abdominal pain, constipation, diarrhea, dry mouth, dyspepsia, nausea, vomiting.
Musculoskeletal: arthralgia, myalgia.
Skin: rash.
Other: *anaphylaxis, angioedema,* back or chest pain, flulike syndrome, hypersensitivity reactions.

INTERACTIONS
Drug-drug. *CNS depressants:* May cause excessive CNS depression. Use together cautiously.
Rifampin: May decrease effects of zolpidem. Avoid using together, if possible. Consider another hypnotic.
Drug-lifestyle. *Alcohol use:* May cause excessive CNS depression. Discourage use together.

EFFECTS ON LAB TEST RESULTS
None reported.

CONTRAINDICATIONS & CAUTIONS
• No known contraindications.
• Use cautiously in patients with compromised respiratory status.

NURSING CONSIDERATIONS
• *Alert:* Anaphylaxis and angioedema may occur as early as the first dose. Monitor patient closely.
• Use drug only for short-term management of insomnia, usually 7 to 10 days.
• Use the smallest effective dose in all patients.

- Take precautions to prevent hoarding by patients who are depressed, suicidal, or drug-dependent, or who have a history of drug abuse.
- *Look alike–sound alike:* Don't confuse Ambien with Amen.

PATIENT TEACHING
- *Alert:* Warn patient that drug may cause allergic reactions, facial swelling, and complex sleep-related behaviors, such as driving, eating, and making phone calls while asleep. Advise patient to report these adverse effects.
- For rapid sleep onset, instruct patient not to take drug with or immediately after meals.
- Instruct patient to take drug immediately before going to bed; onset of action is rapid.
- Tell patient to avoid alcohol use while taking drug.
- For ODTs, tell patient to place the tablet in the mouth, allow the tablet to disintegrate, and then tell the patient to swallow. The tablet may be taken with or without water. Tell the patient not to chew, break, or split the tablet.
- *Alert:* Tell patient not to crush, chew, or divide the extended-release tablets.
- Caution patient to avoid performing activities that require mental alertness or physical coordination during therapy.

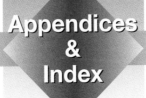

Appendices & Index

Preventing miscommunication
in drug administration

Common combination drugs:
Indications and dosages

◆

Drugs by therapeutic class

◆

Selected references

◆

Index

Preventing miscommunication in drug administration

Nurses carry a great deal of responsibility for administering drugs safely and correctly, for making sure the right patient gets the right drug, in the right dose, at the right time, and by the right route. By staying aware of potential trouble areas, you can minimize your risk of making medication errors and maximize the therapeutic effects of your patient's drug regimens.

Name game

Drugs with similar-sounding names can be easily confused. Even different-sounding names can look similar when written rapidly by hand on a prescription form. An example is Soriatane and Loxitane, which are both capsules. If the patient's drug order doesn't seem right for his diagnosis, call the prescriber to clarify the order.

Allergy alert

Once you've verified your patient's full name, check to see if he's wearing an allergy bracelet. If he is, the allergy bracelet should conspicuously display the name of the allergen. The allergy information should also be labeled on the front of the patient's chart and on his medication record. Whether the patient is wearing an allergy bracelet or not, take the time to double-check and ask the patient whether he has any allergies—even if he is in distress.

A patient who is severely allergic to peanuts could have an anaphylactic reaction to ipratropium bromide (Atrovent) aerosol given by metered-dose inhaler.

Ask your patient or his parents whether he's allergic to peanuts before you give this drug. If you find that he's allergic, you need to use the nasal spray and inhalation solution form of the drug. Because it doesn't contain soy lecithin, it's safe for patients allergic to peanuts.

Compound errors

Many medication errors occur because of a compound problem—a mistake or group of mistakes that could have been caught at any of several steps along the way. For a drug to be given correctly, each member of the health care team must fill the appropriate role:
- The prescriber must write the order correctly and legibly.
- The pharmacist must evaluate whether the order is appropriate and fill it correctly.
- The nurse must evaluate whether the order is appropriate and give it correctly.

A breakdown anywhere along this chain of events can lead to a medication error. That's why it's important for members of the health care team to act as a real team so that they can check each other and catch any problems that might arise before these problems affect the patient's health. Encourage an environment in which professionals double-check each other.

Route trouble

Many drug errors happen, at least in part, from problems related to the route of administration. The risk of error increases when a patient has several I.V. lines running for different purposes.

Risky abbreviations

Abbreviating drug names is risky. Abbreviations may not be commonly known and, in some cases, the same abbreviation may be used for different drugs or compounds. For example, epoetin alfa is commonly abbreviated EPO; however, some use the abbreviation EPO to stand for "evening primrose oil." Ask all prescribers to spell out drug names.

Unclear orders

A patient was supposed to receive one dose of the antineoplastic lomustine to treat brain cancer. (Lomustine is typically given in a single dose once every 6 weeks.) The doctor's order read, "Administer h.s." Because a nurse misinterpreted the order to mean every night, the patient received nine daily doses, developed severe thrombocytopenia and leukopenia, and died.

If you are unfamiliar with a drug, check a drug book before giving it. If a prescriber uses "h.s." and doesn't specify the frequency of administration, ask him to clarify the order. When documenting orders, note "at bedtime nightly" or "at bedtime one dose today."

Color changes

If a familiar drug seems to have an unfamiliar appearance, investigate the cause. If the pharmacist cites a manufacturer change, ask him to double-check whether he has received verification from the manufacturer. Always document the appearance discrepancy, your actions, and the pharmacist's response in the patient record.

Stress levels

Committing a serious error can cause enormous stress and cloud your judg-

ment. If you're involved in a drug error, ask another professional to give the antidote.

Reconciling medications

Medication reconciliation is the process of comparing a patient's medication orders to all of the medications that the patient has been taking. This reconciliation is done to avoid medication errors, such as omissions, duplications, dosing errors, or drug interactions. Medication errors related to medication reconciliation are more likely to occur at admission, upon transfer to another unit, or when discharged from a facility. Studies have shown that a medication reconciliation process can successfully reduce medication errors.

At discharge, it is important to provide both the patient and the next care provider a complete list of current medications, including all prescription and over-the-counter medications, as well as any vitamins, herbal medications, and nutraceuticals.

Be sure to provide a clearly written list that includes:
• the name of each medication and the reason for taking it
• all new medications and pre-hospital medications that the patient is to discontinue
• the correct dose and frequency, highlighting changes from the pre-hospital instructions
• a list of over-the-counter drugs that shouldn't be taken.

In addition to the reconciled list, it's important to ensure the availability of medications upon discharge to the patient and to determine if the patient can read their medication labels correctly, can afford the necessary medications, and is able to get to the pharmacy.

Common combination drugs: Indications and dosages

AMPHETAMINES

Adderall
Adderall XR
Controlled Substance Schedule (CSS) II

Generic components
Tablets
5 mg: 1.25 mg dextroamphetamine sulfate, 1.25 mg dextroamphetamine saccharate, and 1.25 mg amphetamine aspartate, and 1.25 mg amphetamine sulfate
7.5 mg: 1.875 mg dextroamphetamine sulfate, 1.875 mg dextroamphetamine saccharate, 1.875 mg amphetamine aspartate, and 1.875 mg amphetamine sulfate
10 mg: 2.5 mg dextroamphetamine sulfate, 2.5 mg dextroamphetamine saccharate, 2.5 mg amphetamine aspartate, and 2.5 mg amphetamine sulfate
12.5 mg: 3.125 mg dextroamphetamine sulfate, 3.125 mg dextroamphetamine saccharate, 3.125 mg amphetamine aspartate, and 3.125 mg amphetamine sulfate
15 mg: 3.75 mg dextroamphetamine sulfate, 3.75 mg dextroamphetamine saccharate, 3.75 mg amphetamine aspartate, and 3.75 mg amphetamine sulfate
20 mg: 5 mg dextroamphetamine sulfate, 5 mg dextroamphetamine saccharate, 5 mg amphetamine aspartate, and 5 mg amphetamine sulfate
30 mg: 7.5 mg dextroamphetamine sulfate, 7.5 mg dextroamphetamine saccharate, 7.5 mg amphetamine aspartate, and 7.5 mg amphetamine sulfate
Capsules (extended-release)
5 mg: 1.25 mg dextroamphetamine sulfate, 1.25 mg dextroamphetamine saccharate, 1.25 mg amphetamine aspartate, and 1.25 mg amphetamine sulfate

10 mg: 2.5 mg dextroamphetamine sulfate, 2.5 mg dextroamphetamine saccharate, 2.5 mg amphetamine aspartate, and 2.5 mg amphetamine sulfate
15 mg: 3.75 mg dextroamphetamine sulfate, 3.75 mg dextroamphetamine saccharate, 3.75 mg amphetamine aspartate, and 3.75 mg amphetamine sulfate
20 mg: 5 mg dextroamphetamine sulfate, 5 mg dextroamphetamine saccharate, 5 mg amphetamine aspartate, and 5 mg amphetamine sulfate
25 mg: 6.25 mg dextroamphetamine sulfate, 6.25 mg dextroamphetamine saccharate, 6.25 mg amphetamine aspartate, and 6.25 mg amphetamine sulfate
30 mg: 7.5 mg dextroamphetamine sulfate, 7.5 mg dextroamphetamine saccharate, 7.5 mg amphetamine aspartate, and 7.5 mg amphetamine sulfate

Dosages
Narcolepsy
Adults and children age 12 and older: Initially, 10 mg immediate-release tablet daily. Increase by 10 mg weekly to maximum dose of 60 mg in 2 or 3 divided doses every 4 to 6 hours.
Children ages 6 to 12: Initially, 5 mg immediate-release tablet P.O. daily. Increase by 5 mg at weekly intervals to maximum dose of 60 mg in divided doses.
Attention deficit hyperactivity disorder
Adults: 20 mg extended-release capsules P.O. daily.
Adolescents ages 13 to 17: Initially, 10 mg extended-release capsule P.O. daily. Increase after 1 week to 20 mg daily if needed.
Children age 6 and older: Initially, 5 mg immediate-release tablet P.O. daily or b.i.d. Increase by 5 mg at weekly intervals until optimal response. Dosage should rarely exceed 40 mg.

Children ages 6 to 12: Give 10 mg extended-release capsule P.O. daily in a.m. Increase by 5 to 10 mg in weekly intervals to a maximum dose of 30 mg.
Children ages 3 to 5: Initially, 2.5 mg immediate-release tablet P.O. daily. Increase by 2.5 mg at weekly intervals until optimal response. Divide total daily dose into 2 or 3 doses and give 4 to 6 hours apart.

ANTIPLATELET DRUGS
Aggrenox

Generic components
Capsules
25 mg aspirin and 200 mg dipyridamole

Dosages
Adults: To decrease risk of stroke, 1 capsule P.O. b.i.d. in the morning and evening. Swallow capsule whole; may be taken with or without food.

MENOPAUSE DRUGS
Activella
femhrt

Generic components
Tablets
2.5 mcg ethinyl estradiol and 0.5 mg norethindrone acetate (femhrt)
5 mcg ethinyl estradiol and 1 mg norethindrone acetate (femhrt)
0.5 mg ethinyl estradiol and 0.1 mg norethindrone acetate (Activella)
1 mg ethinyl estradiol and 0.5 mg norethindrone acetate (Activella)

Dosages
Signs and symptoms of menopause; to prevent osteoporosis. Women with intact uterus: 1 tablet P.O. per day.

Prefest

Generic components
Tablets
1 mg estradiol and 0.09 mg norgestimate

Dosages
Moderate to severe symptoms of menopause; to prevent osteoporosis. Women with intact uterus: 1 tablet P.O. per day (3 days of pink tablets: estradiol alone; followed by 3 days of white tablets: estradiol and norgestimate combination; continue cycle uninterrupted).

Premphase

Generic components
Tablets
0.625 mg conjugated estrogens; 0.625 mg conjugated estrogens with 5 mg medroxyprogesterone

Dosages
Moderate to severe symptoms of menopause; to prevent osteoporosis. Women with intact uterus: 1 tablet P.O. per day. Use estrogen alone on days 1 to 14 and estrogen-medroxyprogesterone tablet on days 15 to 28.

Prempro

Generic components
Tablets
0.3 mg conjugated estrogen and 1.5 mg medroxyprogesterone
0.45 mg conjugated estrogen and 1.5 mg medroxyprogesterone
0.625 mg conjugated estrogen and 2.5 mg medroxyprogesterone
0.625 mg conjugated estrogen and 5 mg medroxyprogesterone

Dosages
Symptoms of menopause; to prevent osteoporosis. Women with intact uterus: 1 tablet P.O. per day.

OPIOID AGONISTS
Suboxone
CSS III

Generic components
Sublingual tablets
2 mg buprenorphine and 0.5 mg naloxone

8 mg buprenorphine and 2 mg naloxone

Dosages
Opioid dependence
Adults: 12 to 16 mg S.L. once daily, after induction with S.L. buprenorphine.

PSYCHOTHERAPEUTICS

Limbitrol
Limbitrol DS

Generic components
Tablets
5 mg chlordiazepoxide and 12.5 mg amitriptyline
10 mg chlordiazepoxide and 25 mg amitriptyline

Dosages
Adults: 10 mg chlordiazepoxide with 25 mg amitriptyline 3 to 4 times per day up to 6 times daily. For patients who don't tolerate the higher doses, 5 mg chlordiazepoxide with 12.5 mg amitriptyline 3 to 4 times per day. Reduce dosage after initial response.

Perphenazine and Amitriptyline

Generic components
Tablets
2 mg perphenazine and 10 mg amitriptyline
2 mg perphenazine and 25 mg amitriptyline
4 mg perphenazine and 10 mg amitriptyline
4 mg perphenazine and 25 mg amitriptyline
4 mg perphenazine and 50 mg amitriptyline

Dosages
Adults: 2 to 4 mg perphenazine with 10 to 50 mg amitriptyline 3 to 4 times daily. Reduce dosage after initial response.

Symbyax

Generic components
Capsules
6 mg olanzapine and 25 mg fluoxetine
6 mg olanzapine and 50 mg fluoxetine
12 mg olanzapine and 25 mg fluoxetine
12 mg olanzapine and 50 mg fluoxetine

Dosages
Adults: 1 capsule daily in the evening. Begin with 6 mg/25 mg capsule and adjust according to efficacy and tolerability.

Drugs by therapeutic class

Alzheimer's disease drugs
- donepezil hydrochloride
- galantamine hydrobromide
- memantine hydrochloride
- rivastigmine tartrate
- tacrine hydrochloride

Androgens and anabolic steroids
- fluoxymesterone
- methyltestosterone
- testosterone
- testosterone cypionate
- testosterone enanthate
- testosterone propionate
- testosterone transdermal

Antagonists and antidotes
- acamprosate calcium
- activated charcoal
- disulfiram
- flumazenil
- naloxone hydrochloride
- naltrexone
- naltrexone hydrochloride
- physostigmine salicylate

Antianginals
- propranolol hydrochloride

Anticonvulsants
- carbamazepine
- clonazepam
- divalproex sodium
- iamotrigine
- magnesium sulfate
- phenobarbital
- topiramate
- valproate sodium

Antidepressants
- amitriptyline hydrochloride
- bupropion hydrochloride
- citalopram hydrobromide
- clomipramine hydrochloride
- desipramine hydrochloride
- doxepin hydrochloride
- duloxetine hydrochloride
- escitalopram oxalate
- fluoxetine hydrochloride
- fluvoxamine maleate
- imipramine hydrochloride
- imipramine pamoate
- mirtazapine
- nefazodone hydrochloride
- nortriptyline hydrochloride
- paroxetine hydrochloride
- sertraline hydrochloride
- trazodone hydrochloride
- venlafaxine hydrochloride

Antiemetics
- prochlorperazine
- prochlorperazine edisylate
- prochlorperazine maleate

Antihistamines
- diphenhydramine hydrochloride
- promethazine hydrochloride

Antineoplastics that alter hormone balance
- goserelin acetate
- leuprolide acetate

Antipsychotics
- aripiprazole
- chlorpromazine hydrochloride
- clozapine
- fluphenazine decanoate
- fluphenazine hydrochloride
- haloperidol
- haloperidol decanoate
- haloperidol lactate
- lithium carbonate
- lithium citrate
- loxapine succinate
- olanzapine
- paliperidone
- perphenazine
- quetiapine fumarate
- risperidone
- thioridazine hydrochloride

- thiothixene
- thiothixene hydrochloride
- trifluoperazine hydrochloride
- ziprasidone

Anxiolytics

- alprazolam
- buspirone hydrochloride
- chlordiazepoxide hydrochloride
- clorazepate dipotassium
- diazepam
- hydroxyzine hydrochloride
- hydroxyzine pamoate ch
- lorazepam
- oxazepam

Attention deficit hyperactivity disorder drugs

- atomoxetine hydrochloride
- dexmethylphenidate hydrochloride
- dextroamphetamine sulfate
- lisdexamfetamine dimesylate
- methylphenidate hydrochloride

Benign prostatic hyperplasia drugs

- finasteride

CNS stimulants

- doxapram hydrochloride
- modafinil

Diuretics

- spironolactone

Erectile dysfunction drugs

- sildenafil citrate
- tadalafil
- vardenafil hydrochloride

Estrogens and progestins

- esterified estrogens
- estradiol
- estrogens, conjugated
- estropipate

Nonopiod analgesics and pyretics

- aspirin

Sedative–hypnotics

- chloral hydrate
- eszopiclone
- flurazepam hydrochloride
- midazolam hydrochloride
- pentobarbital sodium
- propofol
- ramelteon
- secobarbital sodium
- temazepam
- triazolam
- zaleplon
- zolpidem tartrate

Skeletal muscle relaxants

- dantrolene sodium

Uncategorized drugs

- varenicline

Vitamins and minerals

- folic acid
- thiamine hydrochloride

American Psychiatric Association: *Diagnostic and Statistical Manual of Mental Disorders,* 4th ed., Text Revision. Washington, D.C.: American Psychiatric Association, 2000.

Beau, A., and Ellis, R.J. "Dementia and Neurocognitive Disorders Due to HIV-1 Infection," *Seminars in Neurology* 27(1):86–92, 2007.

Benisty, S., et al. "Diagnostic Criteria of Vascular Dementia in CADASIL," *Stroke* 39(3):838–44, 2007.

Birkenaes, A.B., et al. "The Level of Cardiovascular Risk Factors in Bipolar Disorder Equals that of Schizophrenia: A Comparative Study," *Journal of Clinical Psychiatry* 68(6):917–23, June 2007.

Black, J.M., and Hawks, J.H. *Medical-Surgical Nursing.* St. Louis: Elsevier Saunders, 2005.

Bodenmann, G., et al. "Associations among Everyday Stress, Critical Life Events, and Sexual Problems," *Journal of Nervous & Mental Disease* 194(7): 494–501, July 2006.

Bourget, D., et al. "Evidential Basis for the Assessment and Treatment of Sex Offenders," *Brief Treatment & Crisis Intervention* 8(1):130–146, February 2008.

Boyd, M.A., *Psychiatric Nursing Contemporary Practice,* 4th ed. Philadelphia: Wolters Kluwer Health, 2008.

Briken, P., and Kafka, M. "Pharmacological Treatments for Paraphilic Patients and Sexual Offenders," *Current Opinion in Psychiatry* 20(6):609-13, November 2007.

Cassels, C., and Murata, P. "New Pharmacologic Guideline Issued for Treatment of Dementia." [Online]. Available at *www.medscape.com/viewarticle/571146.* Accessed 03/31/2008.

Clayton, A.H., and Montejo, A.L. "Major Depressive Disorder, Antidepressants, and Sexual Dysfunction," *Journal of Clinical Psychiatry* 2006:67 Suppl 6:33–37, 2006.

Conlon, K.E., et al. "Family Management Styles and ADHD: Utility and Treatment Implications," *Journal of Family Nursing* April 2008. Available at *http://jfn.sagepub.com/cgi/content/short/1074840708315673v1.*

Day, E., et al. "Thiamine for Wernicke-Korsakoff Syndrome in People at Risk from Alcohol Abuse (Review)." *The Cochrane Collaboration* Issue 1:1–12, 2008. [Online]. Available at *www.thecochranelibrary.com.* Accessed 03/31/2008.

Focardi, M., et al. "Accidental Death in Autoerotic Maneuvers," *American Journal of Forensic Medicine & Pathology* 29(1):64–68, March 2008.

Franko, D.L., and Keel, P.K. "Suicidality in Hearing Disorders: Occurrence, Correlates, and Clinical Implications," *Clinical Psychological Review* 26(6):769–82, October 2006.

Frederick, J. "Pick Disease: A Brief Overview," *Archives of Pathology & Laboratory Medicine* 130:1063–66, 2006.

Gottheil, E., et al. "Pathologic Gambling: A Nonsubstance, Substance-Related Disorder?" *Journal of Addiction Medicine* 1(2):53–61, June 2007.

Hellings, J.A., et al. "A Crossover Study of Risperidone in Children, Adolescents and Adults with Mental Retardation," *Journal of Autism and Developmental Disorders* 36(3):401–11, April 2006.

Jakubietz, M., et al. "Body Dysmorphic Disorder: Diagnosis and Approach," *Plastic & Reconstructive Surgery* 119(6):1924–30, May 2007.

Jankovic, J. "Parkinson's Disease: Clinical Features and Diagnosis," *Journal of Neurology and Neurosurgical Psychiatry* 79:368–76, 2008.

Kane, R.L., et al. *Essentials of Clinical Geriatrics,* 5th ed. Chicago: McGraw-Hill, 2004.

Nance, M.A. "Comprehensive Care in Huntington's Disease: A Physician's Perspective," *Brain Research Bulletin* 72:175–78, 2007.

National Institute on Alcohol Abuse and Alcoholism (2006). "Five Year Strategic Plan FY08-13: Alcohol across the Lifespan" [Online]. Available at *http://pubs.niaaa.nih.gov/ publications/StrategicPlan/ NIAAASTRATEGICPLAN.htm.*

Olfson, M., et al. "National Trends in the Outpatient Treatment of Children and Adolescents with Antipsychotic Drugs," *Year Book of Psychiatry & Applied Mental Health 2007*:55–56, 2007.

Pull, C. "Recent Trends in the Study of Specific Phobias," *Current Opinion in Psychiatry* 21(1):43–50, January 2008.

Sadock, B., and Sadock, V., eds. *Kaplan and Sadock's Comprehensive Textbook of Psychiatry,* 8th ed., Volumes 1 and 2. Philadelphia: Lippincott Williams & Wilkins, 2005.

Sparks, M.B. "Inpatient Care of Persons with Alzheimer's Disease," *Critical Care Nursing Quarterly* 31(1):65–72, 2008.

Spencer, T.J., et al. "Efficacy and Safety of Mixed Amphetamine Salts Extended Release (Adderall XR) in the Management of Attention-Deficit/Hyperactivity Disorder in Adolescent Patients: A 4-Week, Randomized, Double-Blind, Placebo-Controlled, Parallel-Group Study," *Clinical Therapy* 28(2): 266–79, February 2006.

Stuart, G., and Laraia, M. *Principles and Practice of Psychiatric Nursing,* 8th ed. St. Louis: Elsevier Mosby, 2005.

Swann, A.C., et al. "Increased Impulsivity Associated with Severity of Suicide Attempt History in Patients with Bipolar Disorder," *American Journal of Psychiatry* 162:1680–87, September 2005.

Tse, J., et al. "Social Skills Training for Adolescents with Asperger Syndrome and High Functioning Autism," *Journal of Autism and Developmental Disorders,* 37(10):1690–69, November 2007.

Walsh, B., et al. "Fluoxetine after Weight Restoration in Anorexia Nervosa: A Randomized Control Trial," *JAMA* 295(22):2605–12, June 2006.

Weintraub, D., and Hurtig, H.I., "Presentation and Management of Psychosis in Parkinson's Disease and Dementia with Lewy Bodies," *American Journal of Psychiatry* 164:1491–98, 2007.

Index

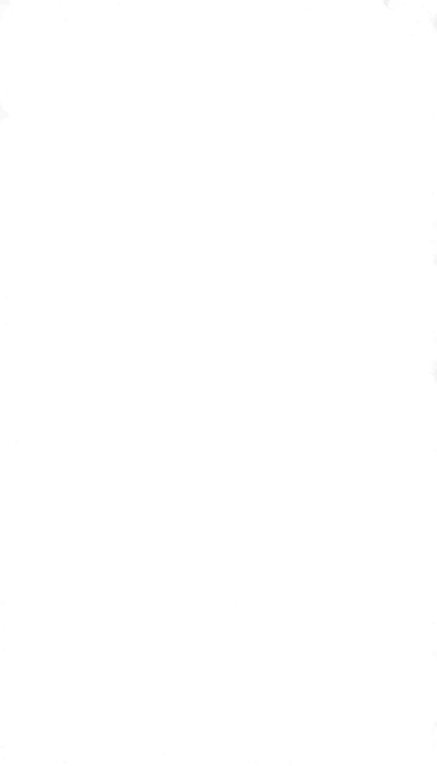